# jamie athome

## Cook Your Way to the Good Life

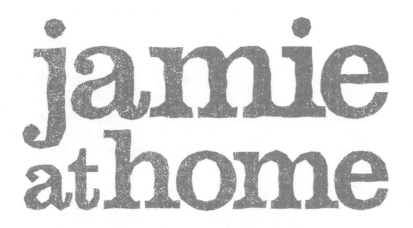

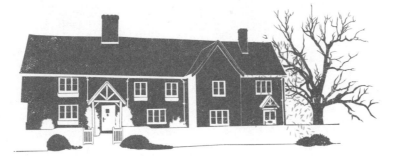

# Jamie Oliver

Photography by David Loftus

Illustrations by The Plant

Michael Joseph
*an imprint of* Penguin Books

Dedicated to
# Steve Irwin
1962–2006

I was so inspired by his verve for life and his ability to connect with people of all ages around the world. And, most importantly, how he taught us all to appreciate this incredible planet we live on! Love and respect to his family and friends.

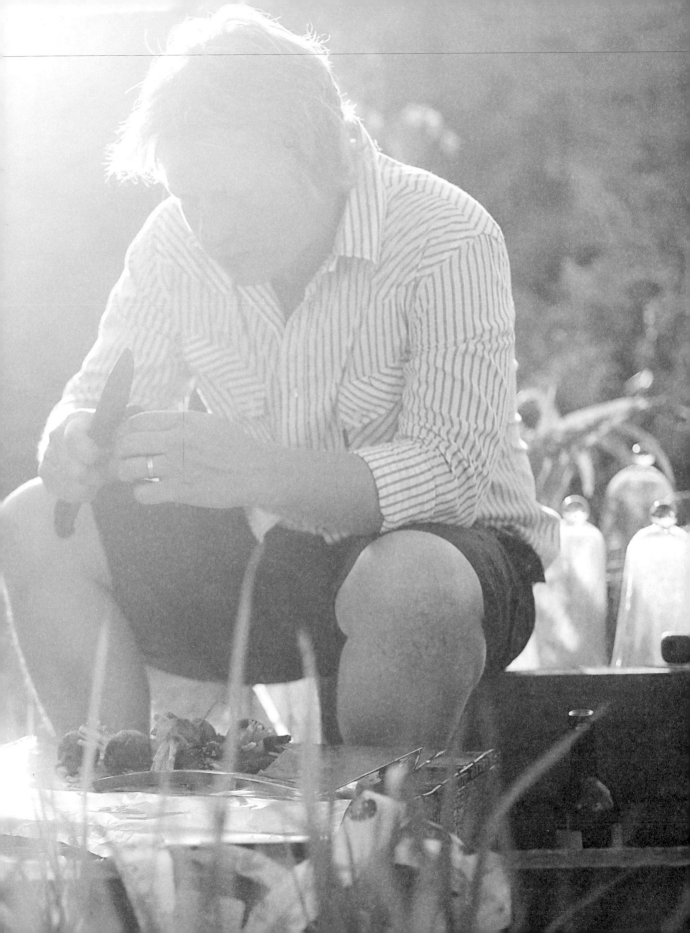

MICHAEL JOSEPH

Published by the Penguin Group
Penguin Books Ltd, 80 Strand, London WC2R 0RL, England
Penguin Group (USA) Inc., 375 Hudson Street, New York, New York 10014, USA
Penguin Group (Canada), 90 Eglinton Avenue East, Suite 700, Toronto, Ontario, Canada M4P 2Y3
(a division of Pearson Penguin Canada Inc.)
Penguin Ireland, 25 St Stephen's Green, Dublin 2, Ireland (a division of Penguin Books Ltd)
Penguin Group (Australia), 250 Camberwell Road,
Camberwell, Victoria 3124, Australia (a division of Pearson Australia Group Pty Ltd)
Penguin Books India Pvt Ltd, 11 Community Centre,
Panchsheel Park, New Delhi – 110 017, India
Penguin Group (NZ), 67 Apollo Drive, Rosedale, North Shore 0632, New Zealand
(a division of Pearson New Zealand Ltd)
Penguin Books (South Africa) (Pty) Ltd, 24 Sturdee Avenue,
Rosebank, Johannesburg 2196, South Africa

Penguin Books Ltd, Registered Offices: 80 Strand, London WC2R 0RL, England

www.penguin.com
jamieoliver.com

First published 2007
9

Copyright © Jamie Oliver, 2007
Photographs copyright © David Loftus, 2007 | www.davidloftus.com
Illustrations copyright © The Plant, 2007 | www.theplant.co.uk
Battery hens image on page 41 copyright © PA Photos
Lamb image on page 55 copyright © Jake Eastham / Alamy
Mushroom log images on page 295 copyright © Adrian Ogden
at Gourmet Woodland Mushrooms

Set in Clarendon
Printed in Germany by Mohn
Colour reproduction by Altaimage Ltd
Printed on Shiro Bright White

A CIP catalogue record for this book is available from the British Library

ISBN: 978-0-718-15243-7

Also by Jamie Oliver

The Naked Chef / The Return of the Naked Chef /
Happy Days with the Naked Chef / Jamie's Kitchen /
Jamie's Dinners / Jamie's Italy / Cook with Jamie

# contents

# a nice little chat

Look, I thought this would be a good opportunity to get you all up to speed, because it will come out in the press eventually anyway, so I'm going to tell you straight: basically, my wife has accused me of having an affair. She'll tell anyone she meets that I've been nipping out of the house for an hour here, an hour there, and coming back looking refreshed, rosy-cheeked and guilty, with grass stains on my knees. Now you might be thinking that a cookbook is not the right place at all to be talking about my personal life, but before you jump to conclusions, let me explain . . .

All I've done is fallen in love with my garden, and with my veg patch in particular! Yes, I *have* kissed a few of my more beautiful, prized vegetables, I might have hugged a couple of trees and on hot days put my ear to the ground to listen to things growing – I'm just going through what many men go through at this point in their lives, when they become one with Mother Nature. And if you think I'm guilty, then lock me up and throw away the key! I can promise you, I've not been having an affair. I just like spending time with my veg. And I'll tell you something, this has been the best cooking year of my life. I've had brilliant fun coming up with the recipes because I've been so inspired by everything that's come out of my garden over the past year.

I spent my childhood growing up in a village in Essex and I moved back there three or four years ago with my wife and kids. Like most people these days, with a busy family life and a hectic working schedule, I began to struggle with finding a balance between the two. I seem to have evened things up a bit now, and it's all thanks to my veg garden, believe it or not. I love spending the odd hour out there, as it really relaxes me. You might think I sound like a complete hippy now, but growing my own veg for these past few years has filled me with such pride, pleasure and passion. Witnessing changes in the garden through the year, having successes and failures, realizing that certain types of fruit or veg can have certain personalities and you have to work with them in different ways, it's all just fascinating to me!

The garden has also made me think about food in a different way: about how it grows and what it stands for. To me, growing food at home means eating outside in the summer, at family get-togethers and occasions, or cosying up next to a fire tucking into an amazing, comforting stew or soup made with stuff from the garden which you've had to go outside and pull up in the pouring rain! It might seem odd, but during the last sixteen years of training and working as a chef, I never thought I would ever grow stuff properly. I'd always made an effort to buy local, seasonal and really fresh produce but for some reason never thought I could do it myself. It just never occurred to me that it might be as easy as taking some seeds out of a packet and popping them into the ground. But it is!

To begin with, and without knowing what on earth I was doing, I simply ordered a few Italian seeds off the Internet. I couldn't understand the instructions for how to plant them because they were in Italian, so I just chucked them into the ground and hoped for the best. Give or take things growing too close together, or pulling up stuff I wasn't supposed to, the first year was just incredible. Complete havoc, but incredible! I grew so much, and I also experimented with using tomato bags, pots, buckets, troughs, any containers I could get hold of really – even old welly boots! It just puts a smile on my

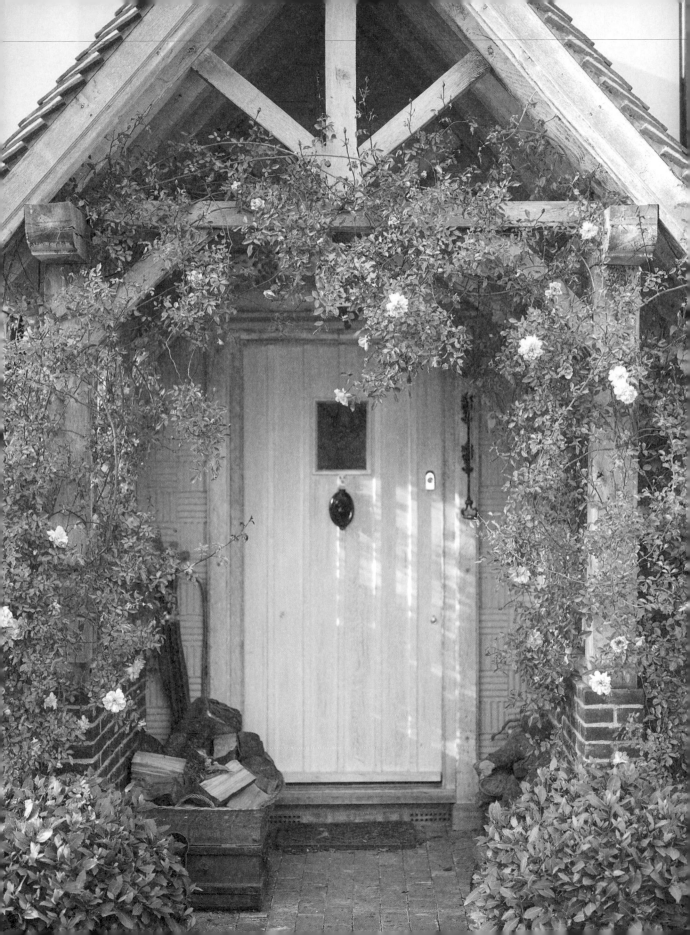

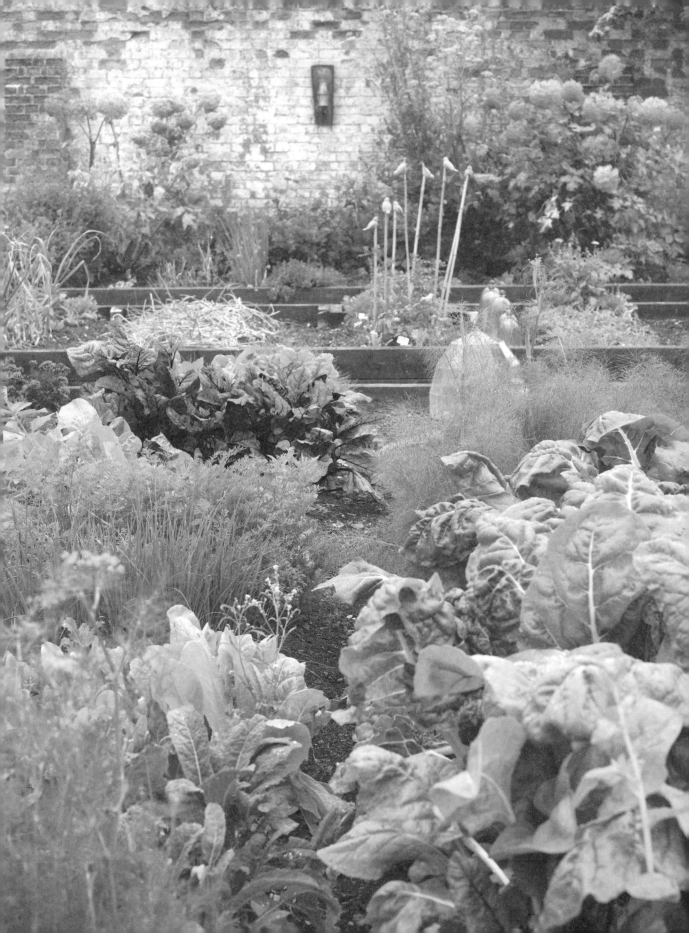

face to see things happening in the garden and to know that I've got loads of lovely food ready to be picked all through the year. I've also been incredibly inspired to come up with cracking new recipes for this book – not based on different celebrations and themes, but simply on whatever ingredients have been popping up in the garden.

I grew up watching that TV programme *The Good Life*, about Barbara and Tom, the couple who didn't have much but grew everything themselves. They lived next to the posh couple called Margo and Jerry, who had everything but weren't all that happy. Thinking back, which one of the couples did we all aspire to be? And would it be the same couple these days? My view is that we're all pretty spoilt now, as far as luxuries are concerned, but I reckon that the best luxury in life comes from experience ('luxuriance' as a mate of mine recently called it!) and knowledge, and I think food and cooking are among the most important things out there for us to learn about.

This book has been such a pleasure to write. It is essentially a cookbook divided into the four seasons, to give you an idea of when each kind of garden produce is ready. Each season contains a whole load of mini chapters based on different ingredients, giving you a mixture of really quick, light and tasty recipes. I've also included some little bits of growing information at the end of each chapter, which I hope will encourage you to have a go at growing some of the same fruit and veg I've had in my garden for the past year or so. Even if you live on the twentieth floor of a block of flats you can still use a windowsill. Or you can turn the flat roof of your garage into a roof garden, or put some pots around your back yard – wherever you live, you can have a go. Just growing a little selection of fruit and veg will give you massive inspiration.

If, like I did, you start off growing just five or six kinds that are well behaved and don't give any trouble, you can't go wrong. A brilliant thing to try at first is mixed salad leaves. I used to sprinkle the seeds into a tomato bag that I kept outside on my flat roof in London, and this gave me interesting salad leaves for four months of the year, without ever having to buy any! New potatoes are absolute heaven when cooked and eaten straight out of the ground. You can grow them in buckets or bags, or plant them straight into the soil. Try a nice selection of herbs – things like thyme, rosemary, sage and bay are pretty reliable all year round and add such dimension to your cooking. And have a go at planting some lovely little strawberry varieties in your hanging baskets this year, instead of flowers (more about that in the strawberries chapter!).

You'll find a section at the end of the book which lists the exact seed and plant varieties I've been using in my garden that I've had real success with, so whether you're interested in growing salad leaves or courgettes, heirloom tomatoes or good old potatoes, have a flick to the back and try some of them out. You'll also find a list of companies that offer a mail order service for great seeds and kit.

Whether you do have a go at growing your own, or whether you never will, nearly all the ingredients I've used in the recipes can be bought from a local farmers' market or good supermarkets. But if you do have a go at doing it yourself, or you feel inspired to do so once you've had a look at the book, I'll feel like I've done my job. I'm really proud of the recipes in this book. As far as the growing information is concerned, I have tried to make each bit read like a recipe to keep it simple. If you want to go further into the whole thing, there are some great gardening books around. So get stuck in!

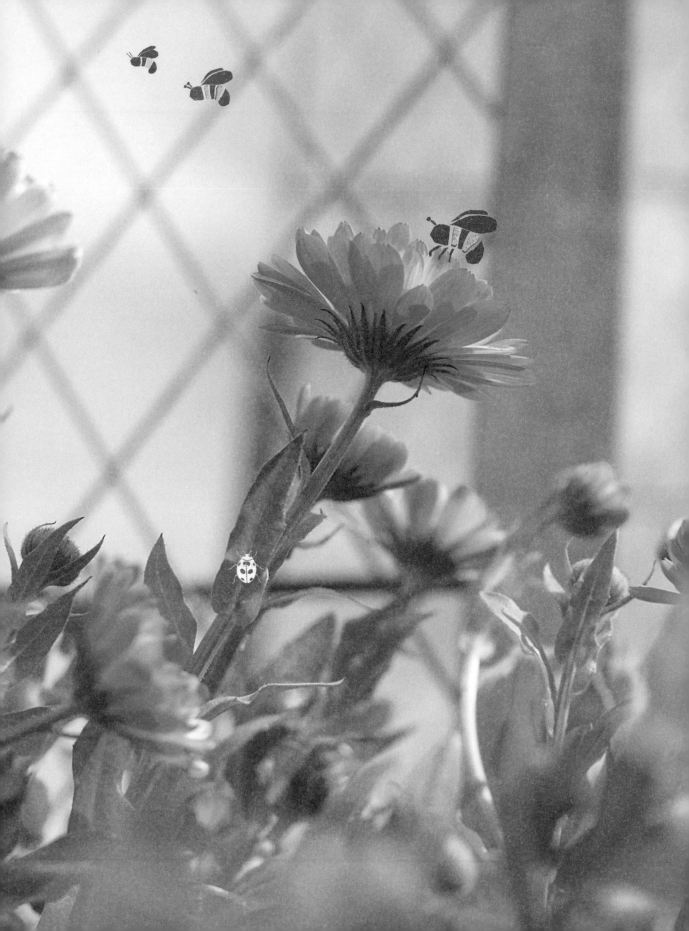

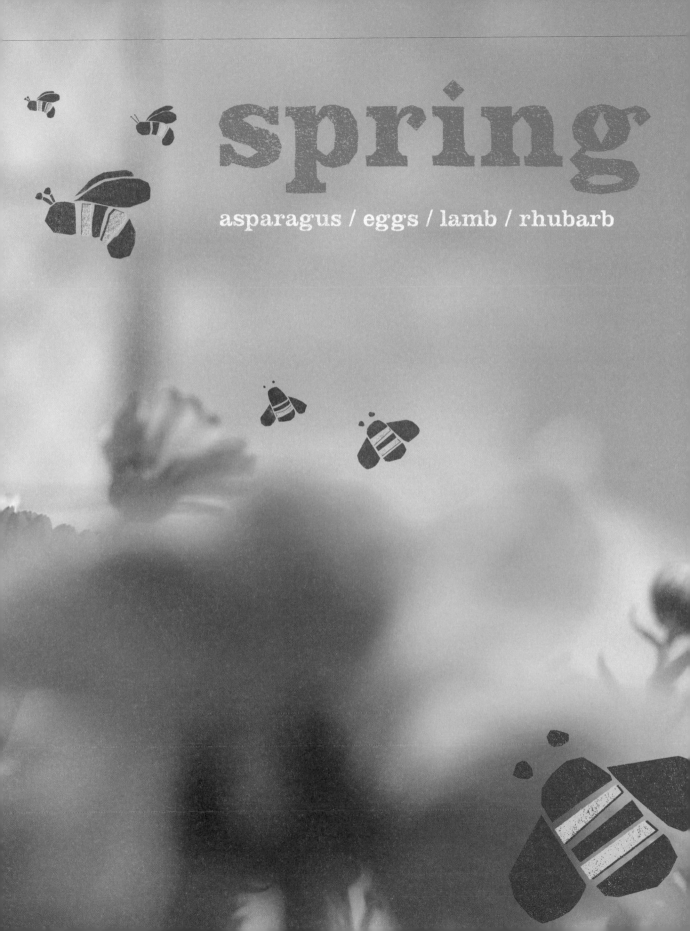

# spring

asparagus / eggs / lamb / rhubarb

I've been eating my own home-grown asparagus for two years now, and I love having it in the garden. It's been kind of painful in some respects, though, because to grow it successfully you need to have patience – something I don't really have! With most of the growing I'm talking about in this book, you'll get to plant and eat something within the first few months, but asparagus isn't like that. It won't produce properly for the first three years, as the plants have to build their network of roots and store huge quantities of nutrients and energy in order to produce their lovely spears. It's this initial investment in time, as well as its low weight yield per square metre and the fact that it can't be churned out, that makes asparagus a more expensive vegetable to buy in the shops. Understanding all this has just made me love and respect this delicate and luxurious vegetable even more. Just remember to pick and cook it as quickly as possible to get the most flavour out of it.

It goes without saying that you don't have to grow your own, because it's possible to buy good asparagus from your local supermarket or market, but please only buy it when it's in season and has travelled from field to store as soon as possible after picking. If you're buying out of season from the other side of the world it can be okay, but it definitely won't be a memorable experience. There are loads of different varieties that you can get hold of in good supermarkets – long thin ones, wild straggly ones and beautiful chunky ones.

Asparagus is one of the most nutritious vegetables you can eat. It contains a whole cocktail of nutrients and vitamins, including a large amount of folic acid (this can't be stored in your body so has to be taken daily – it looks after your blood and is especially good for pregnant women as it protects against spina bifida in developing babies). Asparagus is also a wonderful diuretic, which means it cleanses your liver. And if your liver's happy, everything else tends to be happy as well!

So even though growing asparagus can be a labour of love, it all becomes worth it when the spears pop their heads up through the soil. When they're ready, simply click them off at the base (that way you won't get any woody, stringy stalk), give them a quick wash, and the world of asparagus cooking will be at your fingertips. You can steam the spears, boil them or quickly stew them in pasta sauces to exaggerate all their juiciness and sweetness, or you can dry-grill or roast them to bring out their unusual nutty flavour, which you might not have tasted before.

Whichever way you choose to cook asparagus, a squeeze of lemon juice and a drizzle of olive oil or a dot of butter will really make the most of it. Other friends of asparagus are eggs, smoky crispy bacon, lovely mozzarella, Parmesan, any crumbly cheese like Lancashire or Cheshire, chilli, cream, seafood, herbs like mint, parsley, basil, rosemary ... the list goes on.

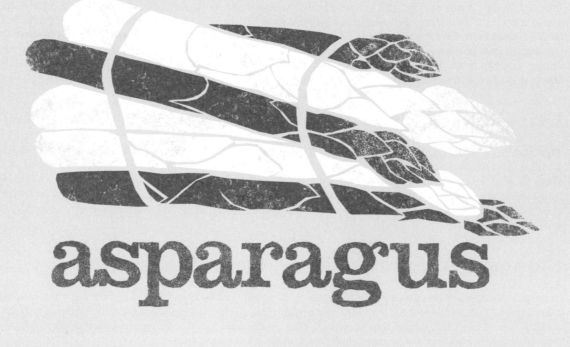

# asparagus

# Three simple ways to cook asparagus

There are many different types of asparagus available these days – thick ones, thin ones, baby, green, wild, white and even absolutely huge ones! Apart from their visual appeal, the real difference between them is their taste. They range from firm and nutty to soft and silky. Here are my three favourite ways of cooking asparagus to serve as side dishes or starters.

For each of these recipes you will need to wash 2 big handfuls or 800g of whichever kind of asparagus you're using, with their woody ends snapped off. Each recipe serves 4 people.

## White asparagus with smashed mint and lemon butter

Using a speed peeler, peel off the outer layer of the asparagus spears, from 5cm below the tip down to the bottom, then tie them in a bundle with a piece of string. Get your deepest saucepan with a lid – the asparagus spears should be able to stand up inside the pan. If they can't, slice the ends off to make them fit. Bring a pan of salted water to the boil and stand the asparagus upright in it. Throw in any sliced-off ends, boil for 5 minutes with the lid on, then turn off the heat. Let the asparagus sit in the pan for another 10 minutes. Meanwhile, smash up 2 small handfuls of mint leaves in a pestle and mortar until you have a pulp, and gently melt 100g of butter with some sea salt and freshly ground black pepper in a frying pan. Add the mint pulp and the juice of 1 large lemon. Stir together and, when it's slowly bubbling, remove from the heat. To test if the asparagus is cooked, take a spear out, slice a bit off and try it. If it's soft, but still holding its shape, they're done, so drain them in a colander. To serve, pour the mint and lemon butter over the asparagus and sprinkle with a few extra mint leaves.

## Grilled asparagus with olive oil, lemon and Parmesan

This is a great combination. Parmesan, olive oil and lemon are wonderful with asparagus. Heat a large griddle pan and dry-griddle the asparagus spears on both sides until nicely marked. As soon as they're ready, put them on to four plates and dress with a good squeeze of lemon juice and three times as much olive oil. Season with sea salt and freshly ground black pepper to taste, then take a block of Parmesan to the table and either grate or shave some over the asparagus with a speed peeler.

## Steamed asparagus with French vinaigrette

Young asparagus is absolutely delicious when steamed. Put the asparagus spears into a colander over a large pan of fast-boiling water, place some tinfoil or a lid on top and allow them to steam until tender but still holding their shape. This should take 5 to 6 minutes but will depend on the size of your asparagus. Use common sense and try them as you go.

To make the vinaigrette, whisk up a heaped teaspoon of French mustard, 3 tablespoons of extra virgin olive oil and a tablespoon of red or white wine vinegar in a little bowl. Add a small swig of white wine or water to loosen it if need be, then whisk again and season with sea salt and freshly ground black pepper to taste. If you can get hold of some chervil, it's particularly good with asparagus, but you can also use flat-leaf parsley, mint or basil. Divide the asparagus between four plates, drizzle generously with vinaigrette and sprinkle with the freshly chopped herbs. Job done – delicious!

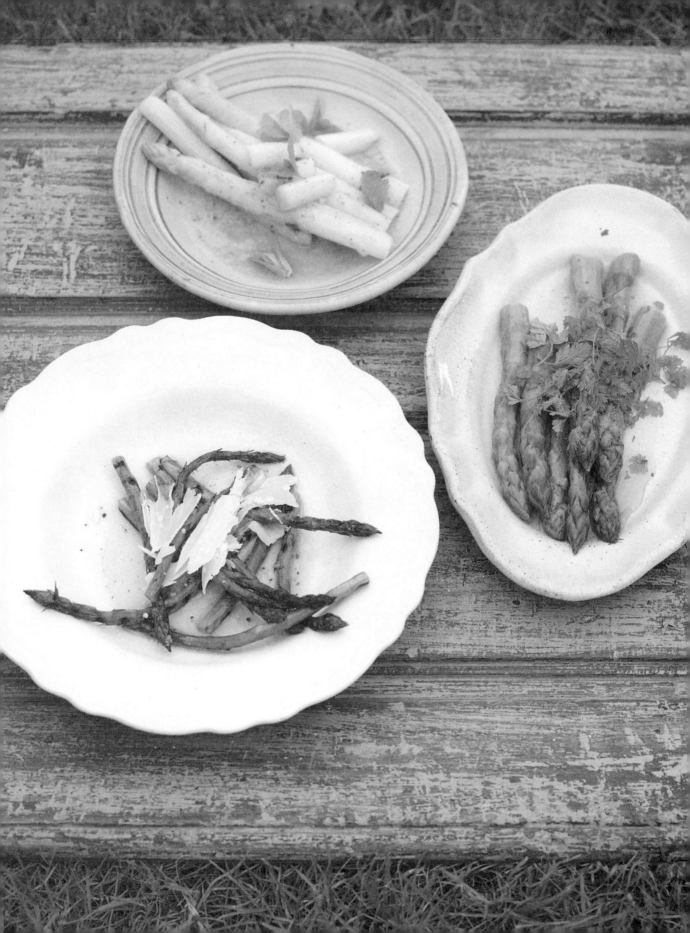

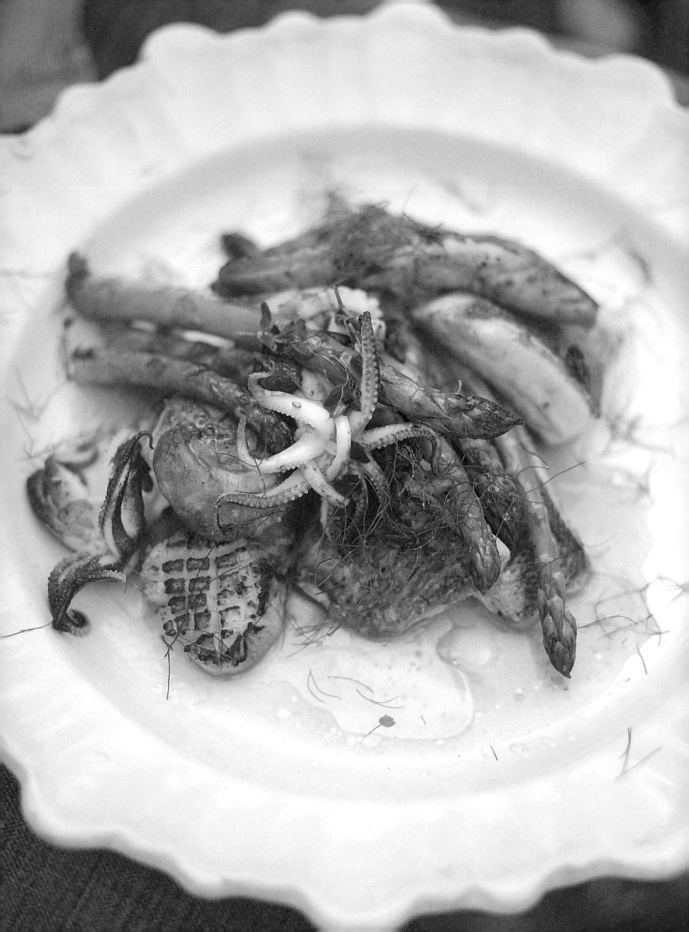

# Pan-cooked asparagus and mixed fish

No matter what your budget, you can make this dish with all different types of fish. It's nice to try to get a mixture of oily and white fish fillets, alongside things like shellfish, prawns and squid. You want everything to cook at the same time, so just make sure that whatever you use is all sliced up into pieces roughly the same size. You can cook it all together in a pan like I'm doing here or on the barbecue or, for a healthier way, you can steam it all – whichever, finish the dish off with extra virgin olive oil, lemon juice and chilli as these flavours all work so well with asparagus and fish.

Get a really large frying pan, or two smaller ones, on the heat and add a glug of olive oil. Score the skin of your fish fillets all over, about 1cm deep, and season. Put the fish fillets into the pan, skin side down, with the squid tentacles. Add the scallops. Run your knife down one side of each squid to open them out, then quickly and lightly score the inside in a criss-cross fashion. Lay them in the pan, scored side down. Add the asparagus and gently shake the pan. Cook for a few minutes, then turn everything over and cook on the other side. Sprinkle over the thyme tips.

You're the one in control of the pan, so if something looks cooked, take it out and keep it warm. Don't watch things burn! When the fish has crispy skin, the scallops are golden brown with caramelized edges and the squid has curled up and is nicely chargrilled, remove the pan from the heat. Put the squid on a chopping board and roughly slice it into pieces at an angle, then return to the pan. Lay the fish fillets on each plate. Toss the asparagus, scallops and squid with half the chilli, a good drizzle of good-quality extra virgin olive oil and the lemon juice. Lightly season and mix together. Divide on top of the plated fish. Sprinkle with the rest of the chopped chilli and the fennel tops, and drizzle with extra virgin olive oil.

serves 2

olive oil
2 small red mullet or snapper fillets, scaled and pinboned
1 royal bream fillet or sea bass fillet, scaled, pinboned and cut in half
sea salt and freshly ground black pepper
2 small squid, gutted and cleaned, tentacles trimmed and reserved
2–4 freshly shelled scallops, cleaned and scored in a criss-cross fashion
10 medium asparagus spears, woody ends removed
a small handful of thyme tips
1 fresh red chilli, deseeded and chopped
extra virgin olive oil
juice of 1 lemon
a small handful of fennel tops

asparagus

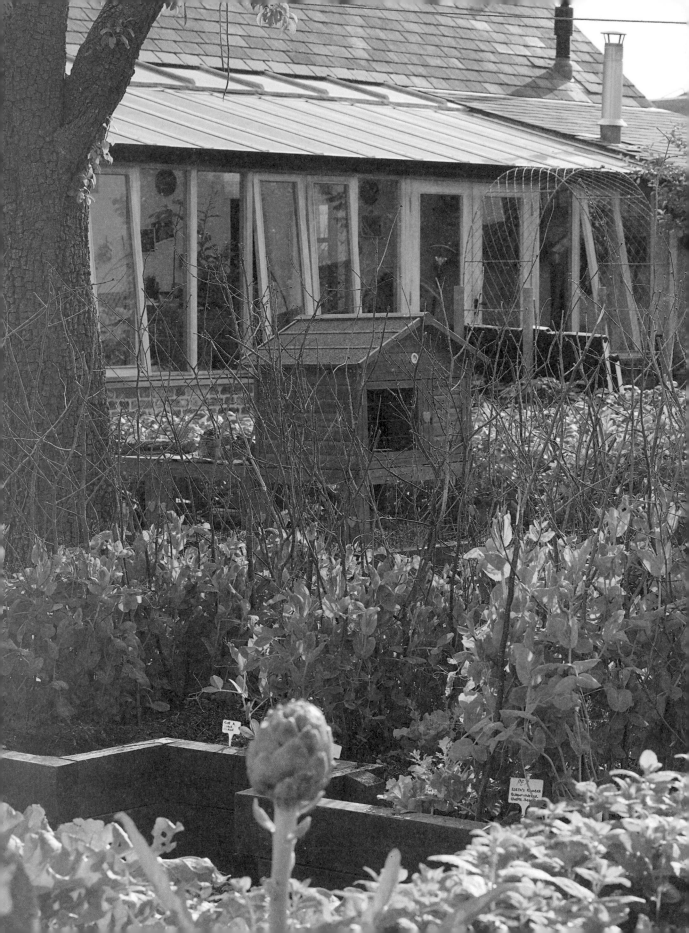

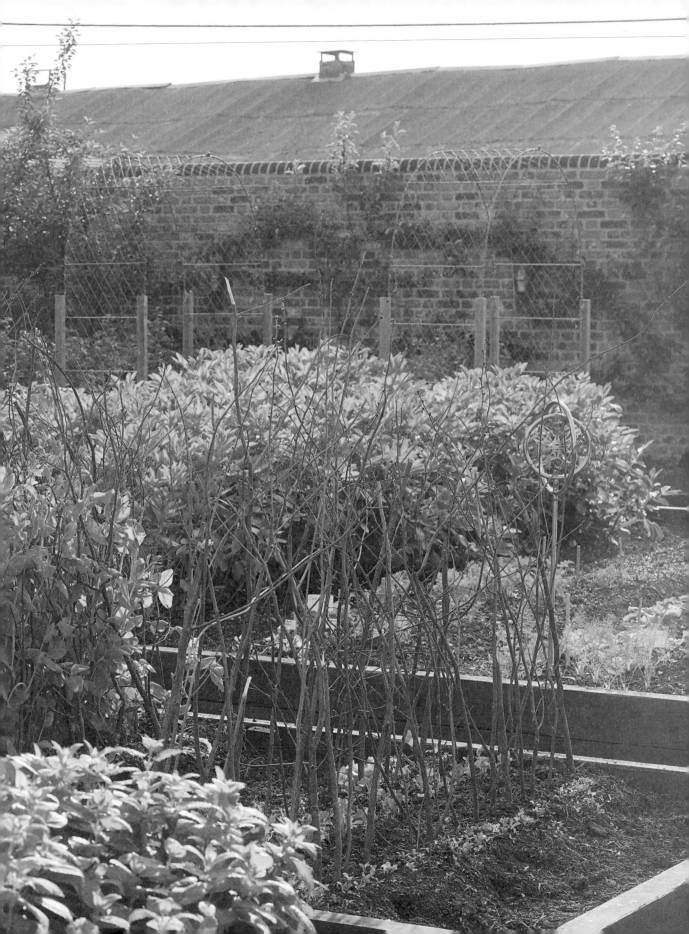

# Crispy asparagus soldiers with soft-boiled eggs

You can serve this dish as a starter, for breakfast, as a snack for lunch, or (dare I say it!) as canapés (as I'm doing here in the picture – I've simply upped the number of eggs). This is a great idea for serving at a party. Everyone gets a little stick of asparagus to dip into a soft-boiled egg. It's like breakfast – bacon and eggs, but rather than toast soldiers you get asparagus ones instead. A great combination.

Preheat the oven to 220°C/425°F/gas 7. Wrap your asparagus stalks in the pancetta with the tips poking out, and place in a roasting tray or earthenware dish. Drizzle with a little olive oil and roast in the preheated oven for 10 minutes, until the pancetta is crispy and golden.

While the asparagus is cooking, you can get on with soft-boiling your eggs. Carefully place them into lightly salted boiling water for 5 minutes, then drain, cut off the lids and put them in eggcups for individual servings, or into an egg box if serving as nibbles at a party. Serve 3 asparagus soldiers each for dipping into your egg, with a good pinch of salt and pepper.

**serves 4**

12 medium asparagus
 stalks, woody ends
 removed
12 rashers of thinly
 sliced pancetta or
 smoked streaky bacon
olive oil
4 large free-range
 or organic eggs
sea salt and freshly
 ground black pepper

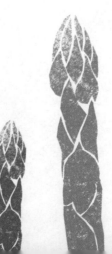

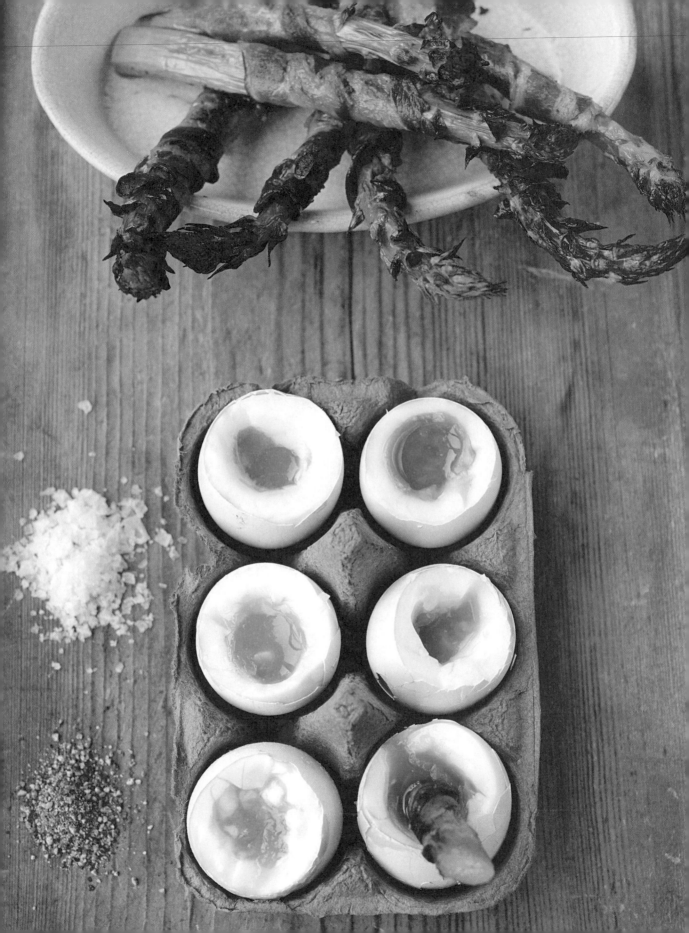

# Creamy asparagus soup with a poached egg on toast

A fantastically simple asparagus soup, puréed till it's silky smooth, is always a winner. Delicious eaten hot (or cold on really hot days with the help of a little lemon juice). The poached egg on toast makes it for me, but of course you don't have to serve the soup with them. I usually poach a couple more eggs than I need in case of breakages in the pan! I've made this for eight, but feel free to halve quantities or freeze soup leftovers.

Chop the tips off your asparagus and put these to one side for later. Roughly chop the asparagus stalks. Get a large, deep pan on the heat and add a good glug of olive oil. Gently fry the onions, celery and leeks for around 10 minutes, until soft and sweet, without colouring. Add the chopped asparagus stalks and stock and simmer for 20 minutes with a lid on. Remove from the heat and blitz with a hand-held blender or in a liquidizer. Season the soup bit by bit (this is important) with salt and pepper until just right. Put the soup back on the heat, stir in the asparagus tips, bring back to the boil and simmer for a few more minutes until the tips have softened.

Just before I'm ready to serve the soup, I get a wide casserole-type pan on the heat with 8 to 10cm of boiling water. Using really fresh eggs, I very quickly crack all 10 into the water. Don't worry about poaching so many at the same time. They don't have to look perfect. A couple of minutes and they'll be done, as you want them to be a bit runny. Toast your ciabatta slices. Using a slotted spoon, remove all the poached eggs to a plate and add a knob of butter to them. To serve, divide the soup between eight warmed bowls and place a piece of toast into each. Put a poached egg on top, cut into it to make it runny, season and drizzle with extra virgin olive oil.

**serves 8**

800g asparagus, woody
  ends removed
olive oil
2 medium white onions,
  peeled and chopped
2 sticks of celery,
  trimmed and chopped
2 leeks, trimmed
  and chopped
2 litres good-quality
  chicken or vegetable
  stock
sea salt and freshly
  ground black pepper
10 small very fresh free-
  range or organic eggs
8 slices of ciabatta bread
a knob of butter
extra virgin olive oil

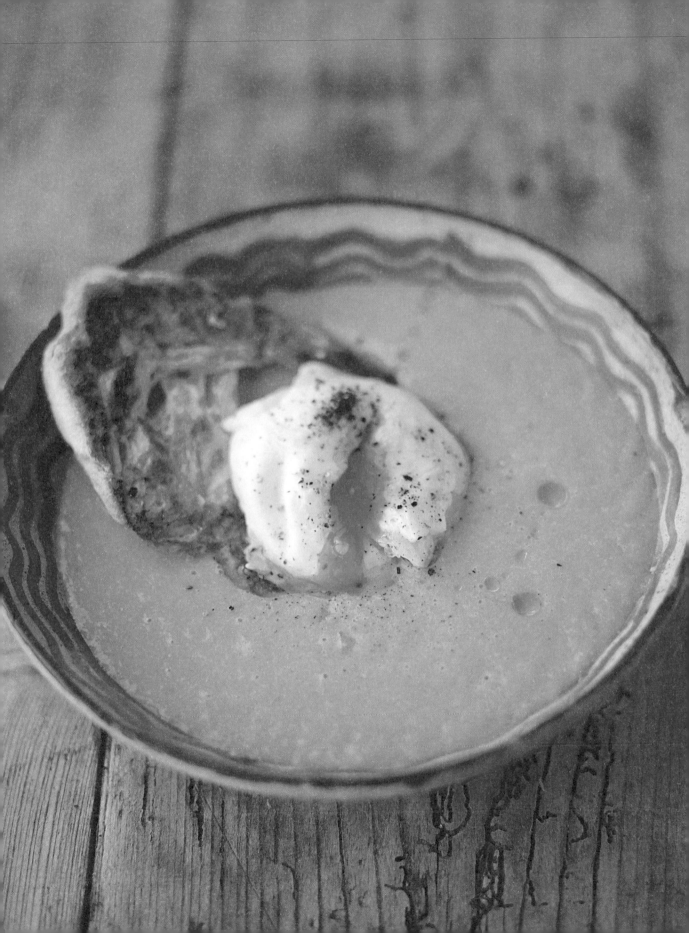

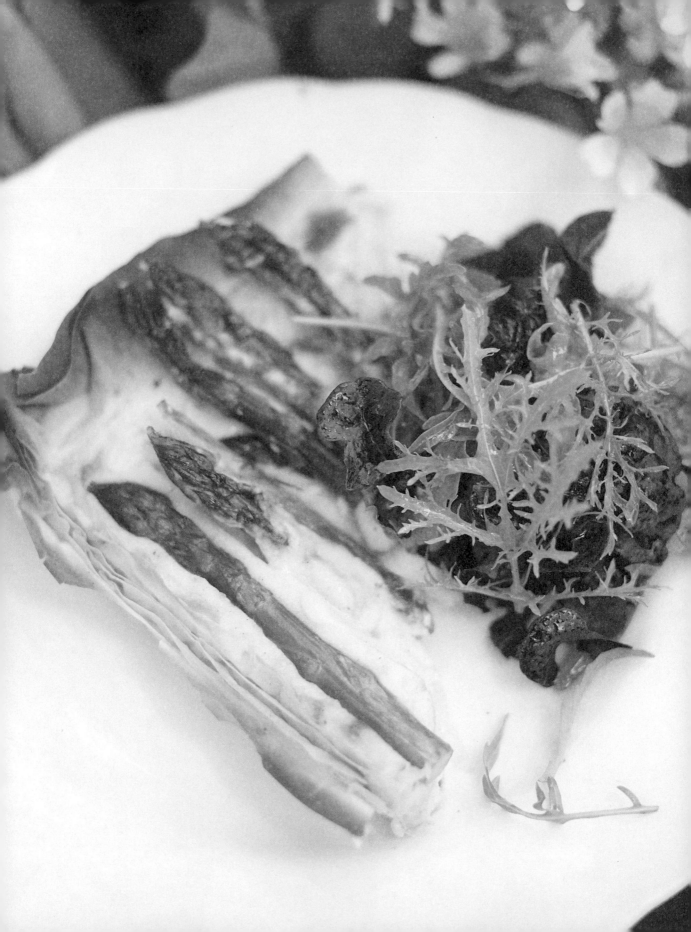

# Crispy and delicious asparagus and potato tart

Filo pastry can be bought in all supermarkets now, yet it often gets forgotten about. You can usually find it in either the fresh or the frozen pastry sections. Next time you're out shopping, pick some up – everyone should keep some at home because it's wonderful to use as a base for sweet and savoury tarts, or to wrap around cheese or spiced meat fillings. It goes really crunchy when cooked, so it's great with softer things. For this recipe, I've used it to make a quick open tart – perfect for a picnic or a simple lunch with a salad. You could even make individual ones and serve them as starters.

Put your potatoes into a pan of salted boiling water and cook for 15 minutes. Meanwhile blanch your asparagus in a separate pan of salted boiling water for 4 minutes, and drain in a colander.

Preheat the oven to 190°C/375°F/gas 5. Get an ovenproof dish – I've used many different shapes and sizes. Layer the sheets of filo pastry in the dish, brushing them with melted butter as you go and letting about 2.5cm hang over the edge. You want to get the pastry about five layers thick. Put a clean, damp tea towel over the top and put to one side.

When the potatoes are done, mash them with the cheeses. In a separate bowl, mix together the eggs and cream and stir into your cheesy mashed potato. Grate in the nutmeg, season well with pepper and mix together. Spread the mashed potato over the filo pastry, then bring up the sides of the filo and scrunch them together to form a rim. Take your blanched asparagus and line them up across the filling, making sure you cover it all. Brush all over with the remaining melted butter and pop into the preheated oven for around 20 minutes, or until golden and crisp. Allow to rest for 10 minutes. Serve just as you would a quiche for a quick lunch or supper, with a salad.

**serves 4**

500g potatoes, peeled
 and cut into chunks
sea salt and freshly
 ground black pepper
500g asparagus spears,
 woody ends removed
200g filo pastry
100g butter, melted
100g freshly grated
 Lancashire cheese
100g freshly grated
 Cheddar cheese
3 large organic or
 free-range eggs
1 x 284ml pot of
 double cream
¼ of a nutmeg

# How I grow asparagus

## Soil

Asparagus can be a fussy plant, but it can also be one of the easiest vegetables to grow if you're patient and give it the right conditions from the very start. It needs a rich, free-draining, slightly sandy soil in a warm, sheltered, sunny part of the garden. However, the soil I have in the garden at home is a thick Essex clay that's cold and soggy in winter and hard and dry in summer – just the conditions asparagus hates! I didn't want to give up at the first hurdle though, so to give mine the best chance I made raised beds for it, filling them with the right soil – a mixture of coarse, sandy grit, rubble, good soil, well-rotted compost, manure and leaf mould. It's definitely worth the effort, because now the beds are established the plants will crop for at least ten years (and possibly even longer). As asparagus is a perennial plant it will come back every year, and it doesn't like to be moved very much. When you've found the right place in the garden the asparagus will need to stay there, so pick a spot you're happy with.

## Planting

Asparagus is cheap to raise from seed, but as I've found out, it can take three years to grow big and strong enough to crop. A good shortcut is to buy one- or two-year-old 'crowns', which are ready-grown plants, from a garden centre or nursery. Ten should be enough to feed an average-sized family. Seeds should be sown individually in 5cm pots or module trays in spring. When the seedlings are a few months old and 10 to 15cm high you can transfer them into larger 10 to 15cm pots, making sure you use good potting compost. Keep them growing until the following spring, when they'll be large enough to plant outside in the ground.

Crowns can be planted outside straight away, bud-side up. All you need to do is bury them about 10 to 15cm deep, spaced 30 to 45cm apart, down the middle of your raised beds. Bare-root crowns may need to have their roots spread out – it's a bit like planting an octopus! Water them well at first, but when established they rarely need extra water. Keep the growing area well weeded and spread a 10cm layer of rotted manure, compost or leaf-mould over it each winter. This will help to protect the crowns from cold weather and enriches their soil – they'll love you for it.

Asparagus grows quite well in big pots (30 to 45cm wide) filled with rich, free-draining potting compost, so if you don't have a garden you can still grow a few spears. They are very pretty plants as well, with fern-like foliage.

## Harvesting

You can start to pick your asparagus in the third year after planting crowns. But only for one month during this first season, as the plant will still be expanding its root system and if too many spears are removed it will weaken the plant. During the fourth year and thereafter, feel free to pick spears from their first appearance in the spring until the middle of June.

Only pick spears that are 12 to 20cm in length and do it by cutting them at the base, or snapping them. Cutting may damage some spear tips that are still below the soil, so, although it's the method preferred by commercial growers, I think it's best to snap them. To do this, grasp your spear near the base and bend it towards the ground. The spear will break off at the lowest point where there's no fibre. As asparagus can deteriorate so quickly after picking, either eat it immediately or blanch it in boiling water before freezing it.

## My growing tips

- Asparagus will develop root rot if allowed to stand in water. This can destroy a complete bed really quickly, so make sure that all water can drain away easily.

- Asparagus roots have a tendency to rise up out of the soil as the bed matures, so it's a good idea to add a covering of soil to keep the crowns under cover if you see this happening.

- Late spring frosts can kill emerging spears, so cover your bed with garden fleece if there's a cold snap.

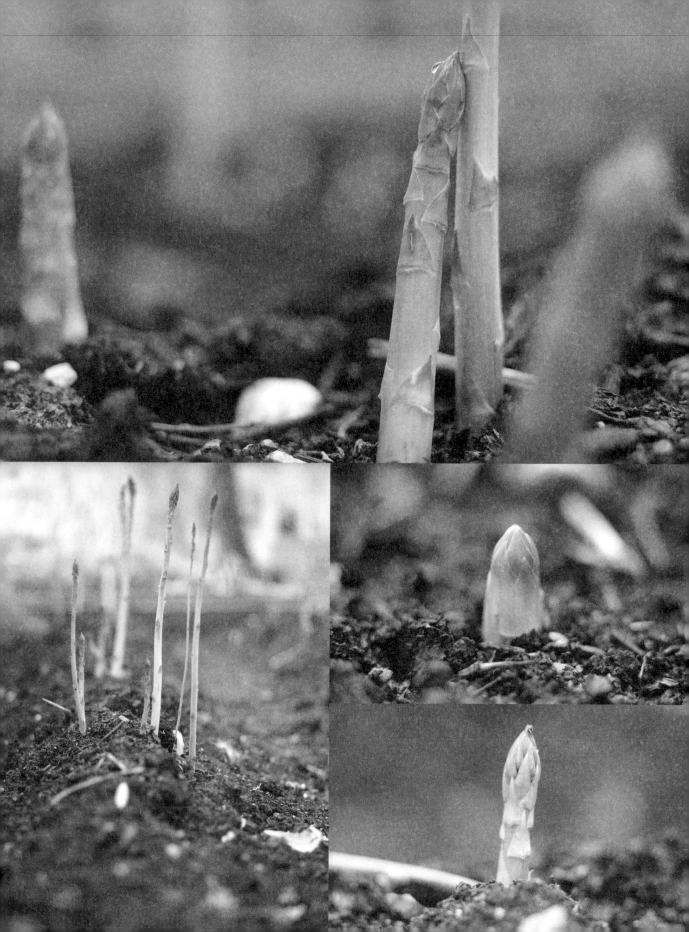

In this chapter I'm going to make some lovely things from the fantastic everyday egg. I've got my own chickens at home now, which is great – not only are they loads of fun but their eggs taste delicious. You only have to see the bright colour of the yolks to know they're something special! I'm pleased to say that recently, in the UK, the supermarkets have upped their game and now you can buy all kinds of different eggs from them – goose, quail, duck and the most incredible gull's eggs. Most of us love to eat eggs one way or another – boiled, scrambled, fried – but there are so many different ways in which they can be used, so I hope you're inspired by my ideas. But before we start cooking, I just want to tell you a bit about where our eggs come from, so that when you're faced with a choice at the shops you'll know what you're buying.

The following types of hen's eggs are now widely available. Sometimes it can be a bit confusing to know exactly where they've come from and under what conditions they've been produced, so here's a brief explanation about the different words used for eggs and how the hens are kept.

### 'Basic' or 'standard' eggs
These are the cheapest eggs and are often referred to as battery eggs. They're produced under the worst kind of conditions. I'm going to cover this in more detail on page 40.

### Barn eggs
Hens are kept in closed barns in pretty squalid conditions where they can move about a little and socialize with each other. There are nine hens per square metre, and they must have access to nests, perches and a litter area. So these eggs are still intensively produced, and the birds will usually have their beaks tipped to stop them pecking at each other, but at least they're not kept in cages.

### Free-range eggs
The hens are kept in a similar way to barn hens, but they are allowed outside during the day. Government regulations state that there must be four square metres of outside space per hen. Good free-range producers will go over and above this to give their hens more access to the outside.

### Woodland eggs
The hens are free-range but with access to established woodland or trees planted to provide natural cover for them. They benefit from being able to forage naturally in the undergrowth.

### Organic eggs
Hens are allowed to roam outside, just like free-range hens, with a natural diet of fresh grass, usually supplemented by organically grown cereals. Flock sizes are smaller, they are not continually fed with antibiotics unless they need them, and genetically modified food is banned. Their feed must be certified organic. With good practice in place, these are generally healthier birds that have more space to move around in their houses, and the result is that they produce much healthier eggs.

# eggs

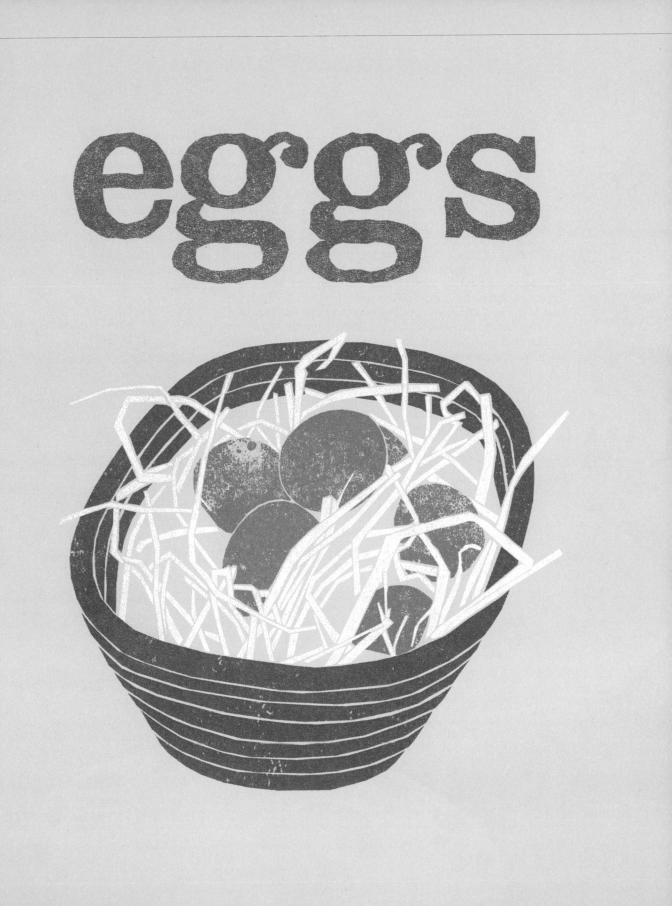

# Eggy breakfast crumpets

This cheeky little version of eggy bread is one of my favourite breakfasts – particularly if I've got a hangover! Brown sauce is great with the eggs but maple syrup is fantastic with the smoky bacon, so take your pick. I got the idea of adding some chilli from a scrambled eggs dish I had in Italy – delicious.

Crack your eggs into a bowl and give them a little whisk with a small pinch of salt and pepper and most of the chopped chilli. Then heat a large, non-stick frying pan over a medium heat and fry the bacon in a tiny amount of olive oil. Let it crisp up on both sides. Meanwhile, get your crumpets and really push them into the egg and chilli mixture. Turn them over a few times – they'll soak it up like a sponge. Push the golden bacon to one side and tilt the pan so the fat runs into the middle. Add the crumpets to the pan and fry them for a few minutes until golden, then turn them over and fry them on the other side.

Serve the eggy crumpets topped with the crispy bacon, with a dollop of brown sauce or a drizzle of maple syrup. To finish, you can sprinkle over the extra chopped chilli, if you're a chilli freak like me. Perfect – heaven on a plate.

**serves 2**

2 large organic eggs
sea salt and freshly
  ground black pepper
1 fresh red chilli, deseeded
  and very finely chopped
6 rashers of good-quality
  smoked bacon
olive oil
4 round crumpets
brown sauce or maple
  syrup, to serve

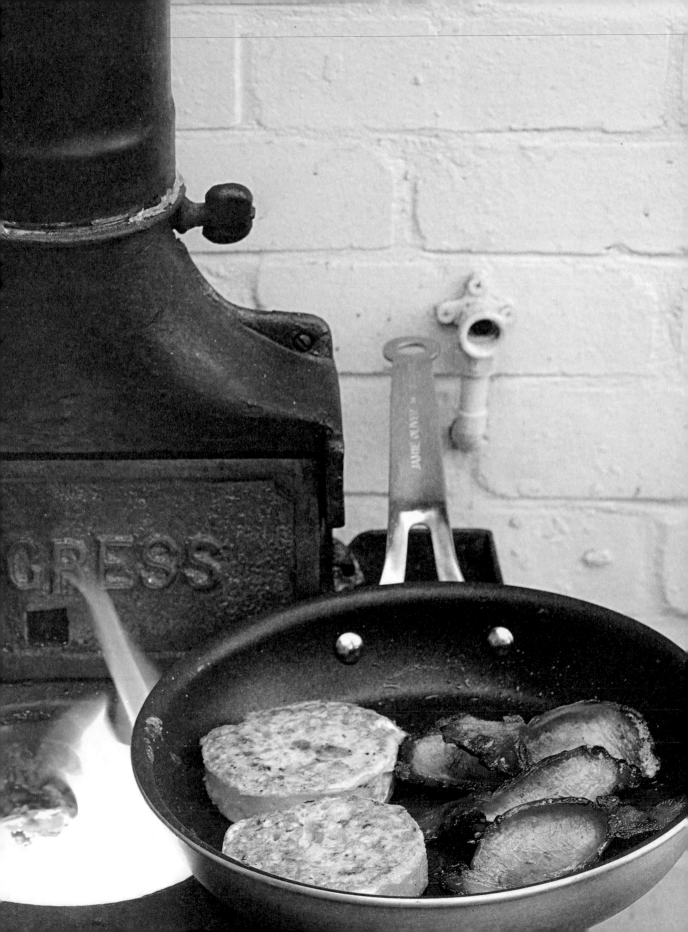

# Fresh tagliatelle with sprouting broccoli and oozy cheese sauce

The hero of this dish (apart from the eggs, of course!) is fontina, a delicious Italian mountain cheese used for melting, available in good cheese shops and delis. But any combination of Parmesan, pecorino, taleggio or Gruyère cheeses will also work well.

You can buy ready-made dried or fresh tagliatelle, but this is a really quick way to make your own. You'll need 1 egg to 100g flour per person as a rule. Crack the eggs into a food processor and add the flour. Whiz it up and listen for the sound changing to a rumble – this means the dough is coming together nicely. Turn the power off and test the consistency by pinching the dough. If it's a bit sticky add a little more flour and pulse again.

Tip the dough mixture on to a floured surface and shape it into a ball using your hands. Give it a little knead till smooth, then divide your dough into four equal parts. Start on the thickest setting of your pasta machine and run the first bit of dough through four or five times, moving the rollers closer together each time until the pasta is silky, smooth and about as thick as a CD. Flour your finished sheet generously, then fold it up and cut across into 1cm strips. Gather all the slices together and toss them through your fingers, with a little flour, to open them up and make your pile of tagliatelle. Place to one side and repeat with the rest of the dough.

Bring a large pan of salted water to the boil. In a bowl large enough to rest on top of the pan, put your crème fraîche, fontina or other melting cheese and your Parmesan with a pinch of salt and pepper. Place the bowl over the pan for the cheeses to slowly melt. It won't take long. Meanwhile, trim any dry ends off the broccoli, then finely slice the stalks diagonally and leave the florets whole (cutting any larger ones in half).

At this point the cheese sauce should be lovely and oozy, so remove the bowl from above the pan and drop the pasta and broccoli into the boiling water. Boil hard for 2 to 3 minutes, until the pasta is just cooked through. Whip up the 2 egg yolks and the marjoram, or other chosen herb leaves, into the sauce. Drain the pasta and broccoli, reserving a little of the cooking water, and quickly toss them with the sauce – the heat from the pasta will be enough to cook the eggs through. If the sauce is a little thick, add a few splashes of cooking water to make it silky and loose. Taste and season if necessary. Serve as quickly as you can, with some extra Parmesan sprinkled over the top and a drizzle of extra virgin olive oil. Grand!

serves 4

freshly grated Parmesan
  for serving
extra virgin olive oil

**for the pasta**
4 large free-range or
  organic eggs
400g Tipo '00' pasta flour,
  plus extra for dusting
sea salt

**for the cheese sauce**
250ml crème fraîche
150g sliced fontina or other
  nice melting cheese
150g freshly grated
  Parmesan cheese
sea salt and freshly
  ground black pepper
400g purple sprouting
  broccoli
2 large free-range or
  organic egg yolks
a small bunch of fresh
  marjoram, oregano or
  thyme tips, leaves picked

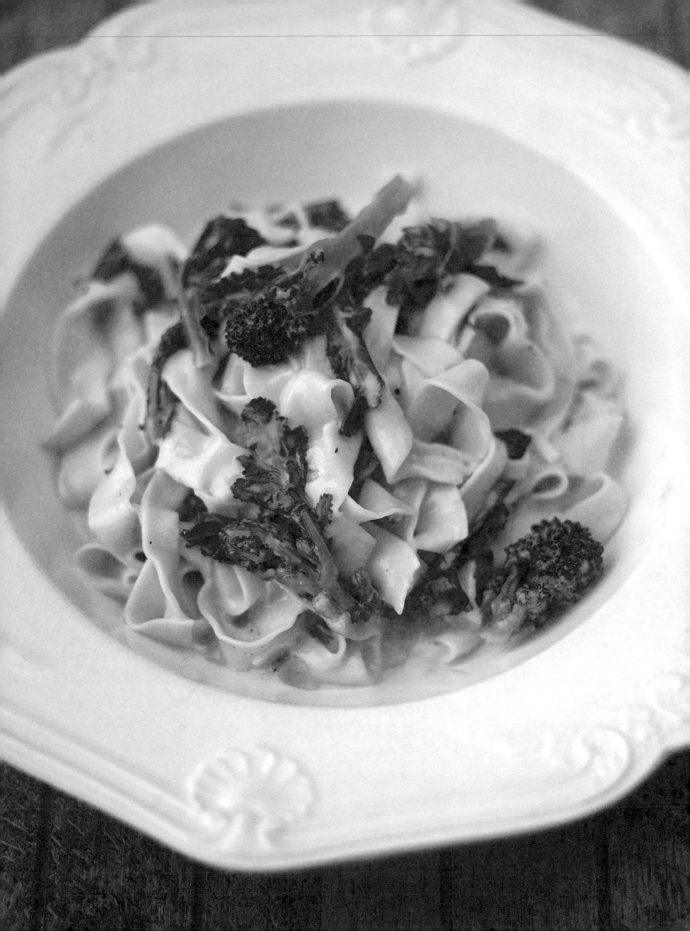

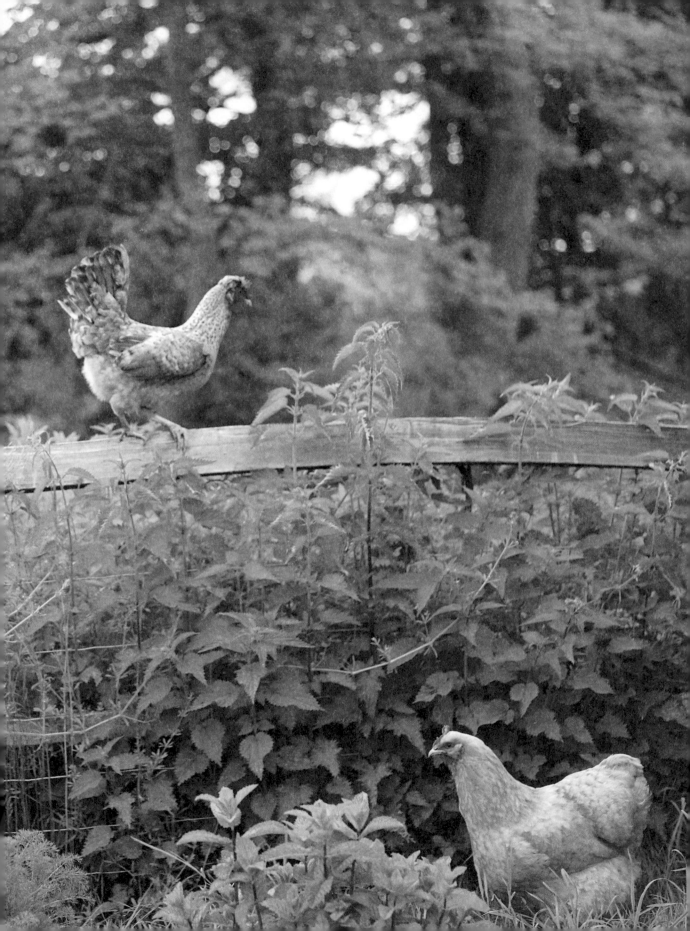

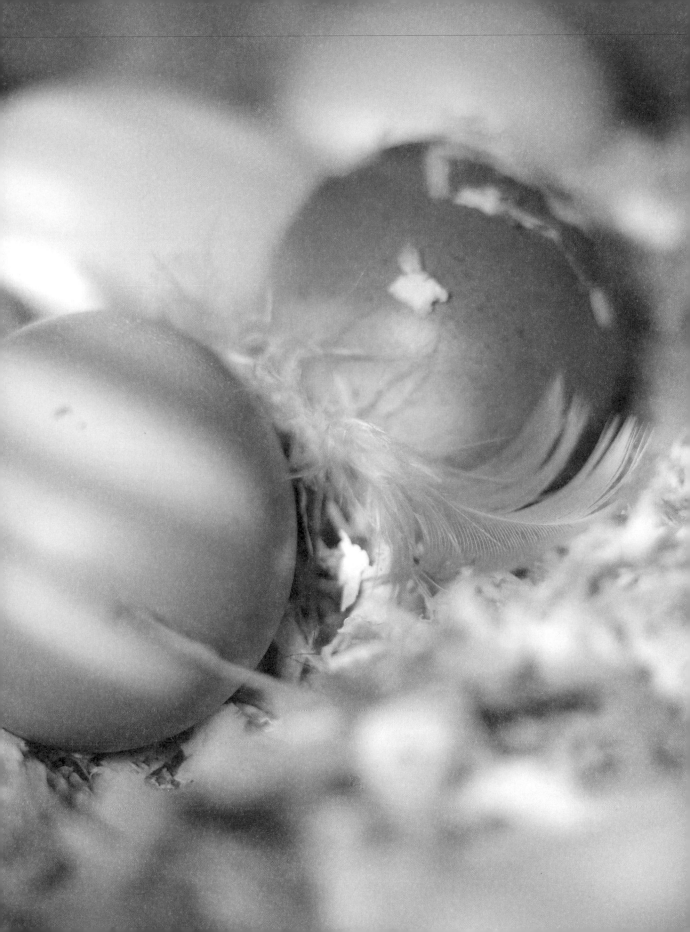

# Delicate egg ribbons with bresaola, crispy fennel and spring leaves

For this dish I wanted to do something a little unusual with eggs, so I decided to turn them into silky ribbons. You can make plain ones or flavour the egg mixture with chilli or chopped delicate herbs. I've suggested finishing the salad off with a few drips of truffle oil, which has a lovely mushroomy taste. Although 'fake' truffle oil still tastes good, try to get the real thing – it's expensive but should last you ages and you can use it in soups, in gratins, on roast potatoes, you name it.

Shave the fennel bulb with a speed peeler or a sharp knife. Put the shavings into iced or very cold water for about a minute – this gives you a lovely crispy texture but the downside is that you lose flavour, so be quick. As soon as the fennel starts to curl up, drain it in a colander, remove any ice cubes, spin it really dry in a salad spinner and put to one side.

Whip up the eggs with a pinch of salt and pepper. Add a splash of water to the mixture as this will give you thin crêpe-like omelettes. Rub a little olive oil over the bottom of a 20cm non-stick frying pan and place it on the heat. Working quickly, pour in a little egg mixture and tilt the pan so it runs all round the bottom. In less than a minute your crêpe will be opaque and cooked through. Touch it lightly to test whether it's done. If it is, hold the pan at an angle and start to peel it away with a spatula. Be gentle and don't rush – if you mess the first one up, don't worry, you'll get the feel for it! When you've made your crêpes, stack them on a board and cover them with tinfoil to keep them warm.

Put the fennel and all the salad leaves into a bowl. Divide the bresaola between four plates and drizzle with a little extra virgin olive oil. Remove the tinfoil from the crêpes. Roll them up one at a time and slice them 1 to 2cm wide. Toss them gently with your fingers to unwind them. Add them to the bowl of fennel and salad leaves with the grated Parmesan. Dress with 6 tablespoons of extra virgin olive oil and the lemon juice. Season with salt and pepper and toss gently but thoroughly. Taste and balance with seasoning and a little extra lemon juice if need be. For a cool tweak, add a teaspoon of truffle oil. Sprinkle the reserved herby fennel tops over the salad. Place the salad bowl in the middle of the table with your plates of bresaola and let everyone help themselves. Lovely finished with an extra grating of Parmesan.

serves 4

1 bulb of fennel, herby tops reserved
4 large free-range or organic eggs
sea salt and freshly ground black pepper
olive oil
1 head of radicchio or treviso, or 2 red chicory, leaves washed, spun dry and torn
2 good handfuls of rocket and/or watercress, washed and spun dry
16 slices of bresaola
extra virgin olive oil
a handful of freshly grated Parmesan cheese, plus extra for serving
juice of ½ a lemon
optional: 1 teaspoon truffle oil (try it!)

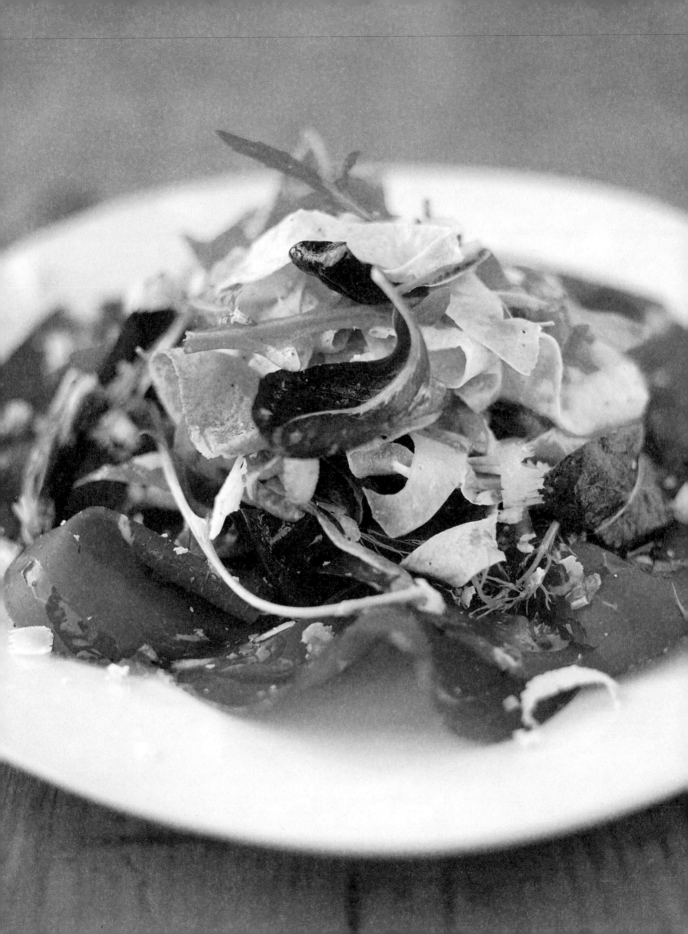

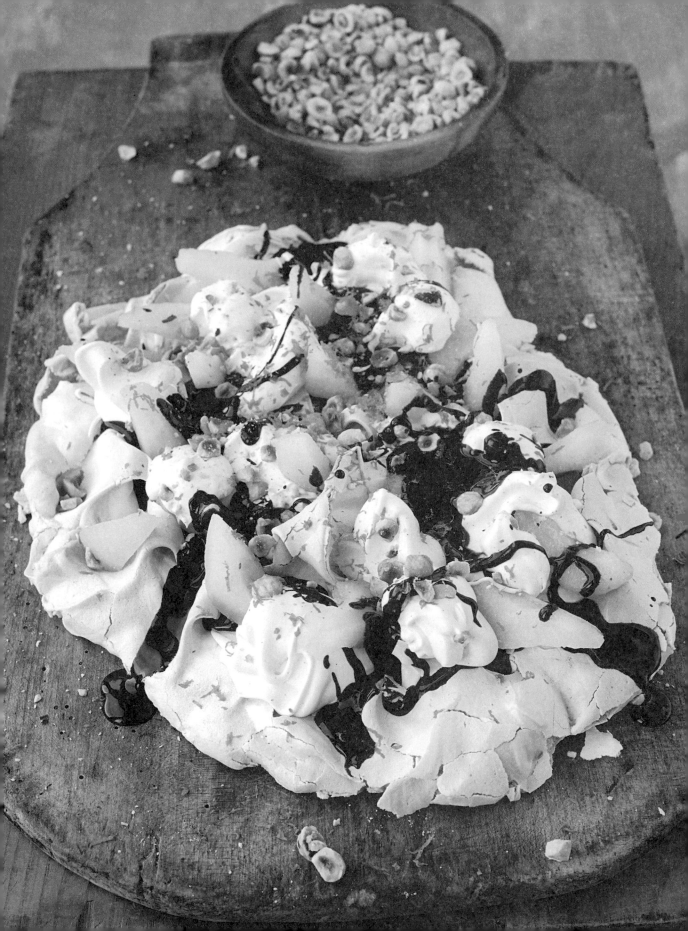

# Tray-baked meringue with pears, cream, toasted hazelnuts and chocolate sauce

This dish, to me, is an assembly of wonderful sweet friends. Having one slab of meringue means serving it is dead easy. Feel free to make up your own topping combinations. Other good ones I really like are chestnut purée mixed with cream and chocolate, or other soft fruits with praline, or mixed toasted nuts and cream.

Preheat your oven to 150°C/300°F/gas 2 and line a 40 x 25cm baking tray with a sheet of greaseproof paper.

Put your egg whites into a squeaky clean bowl, making sure there are absolutely no little pieces of egg shell or egg yolk in them. Whisk on medium until the whites form firm peaks. With your mixer still running, gradually add the sugar and the pinch of salt. Turn the mixer up to the highest setting and whisk for about 7 or 8 minutes, until the meringue mixture is white and glossy. To test whether it's done you can pinch some between your fingers – if it feels completely smooth it's ready; if it's slightly granular it needs a little more whisking.

Dot each corner of the greaseproof paper with a blob of meringue, then turn it over and stick it to the baking tray. Spoon the meringue out on to the paper. Using the back of a spoon, shape and swirl it into an A4 size rectangle. Place in the preheated oven and bake for an hour or until crisp on the outside and a little soft and sticky inside. At the same time, bake the hazelnuts on a separate tray in the oven for an hour or until golden brown.

Drain the tins of pears, reserving the syrup from one tin. Cut each pear half into three slices. Pour the pear syrup into a saucepan with the ginger and warm gently over a medium heat until it starts to simmer. Take off the heat and snap the chocolate into the saucepan, stirring with a spoon until it's all melted.

Take the meringue and hazelnuts out of the oven and leave to cool. Place the meringue on a nice rustic board or platter. Whip the cream with the sifted icing sugar and the vanilla seeds until it forms smooth, soft peaks. Smash the toasted hazelnuts (in a tea towel) and sprinkle half of them over the top of the meringue. Spoon half the whipped cream over the top and drizzle with some of the chocolate sauce (if the sauce has firmed up, melt it slightly by holding the saucepan over a large pan of boiling water). Divide most of the pear pieces evenly over the top. Pile over the rest of the whipped cream and pears. Drizzle with some more chocolate sauce, then sprinkle over the remaining toasted hazelnuts with some grated orange zest. Serve straight away. If you're making this in advance, get everything ready and assemble at the last minute.

serves 6 to 8

4 large free-range or
  organic egg whites
200g unrefined golden
  caster sugar
a pinch of sea salt
100g hazelnuts,
  skins removed
2 x 400g tins of halved
  pears, in syrup
optional: 2 pieces of stem
  ginger, thinly sliced
200g dark chocolate
  (minimum 70%
  cocoa solids)
400ml double cream
50g icing sugar, sifted
1 vanilla pod, halved and
  seeds scraped out
zest of 1 orange

eggs

# The shock of battery farming

Caged battery hens are a sad reality of modern-day farming. In fact, I don't think it can even be referred to as 'farming' as we understand it, because everything about it is horrendous. Who on earth dreamt the idea up? Imagine the scene (because not many people get to see inside these places): the chickens are housed in wire cages (about five in each), having a floor area no bigger than an A4 piece of paper. The cages can be stacked six high, with hundreds crammed along tightly packed rows. This is not natural, because the birds are not free to roam, to scratch about, to dust-bathe themselves to keep fit. Cooped up like this, day in day out, the poor things end up in very bad health.

I recently picked up a load of these chickens from a refuge and brought them home with me to join my free-range hens, so they can enjoy the rest of their lives. Anyone can pick these rescued birds up from the Battery Hen Welfare Trust, either for free or for as little as 50p a bird, which works out cheaper than half a dozen eggs. They were actually the first ones I'd ever seen and I was very shocked by the state they were in. The combs on top of their heads were pale pink, almost white, and flat. They should be red and sticking up. Their feet were in really bad shape, because they didn't have a proper flat surface to stand on – imagine being forced to stand on wire bars for over a year. Instead of being short from scratching about, their claws were long. Their feathers were really dry and in an awful state and their beaks were clipped. In fact, the hens themselves looked almost comatose for the first day or so that I had them at home. This is not respecting an animal while it's alive. This is not giving them a good and natural life. There's absolutely no excuse for treating animals in this way. They may be forced to lay more eggs, to make more profit, but I think the final product is also affected and battery eggs are simply not as good as free-range or organic.

The Battery Hen Welfare Trust has passionately defended the farmers, saying they're not bad people; they're just stuck between a rock and a hard place because farming of recent years has been so tough. And you know what? My little rant in this book is not aimed at the farmers, whether or not I believe that what they're doing is right or wrong, it's more about encouraging you to buy locally and from stock that's been reared as naturally as possible.

From now on, when you buy your eggs, have a look at the box to check they're free-range and feel free to ask at restaurants about the type of eggs they're using. I'm really pleased to say that things *are* changing. More and more of us are choosing free-range or organic eggs, so the message is obviously becoming clearer. However, that's the tip of the iceberg, because in the UK 63% of the eggs we buy come from hens in cages, and 86% of eggs used as ingredients come from hens kept in cages. But while we're consciously making an effort not to buy battery eggs (because we rightly feel uncomfortable about the whole thing), we need to think about all the processed foods we might buy that have eggs in them: quiches, cheap egg sandwiches, biscuits, cakes, mayonnaise, cheap ice cream … this is where the battery eggs are used. So let's all be a bit more aware.

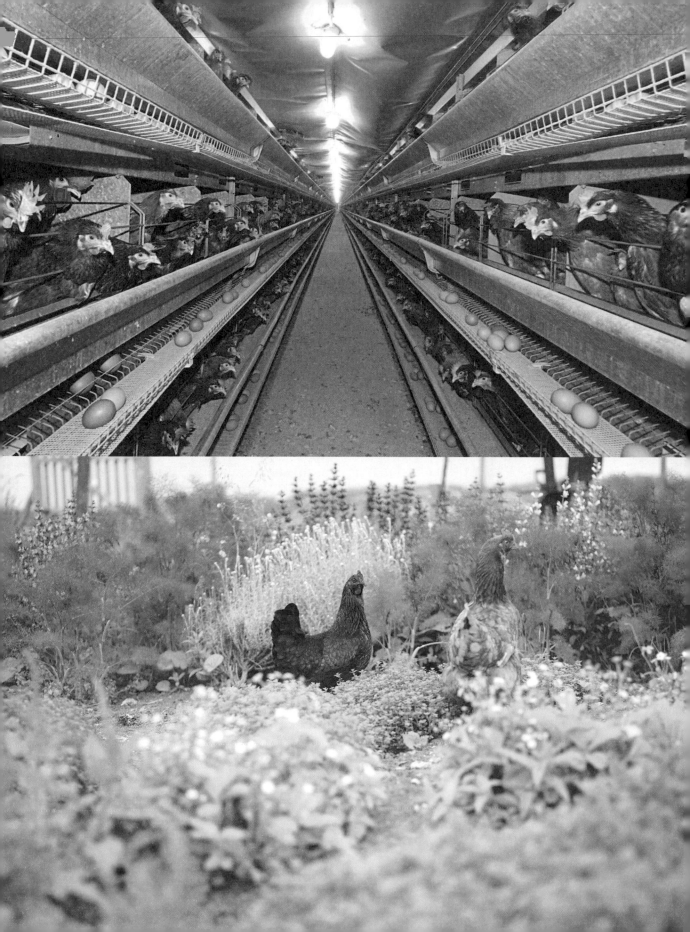

Even though I've got my chickens at home for their eggs, the one thing I haven't had a go at yet, and probably won't do for a while, is keeping animals for food. It doesn't matter though, because wherever you are, if you're excited about food, there's always a way of sourcing meat direct from a local farmer. This is the best alternative to keeping your own and you don't have to buy a whole animal – you can buy half a lamb or part of a lamb. To be able to specify what you want and build a relationship with the farmer, or your local butcher, is a great thing. It can also be much cheaper to buy direct from these places than to buy lamb flown in from halfway around the world. Whatever country we live in, we should all try to buy locally, whether from caring and committed farmers or from good local butchers or quality supermarkets. It's also possible to buy lamb over the internet.

If you have a freezer, and the confidence to buy a whole, half or quarter lamb and break it down, then go for it. Not only will you get really good-quality meat but you'll also know exactly where it's come from, how it's been treated during its life and what it's been fed. It might even encourage you to have a go at cooking the cuts in slightly different ways to get the very best out of your lamb, so you'll be expanding your cooking horizons as well. And the farmer will get a better price, which means he can invest more money back into animal welfare and land management.

Sheep farming is the most natural form of farming there is, because the sheep have to spend most of their time outside in their natural surroundings and it suits them down to the ground! The only time they're brought inside is if the weather's really bad, or before they have their lambs in the spring. My friend Daphne is a sheep farmer in north Wales and her flock are at home up on the mountains, eating the natural herbage. It's where they want to be. And the more contented the animal and the less stress they have, right up to the point of slaughter, the better the meat will be.

Lamb should be hung for four days to a week, depending on age and breed, to allow the meat to tenderize and develop good flavour, and the skin to dry out. Generally speaking, the older the animal, the longer it needs to be hung for. Mutton is normally hung for ten days. A perfectly hung animal should have dark meat with lovely white fat. This goes for beef and venison as well as lamb. When it comes to fat, the supermarkets seem to want to sell us lean meat, but it's actually the fat that gives the flavour. A well-fed, carefully matured animal will have a good marbling of fat, giving a juicy, tasty product.

So what makes really good lamb? Well, it's a combination of things. First, their breeding, second, a caring, capable farmer, and third, the management of the flock. Natural factors like sun and rain, giving plenty of grass, also play a big part. Did you know that spring lamb is actually not the best thing to buy? Yes, it will be tender but the flavour won't have had a chance to develop. The meat from autumn lamb is not only cheaper but it has a better flavour. This is because the lambs have had a chance to mature naturally out on the land and will therefore have benefited from all the food they've eaten through the lush summer months. Worth remembering.

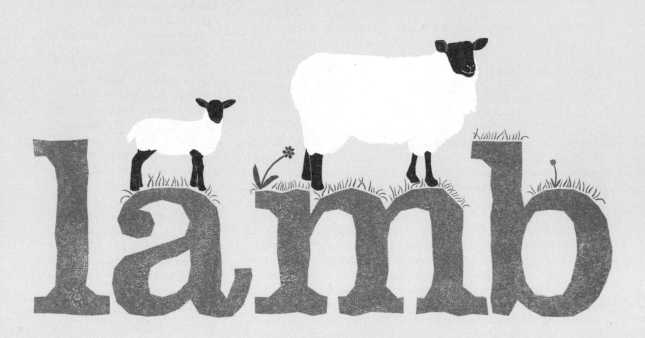

# Grilled lamb kofta kebabs with pistachios and spicy salad wrap

Authentic kebabs are delicious, full of nuts, spices, herbs and fruit, as anyone who's tasted proper Middle Eastern cooking knows. In this recipe I'm using a spice called sumac – it has a lovely flavour – but if you can't find it, try lemon zest instead.

Buy really good minced lamb, or else a cut of trimmed shoulder or neck fillet and mince it up at home in a food processor. If you buy slightly older lamb (hogget or mutton), it's important to ask your butcher to remove the sinews, and that you cook the meat for a few minutes longer.

This dish is best cooked on a barbecue over hot coals, but if that's not possible, put your grill on to its highest setting or heat up a griddle pan. Either way, get your cooking source preheated.

Place the lamb in a food processor with most of the thyme, chilli, cumin and sumac (reserving a little of each for sprinkling over later), a little salt and pepper and all the pistachios. Put the lid on and keep pulsing until the mixture looks like mince.

Divide the meat into four equal pieces and get yourself four skewers. With damp hands, push and shape the meat around and along each skewer. Press little indents in the meat with your fingers as you go – this will give it a better texture when cooked.

In one bowl, mix the salad leaves and mint. In another, combine the sliced onion with a good pinch of salt and pepper and a squeeze of lemon juice (the acidity will take the edge off and lightly pickle the raw onion). Scrunch this all together with your hands, then mix in the parsley leaves.

Grill the kebabs until nicely golden on all sides. Dress your salad leaves and mint with a splash of extra virgin olive oil, a squeeze of lemon juice and some salt and pepper. Meanwhile, warm your flatbreads for 30 seconds on your griddle pan or under the grill, then divide between plates and top each with some dressed salad leaves and onion. When your kebabs are cooked, slip them off their skewers on to the flatbreads – you can leave them whole or break them up as I've done here. Sprinkle with the rest of the sumac, cumin, chilli and fresh thyme, and a little salt and pepper. Now either toss the salads, grilled meat and juices together on top of the flatbreads and drizzle with some of the yoghurt before rolling up and serving; or let your friends toss theirs together at the table, then dress and roll up their own, drizzled with some extra virgin olive oil.

serves 4

500g trimmed shoulder or neck fillet of lamb, chopped into 2.5cm chunks
2 heaped tablespoons fresh thyme leaves
1 level tablespoon ground chilli
1 level tablespoon ground cumin
4 level tablespoons sumac, if you can find any, or finely grated zest of 1 lemon
sea salt and freshly ground black pepper
a good handful of shelled pistachio nuts
a few handfuls of mixed salad leaves, such as romaine or cos, endive and rocket, washed, spun dry and shredded
a small bunch of fresh mint, leaves picked
1 red onion, peeled and very finely sliced
1 lemon
a bunch of fresh flat-leaf parsley, leaves picked
extra virgin olive oil
4 large flatbreads or tortilla wraps
4 heaped tablespoons natural yoghurt

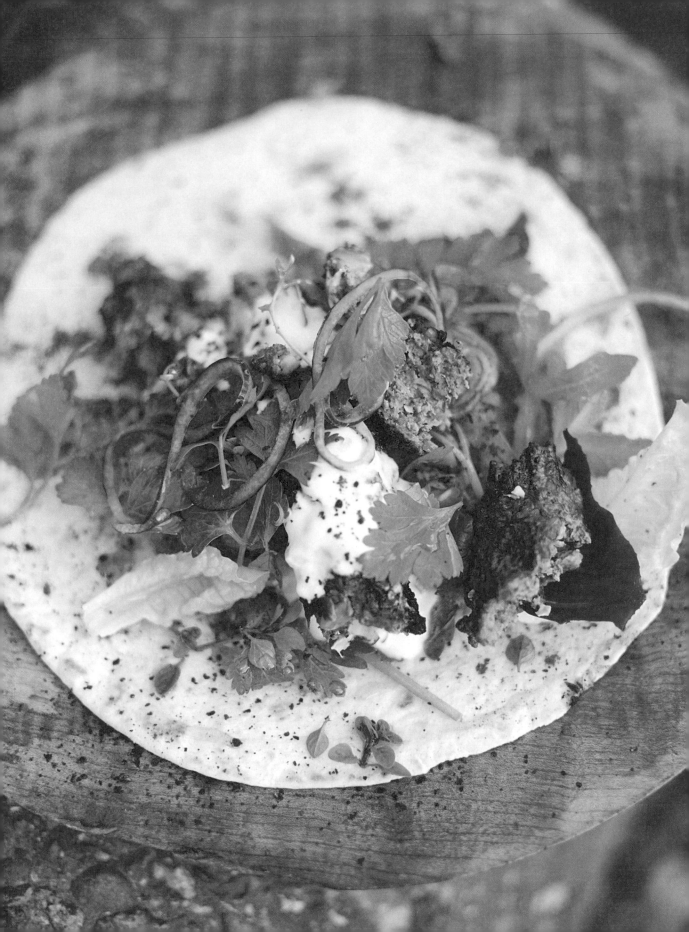

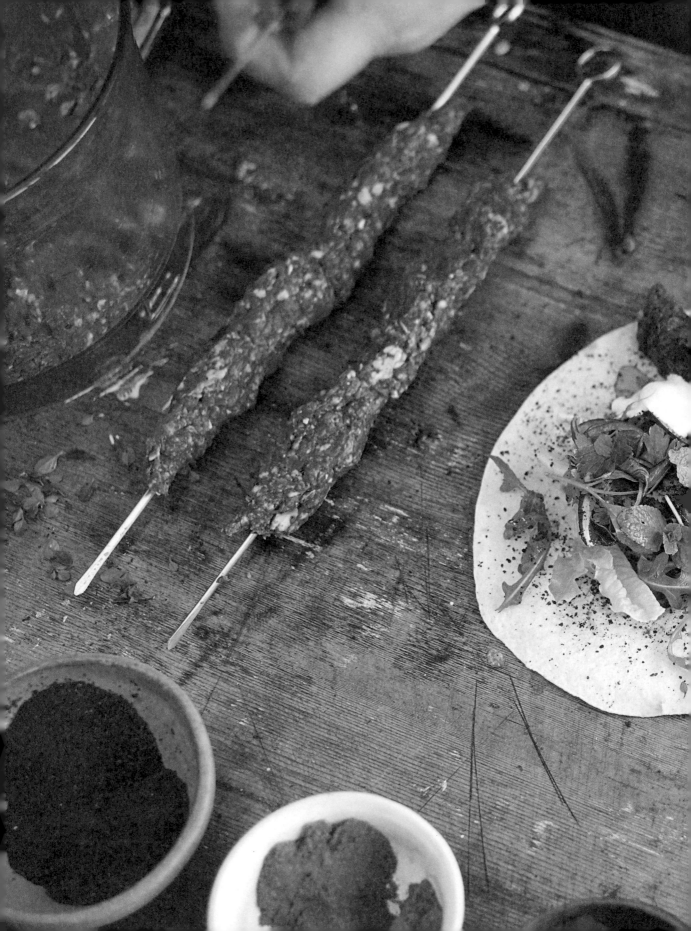

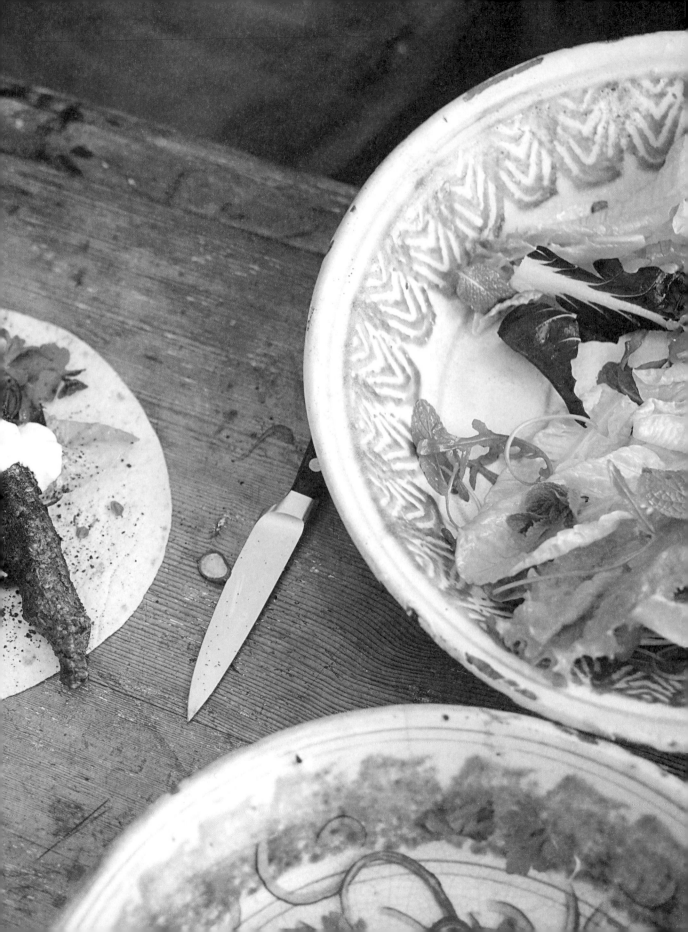

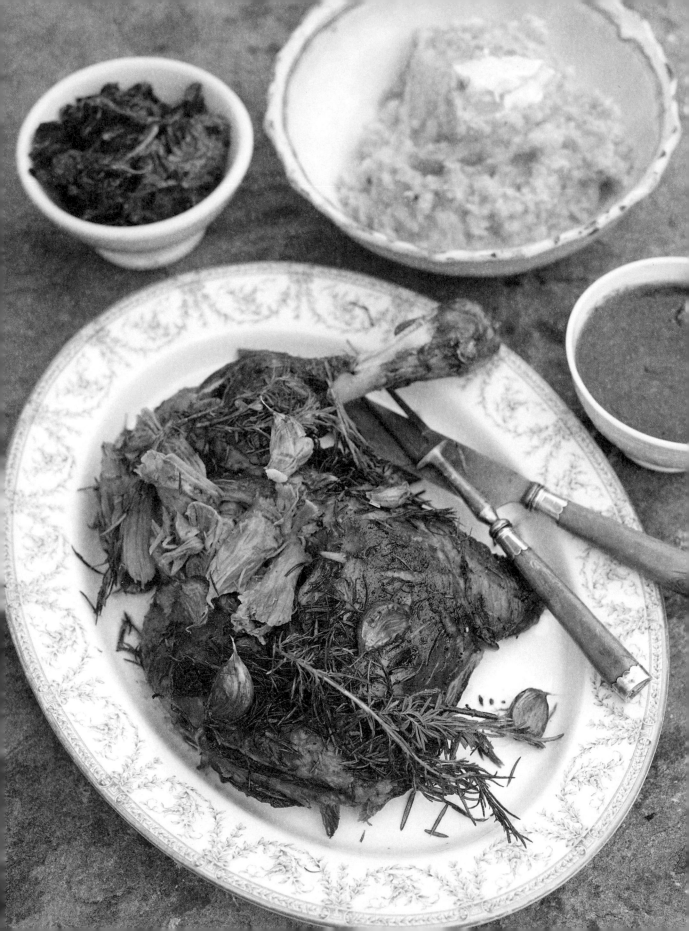

# Incredible roasted shoulder of lamb with smashed veg and greens

In this recipe I'm going to show you how utterly incredible a slow-roasted shoulder of lamb can be. In exchange I'd like you to buy quality local lamb that's had the appropriate amount of hanging time. I'm going to let the meat speak for itself and not add much to it, just a simple sauce made from all the goodness in the tray. You can make this at any time of year served with any seasonal veg.

Preheat your oven to full whack. Slash the fat side of the lamb all over with a sharp knife. Lay half the sprigs of rosemary and half the garlic cloves on the bottom of a high-sided roasting tray, rub the lamb all over with olive oil and season with salt and pepper. Place it in the tray on top of the rosemary and garlic, and put the rest of the rosemary and garlic on top of the lamb. Tightly cover the tray with tinfoil and place in the oven. Turn the oven down immediately to 170°C/325°F/gas 3 and cook for 4 hours – it's done if you can pull the meat apart easily with two forks.

When the lamb is nearly cooked, put your potatoes, carrots and swede into a large pot of boiling salted water and boil hard for 20 minutes or so until you can slide a knife into the swede easily. Drain and allow to steam dry, then smash them up in the pan with most of the butter. If you prefer a smooth texture, add some cooking water. Spoon into a bowl, cover with tinfoil and keep warm over a pan of simmering water.

Remove the lamb from the oven and place it on a chopping board. Cover it with tinfoil, then a tea towel, and leave it to rest. Put a large pan of salted water on to boil for your greens. Pour away most of the fat from the roasting tray, discarding any bits of rosemary stalk. Put the tray on the hob and mix in the flour. Add the stock, stirring and scraping all the sticky goodness off the bottom of the tray. You won't need gallons of gravy, just a couple of flavoursome spoonfuls each. Add the capers, turn the heat down and simmer for a few minutes.

Finely chop the mint and add it to the sauce with the red wine vinegar at the last minute then pour into a jug. Add your greens and stalks to the pan of fast-boiling salted water and cook for 4 to 5 minutes to just soften them. Drain and toss with a knob of butter and a pinch of salt and pepper. Place everything in the middle of the table, and shred the lamb in front of your guests. Absolutely delish!

**serves 6**

500g lovely greens, such as white cabbage, Savoy cabbage, Brussels tops or cavolo nero, leaves separated, stalks finely sliced

*for the lamb*
a large bunch of fresh rosemary
1 x 2kg shoulder of lamb
olive oil
sea salt and freshly ground black pepper
1 bulb of garlic, unpeeled, broken into cloves

*for the smashed veg*
750g peeled potatoes, cut into large chunks
3 large carrots, peeled and cut into small chunks
½ a large swede, peeled and cut into small chunks
75g butter

*for the sauce*
1 tablespoon flour
500ml good-quality hot chicken or vegetable stock
2 heaped tablespoons capers, soaked, drained and chopped
a large bunch of fresh mint, leaves picked
2 tablespoons red wine vinegar

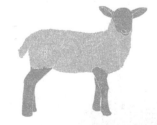

# Pan-fried Barnsley chops with creamy cannellini beans, rainbow chard and salsa verde

A Barnsley chop, also called a butterfly chop, is basically a double lamb chop. For this fantastic dish I'm going to serve them with a cool modern-day salsa verde, some tasty beans and beautiful chard. This is an excellent vegetable to grow as it gives you great stalks, lovely leaves, and delicious shoots that you can use in salads.

Preheat your oven to full whack and bring a large pan of salted water to the boil. For the best salsa verde, finely chop together the garlic, capers, gherkins and anchovies on a large chopping board. Place the herbs on top and carry on chopping and mixing everything until fine. You can use a food processor if you want, but don't leave it running too long – otherwise the sauce will become a purée. Scrape into a bowl, add the red wine vinegar and about 10 tablespoons of extra virgin olive oil. Mix in the mustard and a small swig of water, then stir and season nicely to taste.

Rub the chops with a little olive oil, and season them with salt and pepper. Preheat a large ovenproof griddle pan or frying pan until very hot, and press the chops firmly down on it – don't add oil to the pan because the natural fat from the chops will cook out. After 2 minutes, turn them over and place the whole griddle pan in the preheated oven. Roast them for about 10 to 15 minutes, or until cooked to your liking.

While finishing the meat in the oven, blanch the chard in the pan of boiling water for 3 or 4 minutes, until the stalks are tender, then drain it. Toss in a bowl with a little extra virgin olive oil, a squeeze of lemon juice and some seasoning.

Heat a saucepan and pour in a splash of olive oil. Fry the garlic for a few seconds until lightly golden, then add the chillies and beans. Top with the rosemary, pop the lid on, turn the heat down and warm the cooked beans gently. Season them with a bit of salt and pepper.

When the chops are cooked, lay them on a warm platter and spoon over a large dollop of salsa verde. Pour away any excess fat from the pan and squeeze in the juice of half a lemon, then scrape and stir all the stickiness off the bottom. Feel free to discard the rosemary sprigs from the beans. Pour the beans into a large bowl and top with the chard. Spoon all the meaty goodness from the pan over the top and serve next to the chops.

**serves 4**

sea salt and freshly
  ground black pepper
4 Barnsley lamb chops,
  about 3cm thick
olive oil
300g rainbow chard
1 lemon, halved
1 clove of garlic, peeled
  and sliced
2 small dried chillies,
  crushed
1 x 650g jar of good-quality
  cooked cannellini, borlotti
  or butter beans, drained
3 sprigs of fresh rosemary

*for the salsa verde*
½ a clove of garlic, peeled
1 teaspoon capers, soaked
  and drained
4 little gherkins
2 good-quality anchovy
  fillets in olive oil, drained
a small bunch of fresh flat-
  leaf parsley, leaves picked
a small handful of fresh
  basil, leaves picked
a small handful of fresh
  mint, leaves picked
1–2 tablespoons red wine
  vinegar, to taste
extra virgin olive oil
1 teaspoon Dijon mustard
sea salt and freshly
  ground black pepper

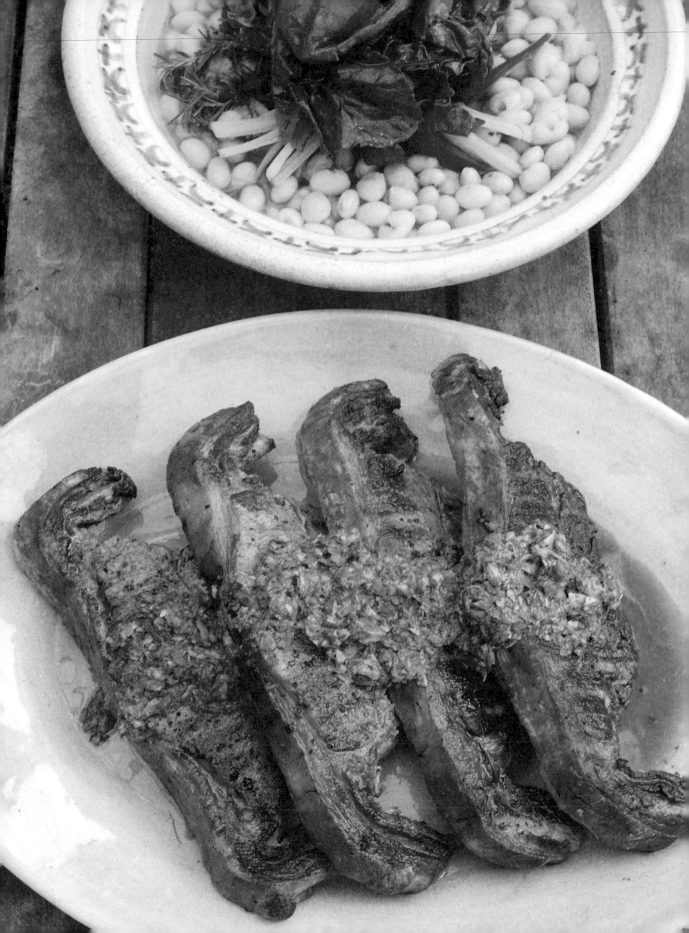

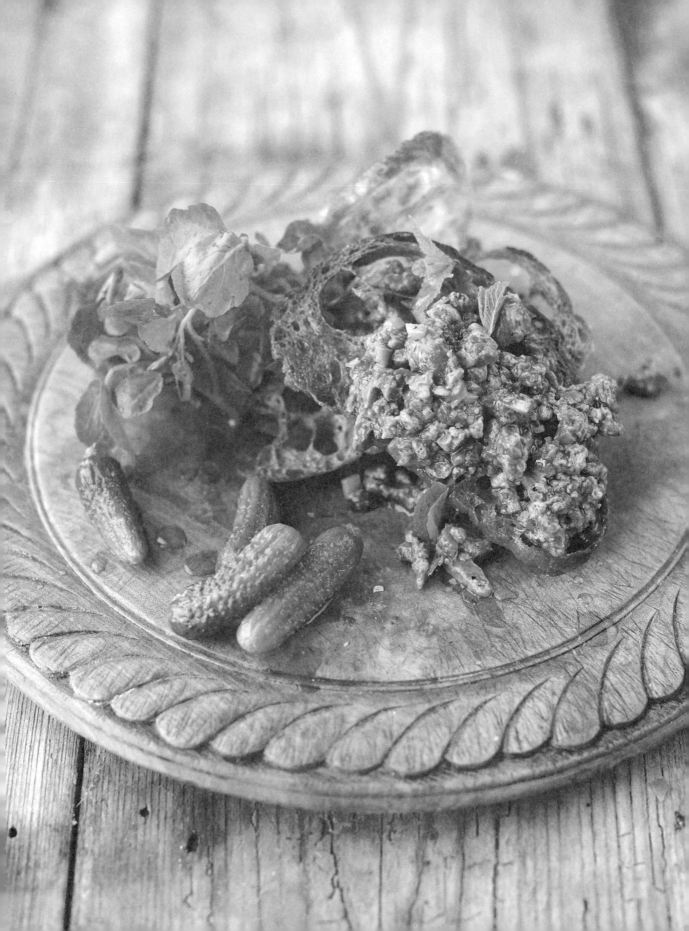

# Really very delicious and simple lamb tartare

You might be surprised to hear this, but there's absolutely nothing wrong with eating raw lamb, just as there's nothing wrong with eating raw beef. Carpaccios and steak tartares are pretty commonplace in France and Italy, and for quite some time now we've been featuring lamb tartare on our menus at Fifteen. It always goes like hot cakes and people clean their plates, so I'd love for you guys to give it a go. It's quick to make, contemporary, slightly restauranty but absolutely delicious.

In Italy I tasted this with new season's olive oil, which was just delicious. Try to get hold of some because a good oil can make all the difference, rather than using cheap gear.

As far as the cut of meat is concerned, the fillet or loin is traditionally used to make tartare, but with lamb you can use slightly tougher and tastier cuts like rump and leg as long as the sinews are removed (this is really important – the butcher can do it for you) and you give the meat a good bash with a tenderizing hammer, or something heavy, before you start chopping it up.

Get yourself a large chopping knife. Put your meat on a chopping board and slice it up, then chop it until you end up with coarse mince. Push this to one end of the board and finely slice your chilli on the other. (I think chilli and lamb work really well together – if you want to use less or more, feel free.) Add the gherkins to the board and chop these up on top of the chilli, then add the mint on top and finely chop again.

Put the meat and all the flavourings from the board into a bowl and stir together, adding the mustard and orange and lemon juice. Mix up and season with salt and pepper to taste. Pour in a few glugs of extra virgin olive oil. Mix everything together so that all the meat is nicely coated and dressed in the lovely flavours – have a taste. This is your opportunity to add a little more heat if you want it, with mustard or chilli, or a little extra lemon juice to cut through. Seasoning it well is also really important.

When the meat is tasting really good, heat up your grill or a griddle pan and toast your ciabatta slices. There are two ways I like to serve this dish. You can give each person a couple of toasted ciabatta slices on their plate, topped with a spoonful of the tartare, a drizzle of extra virgin olive oil and a little lemon-dressed watercress. Or, if you want to be a little more family-style, you can put all the tartare on to a big platter, drizzled with extra virgin olive oil. Place a couple of extra gherkins on the side and scatter over the reserved baby mint leaves. Serve a bowl of lemon-dressed watercress and a basketful of toasted bread next to it and let everyone dive in and help themselves!

serves 4

450g trimmed best-quality lamb meat (see recipe introduction)
1 fresh red chilli, halved and deseeded
a small jar of little gherkins
a small bunch of fresh mint, finely chopped, baby leaves reserved
1 teaspoon French mustard
juice of ½ an orange
juice of ½ a lemon
sea salt and freshly ground black pepper
extra virgin olive oil (new season's if possible!)
8 x 1cm thick slices of ciabatta bread
2 handfuls of watercress, washed and spun dry

lamb

# Lamb

## When is a lamb a 'lamb'?

A lamb is called a 'lamb' during its first year of life. Then in its second year it's called a 'hogget' – still tender and really tasty but a little underrated. And then there's 'mutton', which is any sheep over two years old. Mutton is a fine piece of meat – it's much darker than lamb, and it needs to be cooked slowly to make it really tender but, my God, the flavour is amazing! Two- to three-year-old mutton is usually the best; however, because it has to be matured in a chiller for around two weeks, the supermarkets don't want to know and only the best local butchers will dedicate the space and time to maturing it. After the war people got out of the habit of cooking mutton, which is such a shame! We really should all start asking for mutton in order to get it back into fashion. It would make such a difference, financially, to the farmers as well. Mutton is a by-product of sheep farming because the animal is kept primarily as breeding stock. However, when it comes to selling it, the farmers can't get a good price, so it would make a huge difference to them if there was a demand for it. When you're next at the butcher's please ask for some, and have a look at this website as well, which is a celebration of mutton: www.muttonrenaissance.org.uk.

## The different cuts of lamb

Now, to give you a heads-up, I want to show you where on the animal the cuts come from. Even in a lot of good butcher's shops the lamb on display is very often already broken down into steaks or chops, and they might not be displayed next to the cuts that would naturally come beside them on the animal. And in the supermarkets we see all the cuts packaged up. With a sheep it's really quite easy to get the general gist of things. They have similar cuts to pork, beef and venison, but as those animals grow bigger the butcher creates more cuts and therefore it gets slightly more complicated. When describing these cuts I'm going to be reasonably general, as different countries, and even regions within countries, have their own ways of breaking down animals.

### Shoulder

This is the front leg, but it's quite different from a 'leg' of lamb, which is from the back of the animal. The shoulder is much more toned and muscular as it has to carry the extra weight of the animal's neck and head and constantly supports the weight of the lamb as it bends down to eat. This makes it a tougher cut of meat, but when cooked long and slow at a low temperature it becomes beautifully tender. It's my personal favourite and probably the best-kept secret of all! Try roasting a shoulder instead of a leg next time.

### Neck fillet

These are the muscles that run down from the back of the head into the shoulder and, if trimmed and finely sliced, they're fairly tender with good flavour. Also pretty cheap, so they're ideal for barbecues when you want to feed a lot of people!

### Best end

This is the classic, most fashionable part of the animal. The racks can be French-trimmed and all posh restaurants want to buy this bit. It's very nice, but also very expensive.

### Short loin

This is where you find the fillet, the loin and the short saddle, and when you look at this cut you can see how the fillet, bone and loin fit together – almost like a T-bone steak. This is where chops come from, including the double Barnsley chop (see the recipe on page 50).

### Rump

This is the lamb's bottom! It's a lovely cut and can be pricey. It's got good flavour and is very tender. Best cooked quickly as steaks.

### Leg

Everybody loves the quintessential British Sunday roast and this is the cut of lamb more commonly used for that. You can also get lovely lamb shanks from the bottom of this cut.

### Breast of lamb

This cut is just like belly of pork, but with less meat. It's a bit more fiddly than other cuts, as it has to be trimmed and rolled, but when it's cooked long and slow with some basting it can be a real show-stopper.

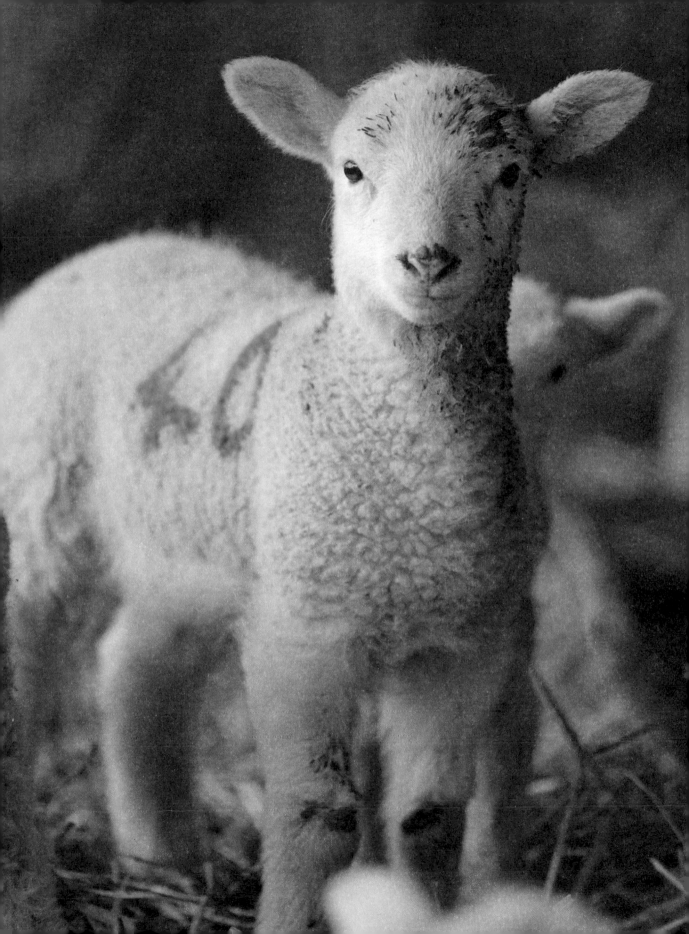

Rhubarb is a funny one. It's usually thought of as a dessert fruit but is actually part of the sorrel family, so it's really more of a herb. If you've got any sort of growing space, it's definitely worth having a plant or two of rhubarb. Not only does it look beautiful, but I love having it in the garden for those times when I fancy making a tart, crumble or pie. It's such a treat to be able to go outside and pull some rhubarb off your own plant! It's extremely sour and very acidic, so regardless of how you cook it, you've got to balance the acidity with sugar. Because of this, it can really never be consumed in a healthy way (but we all need some naughty things in our lives once in a while!).

There are two different types of rhubarb available: forced and naturally grown. In my opinion, each tastes as delicious as the other. The main difference is that forced rhubarb is brighter pink in colour, has delicious spindly shoots and is much more tender, with less stringiness. It also holds its shape better when cooked. And, of course, by forcing it to grow, you get to enjoy rhubarb about six to eight weeks before the natural season's crop.

Rhubarb has been eaten for thousands of years – dating back to 2000 BC in China, where it was used only for medicinal purposes. Funnily enough, it's not actually very nutritious because it's mainly made up of water. It does have a bit of vitamin C, some calcium and fibre, but that's not the point of rhubarb ... Instead, it has an amazing flavour spectrum – one that floats, skips, jumps and crashes right over your tongue, from the front to the sides and back again! It's incredibly refreshing, so eating rhubarb is a great way to finish your meal. As rhubarb goes so well with sweet, rich flavours, it is a favourite ingredient for British desserts. Sponges, puddings, pastries and tarts all go hand in hand with rhubarb, but its classic friendship is with vanilla custard. A genius combination, whether the two flavours are rippled together in ice cream, or are served simply as a bowl of stewed rhubarb and custard.

It only takes five minutes to stew up some rhubarb, so it's a great thing to serve for breakfast, either stirred into cold Greek yoghurt, with lovely toasted mixed nuts and oats sprinkled over the top, or spooned over the top of pancakes – delicious. Recently I've also got into using stewed rhubarb compote alongside meat, as you would an English apple sauce with pork or a Chinese plum sauce with duck, for instance. Or I mix it into my gravy before serving. So in this chapter you'll find some delicious rhubarb desserts as well as one of the nicest Asian-style sticky pork and rhubarb stir-fries that I've ever come across! And the rhubarb bellini is a real winner – you have to try it.

Now I'm thinking about it, as soon as my next lot of rhubarb is ready I'm going to make a load of thick rhubarb jam, so that when it cools down it will set in a solid slab. This will be lovely served with cheeses – a bit like quince paste.

PS Rhubarb leaves are mildly poisonous, so don't cook, eat or smoke them!

# rhubarb

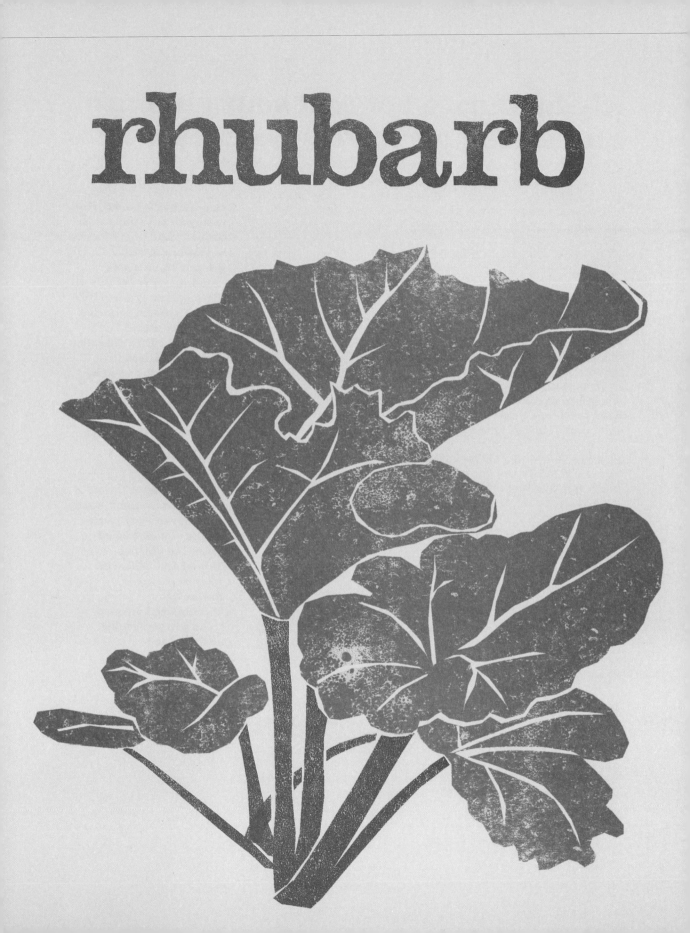

# My favourite hot and sour rhubarb and crispy pork with noodles

This recipe was a total experiment, and I was so pleased that it worked! I wanted to use the acidity and flavour of the rhubarb to produce an incredible sauce in which to stew that tough old bit of pork, the belly, until deliciously tender. The pieces of pork were then wok-fried until crisp and served with the rhubarb sauce and some simply cooked noodles – bloody hell, what a dish! It's a winner.

PS You should be able to get hold of interesting cresses at any good supermarket.

Preheat the oven to 180°C/350°F/gas 4. Place the pork pieces in a roasting tray and put to one side. Chuck all the marinade ingredients into a food processor and pulse until you have a smooth paste, then pour this all over the pork, adding a large wineglass of water. Mix it all up, then tightly cover the tray with tinfoil and place in the preheated oven for about an hour and 30 minutes, or until the meat is tender, but not coloured.

Pick the pieces of pork out of the pan and put to one side. The sauce left in the pan will be deliciously tasty and pretty much perfect. However, if you feel it needs to be thickened slightly, simmer on a gentle heat for a bit until reduced to the consistency of ketchup. Season nicely to taste, add a little extra soy sauce if need be, then remove from the heat and put to one side.

Put a pan of salted water on to boil. Get yourself a large pan or wok on the heat and pour in a good drizzle of groundnut or vegetable oil. Add your pieces of pork to the wok and fry for a few minutes until crisp and golden. (You might need to do this in two batches.) At the same time, drop your noodles into the boiling water and cook for a few minutes, then drain most of the water away. Divide the noodles into four warmed bowls immediately, while they're still moist.

What I love most about this dish is the contrast between the flavours going on in it: from the simple, plain noodles to the zinginess of the spicy rhubarb sauce and the beautifully crispy, yet melt-in-your-mouth pork. To finish, spoon over a good amount of the rhubarb sauce. Divide your crispy pork on top, and add a good sprinkling of spring onions, chilli, cresses and coriander. Serve with half a lime each – perfect.

serves 4

1kg pork belly, boned, rind removed, cut into 3–4cm cubes
sea salt and freshly ground black pepper
groundnut or vegetable oil
375g medium egg noodles
4 spring onions, trimmed and finely sliced
1 fresh red chilli, deseeded and finely sliced
2 punnets of interesting cresses (such as coriander, shiso or basil cress)
a bunch of fresh coriander
2 limes

*for the marinade*
400g rhubarb
4 tablespoons runny honey
4 tablespoons soy sauce
4 garlic cloves, peeled
2 fresh red chillies, halved and deseeded
1 heaped teaspoon five-spice
a thumb-sized piece of fresh ginger, peeled and chopped

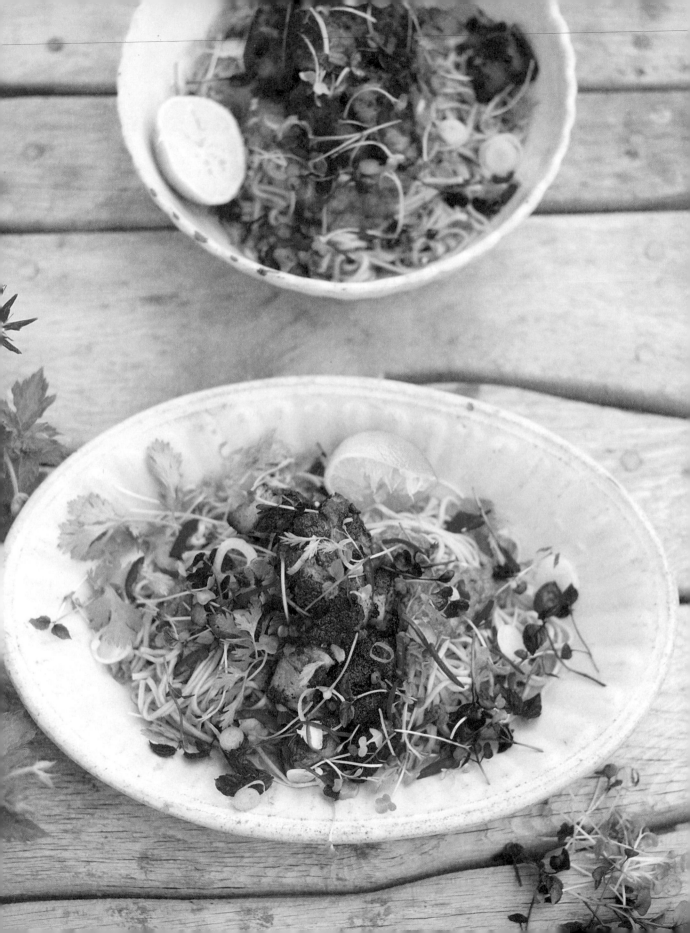

# Rhubarb and custard kinda soufflé

This is like a cross between a soufflé and a light pudding. A soufflé is an old-fashioned classic that I always try to avoid making these days, as I made so many of them when I was at college! Like a good omelette, a soufflé is the test of a really good cook – if you don't get your temperature, speed and stages right you can end up with something as flat as a pancake. But now I've come up with a recipe that's so delicious, with such a beautiful flavour and texture, it doesn't really matter if it sinks. My favourite bit is getting everyone to make a hole in the top of their hot soufflé and pour in some very cold custard. There's nothing better.

Preheat the oven to 180°C/350°F/gas 4 and put in a baking tray to heat up. Put the rhubarb into a saucepan with the 100g of sugar. Put a lid on the pan and simmer gently for about 10 minutes, until the rhubarb is soft. Put to one side and leave to cool completely.

Get yourself six ramekin dishes and rub their insides with the butter. Put the gingersnap biscuits into a sandwich bag, tie a knot in the top and smash the biscuits with a rolling pin or the bottom of a pan to make quite fine crumbs. Dust the insides of the buttered ramekins with the smashed biscuits, then shake out any excess crumbs and keep them for later. (You can put the dishes into the fridge at this point until you're ready to put your soufflés together.)

Blob a tablespoon of the cooled stewed rhubarb into each ramekin dish. Mix the rest of the rhubarb with the custard, the egg yolk and the flour. In a large, clean bowl, using an electric whisk, beat the egg whites with a pinch of salt until you have soft peaks. Add the remaining 2 tablespoons of sugar and whisk on a high speed until the whites are very stiff – this should take about 3 minutes.

Working gently, fold 2 spoonfuls of the stiff egg whites into the rhubarb mixture. Tip this into the bowl containing the remaining egg whites and fold together very carefully. Divide the mixture between the ramekins and level the tops. Wipe the rims of the dishes clean.

Remove the hot baking tray from the oven and place the ramekins on it. Put back into the preheated oven and bake for 18 to 20 minutes, or until the soufflés are a lovely golden colour and have risen nicely. Serve immediately, sprinkled with your leftover gingersnap crumbs.

serves 6

400g rhubarb, cut into
  2.5cm chunks
100g caster sugar,
  plus 2 tablespoons
25g softened butter
6 gingersnap biscuits
150g readymade custard,
  plus extra for serving
1 large free-range or
  organic egg yolk,
  plus 4 egg whites
1 teaspoon plain flour
sea salt

rhubarb

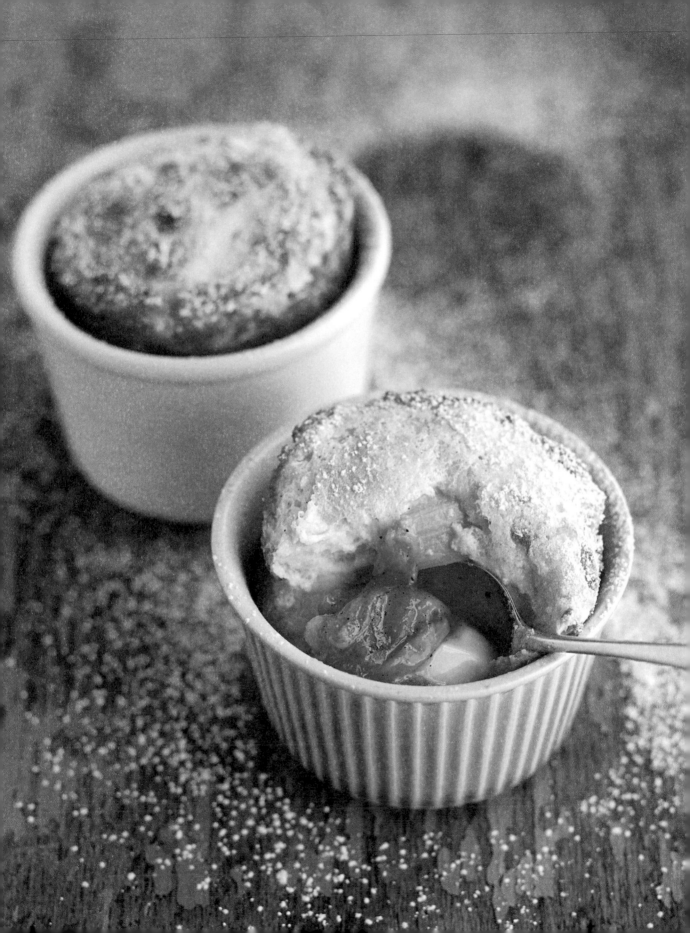

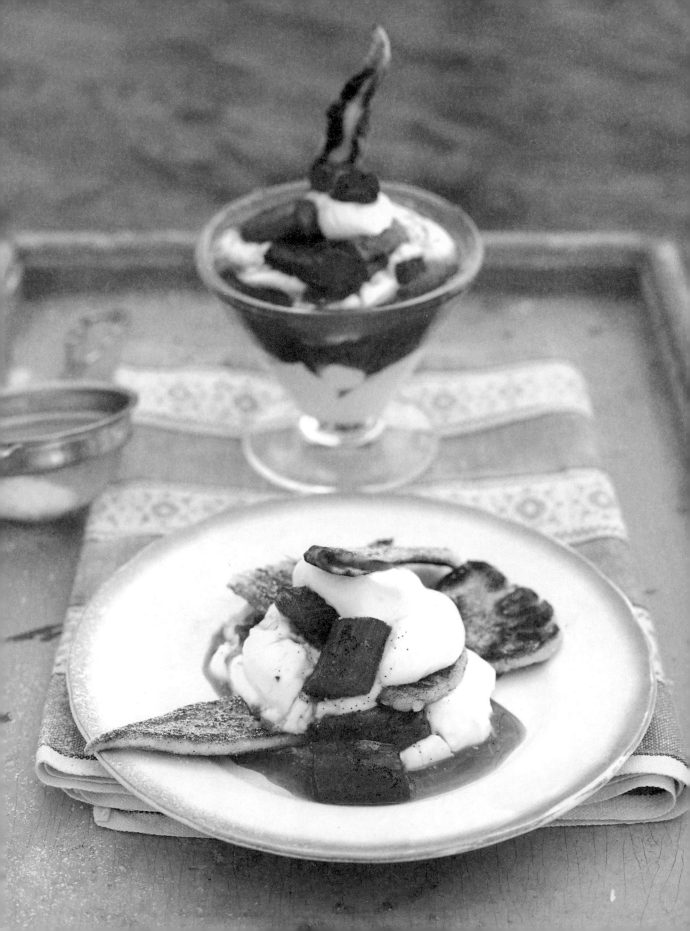

# Speedy rhubarb fool

This is such an easy rhubarb fool to make. It only takes 5 minutes to get the fruit stewed and your puff pastry done, and a couple more to put the whole thing together.

Get yourself a small pan and throw in the rhubarb, sugar and orange juice. Put a lid on top, bring to the boil for a couple of minutes, then remove the lid and simmer for a few more minutes until you get a thick compote consistency.

While the compote is stewing, we'll make some lovely crisp wafers. Sieve the icing sugar and cinnamon on to a clean work surface. Cut 4 slices about 1cm thick off your pastry block and place them flat on your dusted work surface. Pop the rest of your pastry block in the fridge or freezer for another day. Roll each slice out to 0.5cm thick, turning it over as you go so it gets covered in the icing sugar mixture. Cut the strips in half diagonally – you'll end up with long, triangular shapes. Preheat a large, non-stick frying pan and fry the pastry triangles, in two batches, on each side until golden brown. Leave to cool on a rack.

Mix the yoghurt, orange zest and honey together. To serve, dollop a spoonful of yoghurt into each serving glass, followed by a spoonful of rhubarb compote. Continue layering the yoghurt and compote until the glass is full, then stick in a puff pastry triangle in the top. Alternatively, layer up the yoghurt, rhubarb and pastry triangles on individual plates. Now tuck in!

**serves 4**

**for the rhubarb compote**
**500g rhubarb, trimmed
  and chopped**
**100g sugar or vanilla
  sugar**
**juice of ½ an orange**

**for the wafers**
**3 tablespoons icing sugar**
**1 teaspoon ground
  cinnamon**
**500g block of puff pastry**

**for the flavoured yoghurt**
**500ml natural yoghurt**
**zest of 1 orange**
**1 heaped tablespoon
  runny honey**

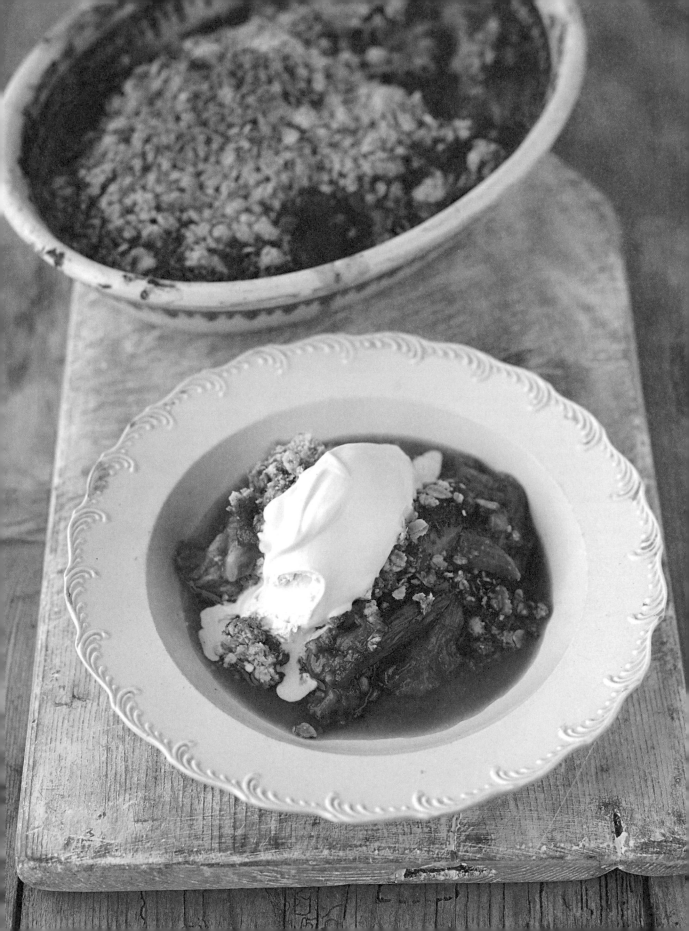

# Rhubarb and sticky stem ginger crumble

This is a classic rhubarb crumble recipe but I've given it a little twist by adding stem ginger and porridge oats to make the best crumble mix ever. It's an absolutely delicious combination of flavours and really nice served with thick Jersey cream or cold custard (Bird's of course – my only vice at the moment).

Preheat your oven to 180°C/350°F/gas 4. Put the rhubarb and half the sugar into a pan. Add the orange juice and zest, put a lid on top, bring to the boil and simmer for a few minutes. Remove the lid and simmer for around 5 more minutes, until the rhubarb has softened slightly. Spoon into an ovenproof baking dish or individual dishes and spread out evenly across the bottom.

To make your crumble topping, use your fingers to lightly rub together the flour and butter until the mixture resembles fine breadcrumbs. Stir in the oats, the rest of the sugar and the stem ginger. (If you like, you can make the crumble topping in a food processor. Just whack in the flour, butter, sugar and stem ginger and whiz up. Add the oats for the last 10 seconds.) Sprinkle the crumble over the rhubarb and bake in the preheated oven for 40 to 45 minutes, or until the rhubarb is bubbling up and the crumble is golden.

**serves 4 to 6**

**1kg rhubarb, trimmed and
   sliced into large chunks
200g soft brown sugar
zest and juice of 1 orange
100g plain flour
100g cold butter
100g oats
2 pieces of stem
   ginger, chopped**

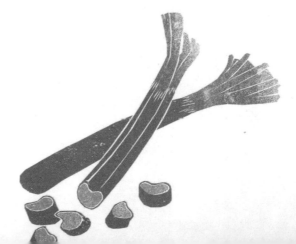

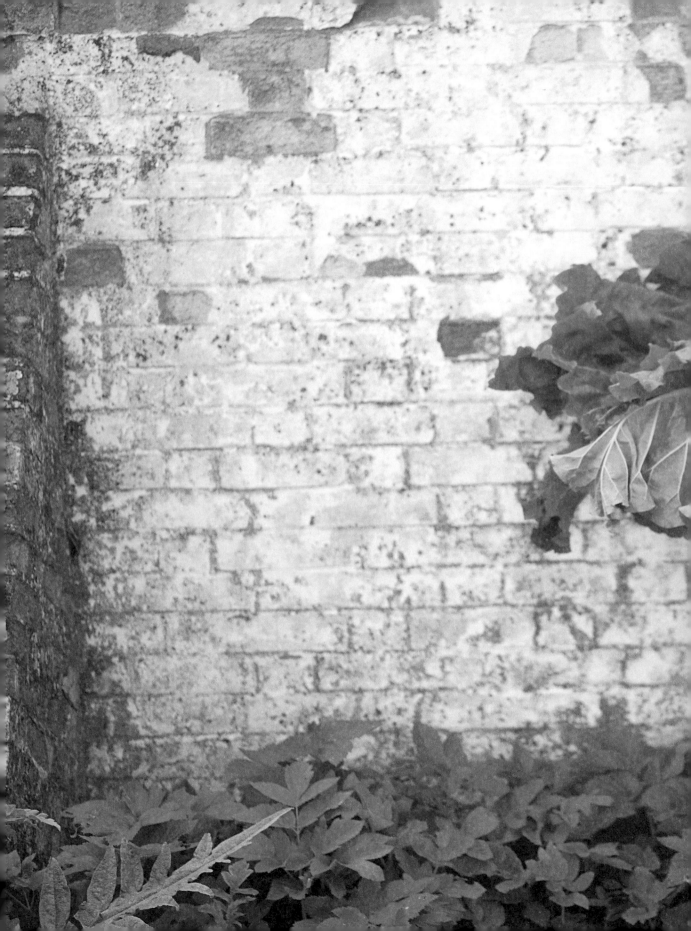

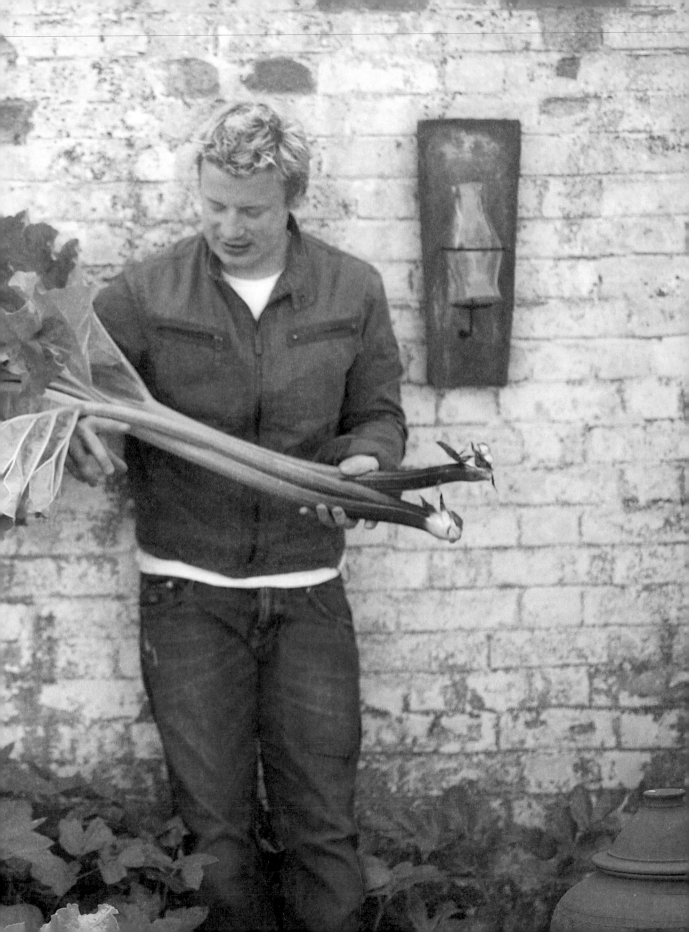

# Creamy rhubarb and vodka cocktail

At Fifteen Cornwall, they have a top cocktail man called Tristan. He used to be a chef, but now he's a cocktail-maker and you can tell from his drinks that he has a really good feel for flavours. He makes a brilliant cocktail using the wonderful liquor that comes out when you stew rhubarb, a bit like the one I've made here.

Place the rhubarb, sugar and orange juice in a small pan and put the lid on. Simmer for a couple of minutes, then remove the lid and simmer for a few minutes more until you get a thick, compote consistency. Pour the rhubarb into a sieve over a bowl and let the liquid drip through. It's this liquid you want (the rhubarb left in the sieve is lovely served with some custard).

Put the vodka, Galliano, cream, milk, ice cubes and 2 shots of the rhubarb liquid into a cocktail shaker and shake it about. Strain into two cocktail glasses. Beautiful.

**makes 2**

500g rhubarb, trimmed
  and chopped
100g sugar
juice of ½ an orange
2 shots of vodka
½ a shot of Galliano
½ a shot of double cream
½ a shot of milk
a handful of ice cubes

# Rhubarb bellini

I recently had this fantastic drink at my mates Arthur and Jamie's restaurant (Acorn House in London, worth a visit). Not only was it a refreshing start to our meal, but it also reflected the rhubarb season brilliantly. You can buy some half-decent sparkling wines and Proseccos with reasonable price tags these days, so this recipe makes you feel like you're having a bit of affordable luxury. It's based on the classic bellini, which is made by mixing Prosecco or Champagne with a peach purée, and you're going to love it.

PS I really like serving this cold cold cold on a hot day, so I put the bubbly into the freezer about 40 minutes beforehand. Don't forget it's there!

**makes 6**

**300g rhubarb, trimmed
and finely sliced**
**75g sugar**
**a bottle of bubbly, such as
Prosecco or Champagne**

Get yourself a small pan and throw in the rhubarb, sugar and a couple of tablespoons of water. Put a lid on top, bring to the boil and simmer for a couple of minutes. Remove the lid and simmer for a few more minutes, stirring occasionally, until you get a thick compote consistency. Whiz up with a hand blender or in a liquidizer until you have a lovely smooth purée. Leave to cool, then stir again and divide the purée between six glasses. Pour over your Prosecco or Champagne, stirring as you pour, with a long spoon or something similar, until the glass is three-quarters full. Top it up with bubbles and you're done. Cheers!

# How I grow rhubarb

## Soil

Rhubarb is really easy to grow and a nice steady character to have in the garden. It's not a temperamental plant, so it won't require much of your attention and, once planted, can last twenty years or more, especially if you split it in half (or more if the plant is really big), cutting through the rootstock every five years or so. You can plant the pieces out to make more plants. As rhubarb is such a 'permanent' plant you want to give it a good start in life by preparing the soil well. Choose some nice sunny or partially shaded areas of the garden and dig in lots of good organic compost, well-rotted manure and a little sprinkling of organic fertilizer.

## Planting

Rhubarb is usually sold as 'bare-rooted crowns'. These are available as named varieties from good nurseries or garden centres in winter or early spring, and they need to be planted straight away. Sometimes you will see pot-grown rhubarb for sale, and this can be planted at any time of the year. I bought several different types of crowns a couple of years ago. I planted them out, waited for them to grow ... and they all died! I don't really know why. Gardening is like that sometimes. So I had to start all over again. I planted my new ones in a sunny place but I've also tried planting some in empty bits of my garden because I love the way it looks – it's quite ornamental, in a chunky sort of way!

Dig a hole in your prepared soil, big enough to fit the bare-rooted crown or pot-grown plant, and place it in the hole. Sprinkle good soil round the roots or rootball and gently firm the soil around it. Make sure the top buds of the crown are level with the soil surface. Plant each individual crown about 90 to 100cm from the next and give them a good soaking of water, as this will help to settle the soil round the roots.

## Harvesting and storing

Whatever you do don't be impatient. Give your new rhubarb plants at least one whole year of growing, preferably two, before cropping them. Remember that you could be harvesting from them for twenty years or more if you treat them well when they're young.

Old established plants can take a bit of rough treatment though! I blagged a whopping great rhubarb plant off my mate Pete, who dug it out of his allotment in the middle of winter for me (it took two people to lift it!). I should be able to take a few shoots off it this year, which I'm looking forward to. It's safe to dig up rhubarb plants between November and March if you want to split them up to make new ones. Just make sure each chunk of root has one or more growth buds.

The right time of year to harvest your rhubarb is between February and May. Select three of the largest stalks, then gently twist the stems and pull them from the base of the plant. Rhubarb stalks are best eaten on the day they are harvested, but they'll keep in reasonable condition in the fridge for one to two weeks. Raw and cooked rhubarb also freeze well.

## My growing tips

- Rhubarb flowers in the spring and summer and it's a spectacular show of tall red and green spires with loads of creamy-yellowy bits. Most people recommend cutting these off as they weaken the plant, but I usually leave a few because they look so good.

- 'Forcing' rhubarb to get an early or particularly tender bunch of stalks is quite easy. All you need to do is stick a dustbin, bucket or terracotta forcing pot over the crown in late winter. Check it regularly until the stalks look big enough to pull. Don't force the same plant every year though, as you'll tire the poor thing out!

- I usually mulch my rhubarb each autumn and spring by spreading a layer of good compost or well-rotted manure around it. This helps to retain moisture in the soil, especially during the summer.

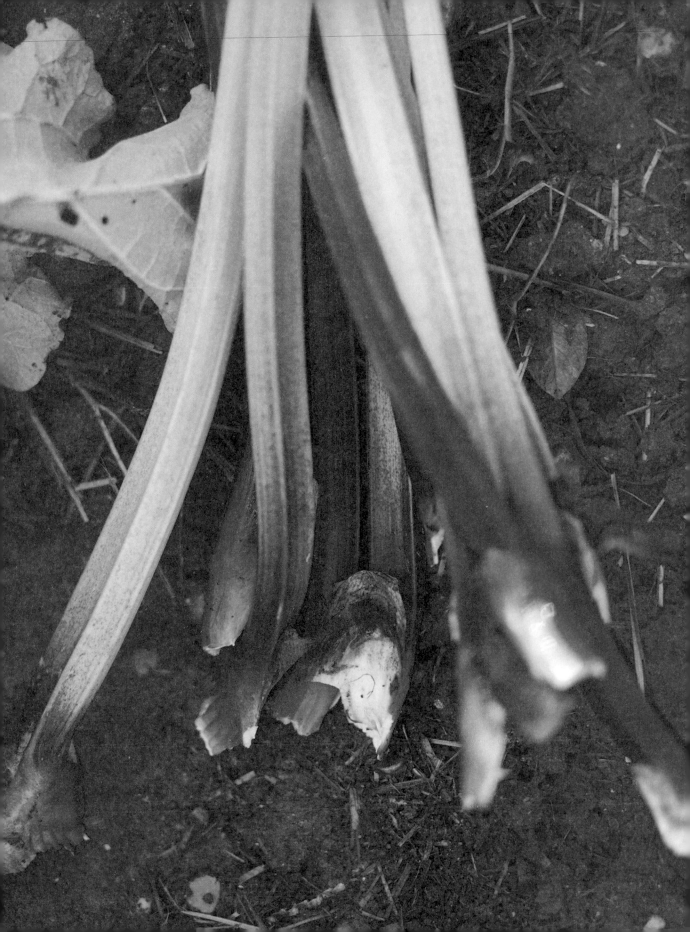

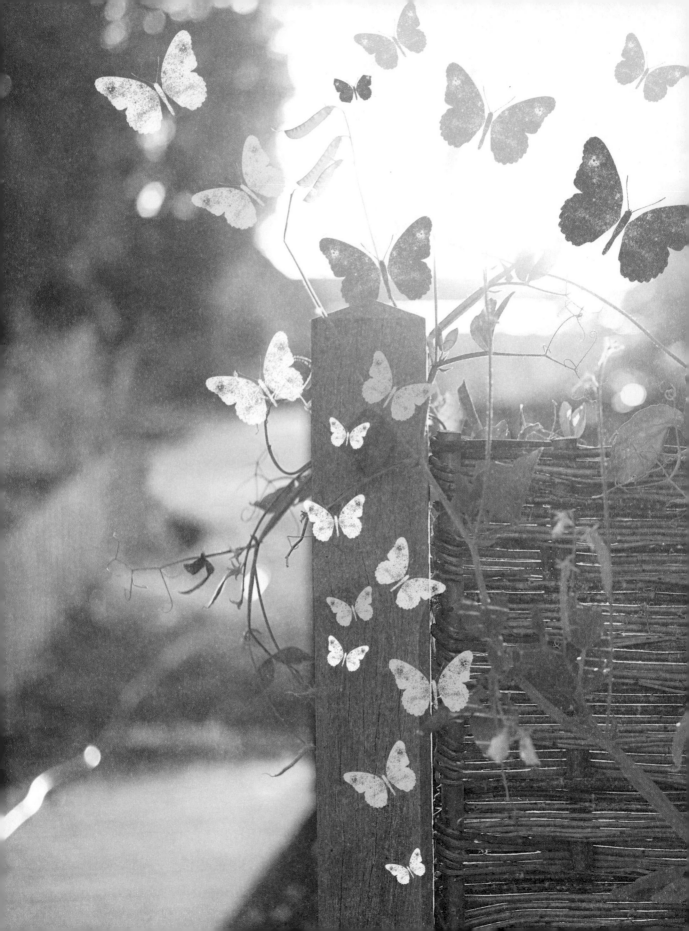

# summer

barbecue / cabbage family / carrots and beets /
climbing beans / courgettes / onions /
peas and broad beans / pizza / potatoes /
strawberries / summer salads / tomatoes

For me, barbecuing is one of the most evocative, honest and natural ways to cook food. It's a method of cooking common to countries and cultures all over the world – South Africans call it 'braai', in Australia electric barbecues are supplied for public use in parks, and Koreans and Mongolians put mini barbecues on their dining tables so that people can cook their own meat, fish or veg. It's a wonderful way to get everyone involved around the table.

When you think about it, we've only been cooking with gas or electricity for a tiny length of time in history but people have been building fires and cooking over hot coals for thousands of years, since we first became civilized. Maybe that's why men always seem to think they should do the cooking on the barbie – it brings out their primeval side, having to provide food for their families! Originally, to barbecue meant to slow-cook meat at a low temperature for a long time over wood or charcoal. In America, this way of cooking originated in the late 1800s at Western cattle drives. Cowboys would be fed the cheapest, toughest cuts of meat, like brisket, which required five to seven hours of cooking to tenderize them.

I've come across a few theories about how the word 'barbecue' came about. I like the one about French pirates in the West Indies who would impale their goats on a spit and roast them on an open fire. They referred to it as 'de la barbe au cul', which literally means 'from beard to butt'! And there's the term used by the Taíno people of the Caribbean, 'Taíno barabicoa', which translates as 'the sticks with four legs and many sticks of wood on top to place the cooking meat'. Pretty much explains a barbecue! The Taíno also used the word 'barabicu', which means 'sacred fire pit'.

A barbecue isn't just for grilling, you know. It can also be used to steam veg over a pan of water or in a tinfoil bag (see page 86), to smoke shellfish under an upside-down bowl or roasting tray (see page 81) or to bake potatoes wrapped in tinfoil straight on the embers. Don't be afraid to try different things!

If you're a real barbecue connoisseur, I hope you enjoy reading the next few pages and that you pick up some good tips. My main advice, though, is not to buy an electric or gas barbie. That's just cheating. The food won't taste as good and I think they are a waste of time – you'll never get that wonderful, smoky, proper barbecued flavour from them. So go for the authentic type, and use different woods and coals. If you have any woody herbs growing in your garden, like bay, rosemary, sage or thyme, cut off some large branches and pop them directly on top of your coals. They'll give off an amazing smell and will flavour whatever you're cooking with a lovely perfumed smokiness.

# barbecue

# Crispy barbecued side of salmon with cucumber yoghurt

I love cooking big pieces of fish on my barbecue, but you must use a medium-hot part of the barbie – if it's too hot, you'll crisp the skin before the inside is cooked. Start the fish off with the skin side down and only turn it over when it's crisp and golden. If you're not keen on eating fish skin, that's probably because you haven't tried it when it's been cooked till it's nice and crispy! It can be as good as pork crackling if done properly.

Brush the bars of the barbie clean to prevent your fish sticking, then light it and get the coals glowing hot. If your barbie is small, feel free to cut the salmon in half to make it more manageable.

Place the salmon skin side down on a plastic board and, using a sharp knife, slash it evenly all over on the fleshy side, making the incisions about 1cm deep. Scatter the lemon zest and most of the chopped fennel tops or basil over the salmon, then push these flavourings into the incisions – don't hold back; really push them in! Rub the fish lightly all over with olive oil then season with salt and pepper, giving the skin side a generous amount as most of this will fall off.

When your barbie's ready, lay the salmon on the bars, skin side down. The flesh will start to colour from the bottom up and after about 4 minutes the skin should be beautifully golden brown. Carefully flip the salmon over with a roasting fork or a spatula and cook for a further 2 to 3 minutes on the other side. While it's cooking, gently ease the skin away from the fish and put it on the barbie alongside to crisp up.

If your salmon is wild it will have slightly less fat in it, so will be a drier fish. You can therefore cook it for a shorter amount of time, even leaving it slightly undercooked – although this might feel unusual to us Brits, who nuke fish beyond belief, this is a really good idea! If it's (organically) farmed, cook it through, but please don't overcook it or it will become too dry. Lift the salmon carefully off the barbecue and place it on a nice serving platter or board. Allow to cool a little, then break the skin into pieces, a bit like poppadums.

Cut the cucumber in half lengthways, remove and discard the seeds, chop it up and mix it in a bowl with the yoghurt. Balance the flavours with the lemon juice, half the chopped chilli, and all the chopped mint or oregano. Drizzle over a little extra virgin olive oil. Season carefully to taste with salt and pepper.

Break the salmon up with a fork into four to six chunks. Serve with the cucumber yoghurt, sprinkled with the rest of the chopped chilli and the remaining fennel tops or basil. Drizzle with extra virgin olive oil and make sure everyone gets a piece of the crunchy fish skin.

**serves 4 to 6**

1 x 1.5kg side of salmon, scaled and pinboned
zest and juice of 1 lemon
a bunch of fresh herby fennel tops or basil, leaves picked and finely chopped
olive oil
sea salt and freshly ground black pepper
1 cucumber, peeled lengthwise at intervals
300ml natural yoghurt
1 fresh red chilli, deseeded and finely chopped
a small bunch of fresh mint or oregano, leaves picked and chopped
extra virgin olive oil

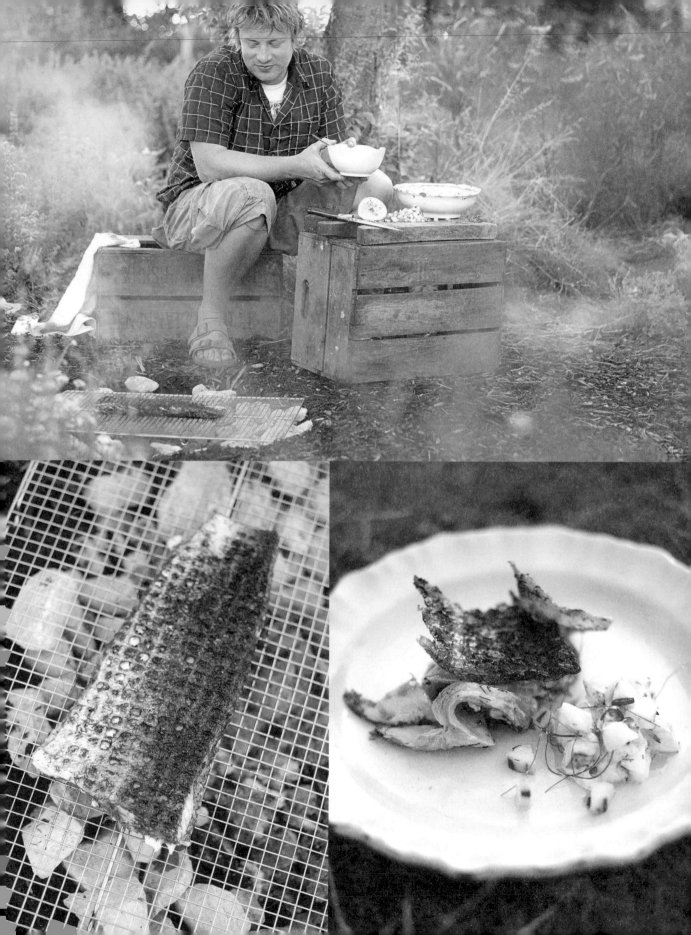

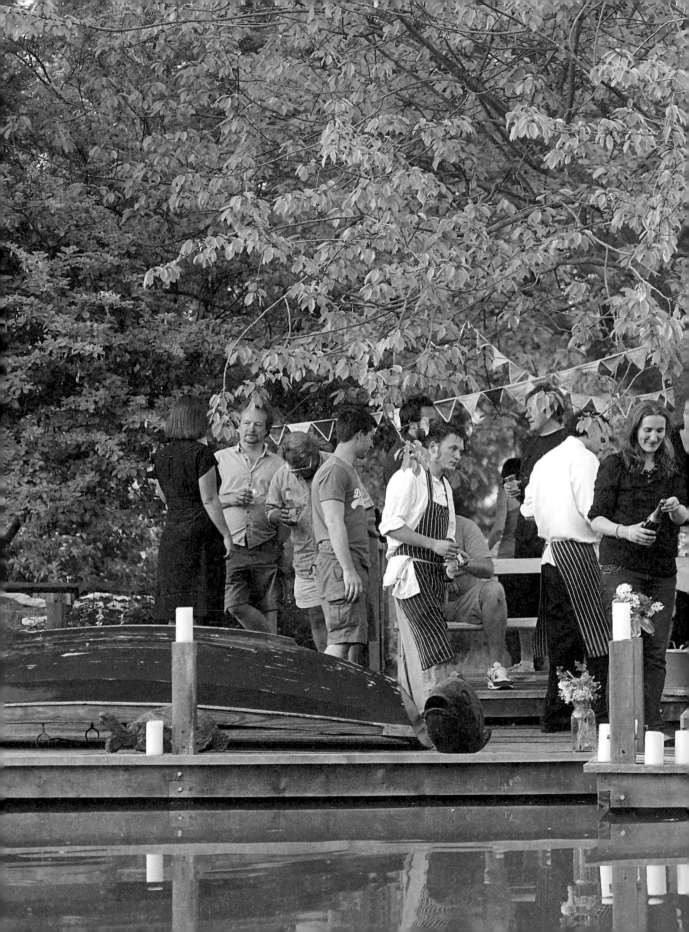

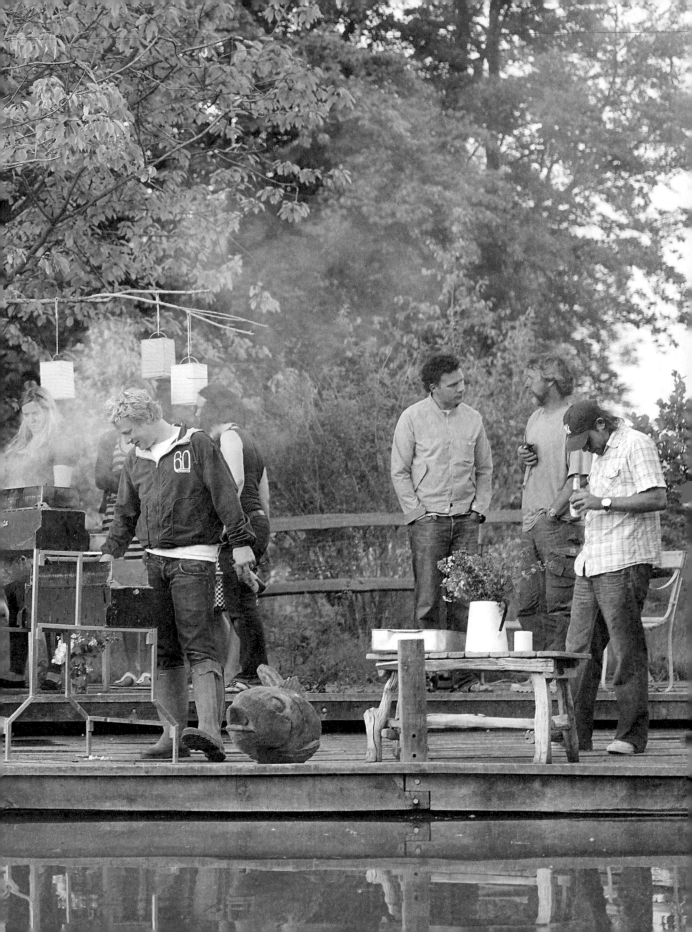

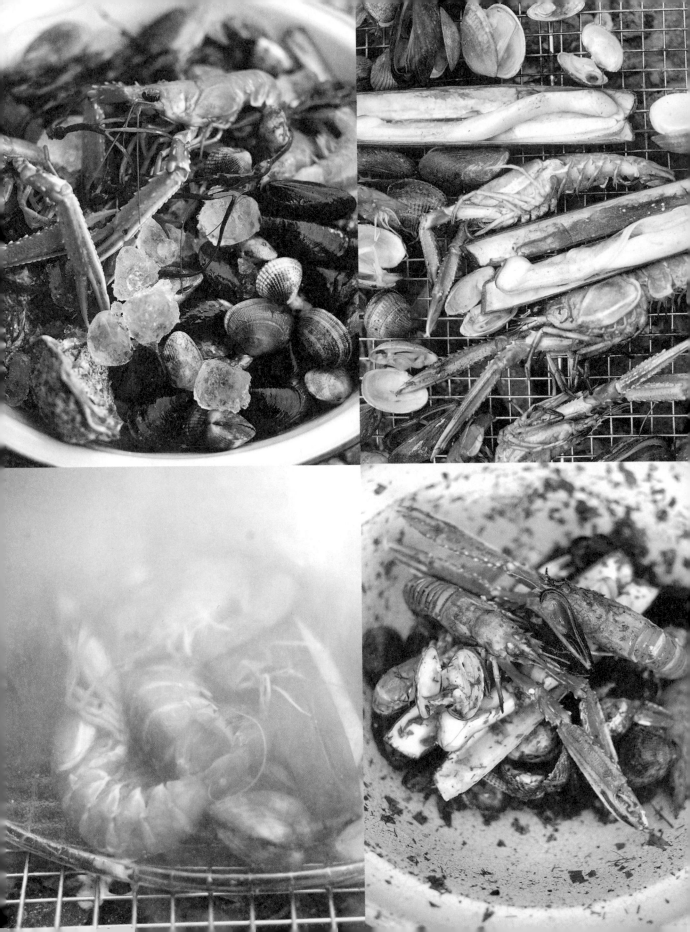

# Smoked barbecued shellfish with a chilli-lime dressing

I love making this dish, especially when I've got friends coming round. It's such a visually attractive thing to make – to see the shellfish cooking, bursting open and smoking through a large glass bowl is quite fascinating and seductive! And that's before you've dressed the whole thing with the delicious zingy dressing. These shellfish are wonderful served hot or cold, tossed with spaghetti or served simply on a piece of garlic-rubbed, toasted bread.

PS Only buy shellfish that are tightly closed so you know they're still alive and fresh and make sure you buy and cook them on the same day.

Light your barbie and get yourself a nice bed of glowing hot coals. If you've got bay, thyme or rosemary growing in your garden, throw some whole branches of these on to the coals so that they start to burn and smoke. By doing this, you'll get some tasty smoke happening.

To make the dressing, put most of the chopped herbs into a nice big bowl (reserving the rest for sprinkling over later) with the chilli, the lime zest and juice, and three times as much extra virgin olive oil as lime juice. Season with a little pepper and have a taste – you want the dressing to be quite limey.

As oyster shells are quite thick, you can carefully lift up the hot bars and put your oysters, flat side of the shell facing up, directly on to the hot coals for 3 to 4 minutes. When they're cooked (you'll know when they're done because they'll open up), remove them to a platter. Place your shellfish directly on to the bars over the hottest part of the barbie. Make sure the biggest ones are at the bottom, as they'll get the most heat. If your bars are wide apart, sit your shellfish on a cooling rack so they don't fall through. Feel free to cook them in batches, as you've got 2kg of shellfish to do! Put a large heatproof glass or metal bowl or a deep roasting tray over the shellfish. You may think this sounds mad, but this will trap all the hot air and smoke around the shellfish, giving them a great smoky flavour.

After a few minutes, carefully lift up the side of the bowl to check that all the shellfish have opened. If most of them have, lift the bowl off. They'll take slightly different times to cook, so just remove them as they're done. Using a pair of tongs, pick up the cooked shellfish and add them to the bowl of dressing. Throw away any shellfish that won't open.

Gently mix the shellfish, oysters and dressing together and serve with the remaining chopped herbs sprinkled over the top. Don't forget paper towels and maybe even a finger bowl.

**serves 4**

optional: a few fresh herb branches, such as bay, thyme or rosemary
4 oysters
2kg shellfish (razor clams, clams, mussels, langoustines and queen scallops are all good)

*for the chilli-lime dressing*
a small bunch of fresh mint, leaves picked and chopped
a small bunch of fresh flat-leaf parsley, leaves picked and chopped
a few sprigs of fresh herby fennel tops, leaves picked and chopped
1–2 fresh red chillies, deseeded and finely chopped
zest and juice of 2–3 limes
extra virgin olive oil
freshly ground black pepper

barbecue

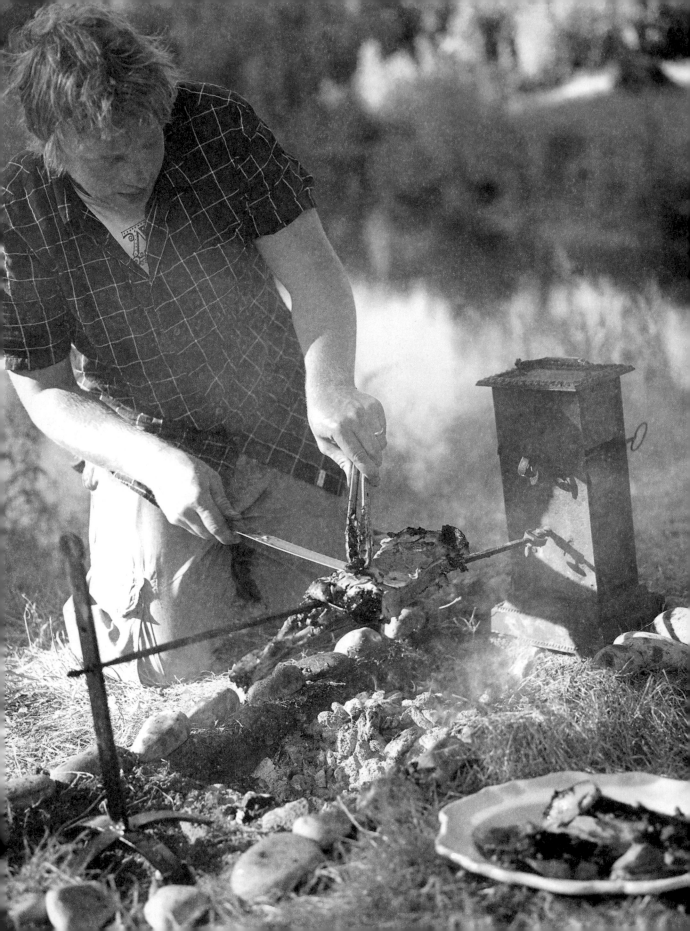

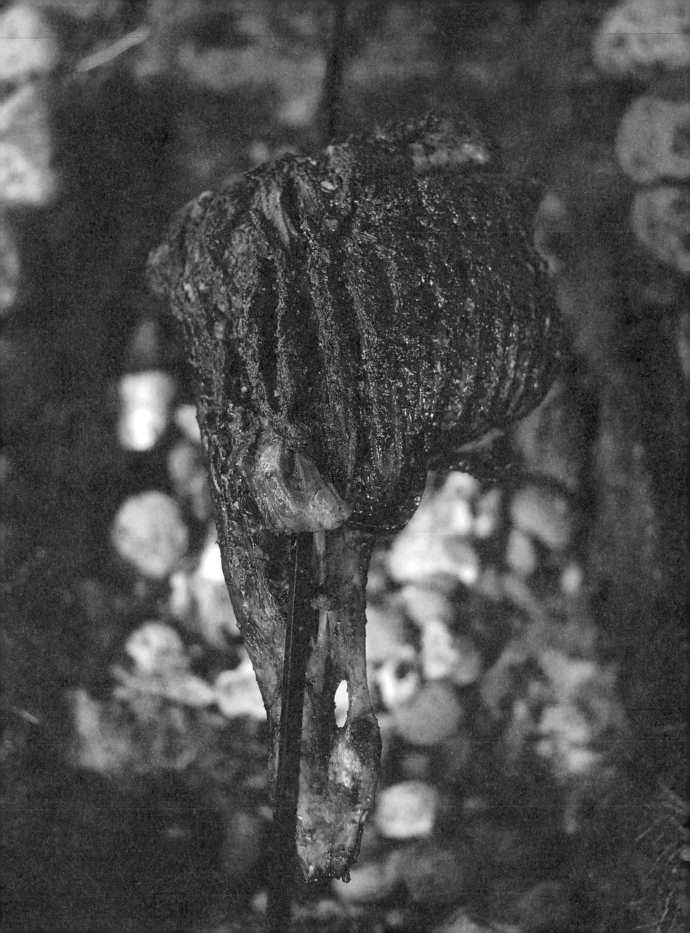

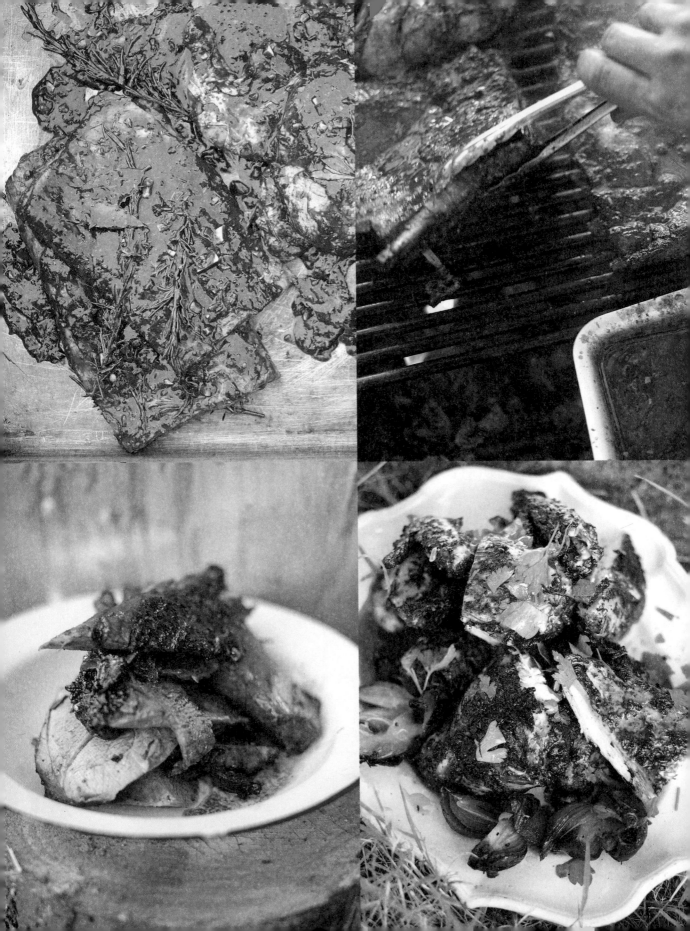

# Best barbecued meat and homemade barbecue sauce

All types of meat can be barbecued, but the various cuts have to be treated differently. For instance, thin steaks, pork chops and chicken legs cook in a very different way from a whole leg of lamb, pork ribs or a large chicken. If you were to cook them all the same way, the larger cuts would end up nicely cooked on the outside but raw in the middle. Here I'm going to show you how to barbecue larger cuts of meat so they're flavoured and moist in the middle and golden and crisp on the outside every time. The thing to remember is to cook the meat through in the oven first, without colouring it, to make it lovely and juicy, then finish it off on the barbecue, basting the meat with the marinade and cooking juices.

PS This recipe makes enough marinade for one of the types of meat listed in the ingredients. However, I love to do three different types of meat at the same time – if you want to do that, make three times the amount of marinade.

Preheat your oven to 180°C/350°F/gas 4 and light your barbecue about 40 minutes later.

To make your marinade, grind the cumin seeds, fennel seeds and cloves in a pestle and mortar with some salt and pepper. Chop the thyme and rosemary leaves, orange zest and garlic together finely. Put into a bowl with the ground spices, then add the rest of the marinade ingredients and mix together.

Rub your chosen meat all over with the marinade, really getting it into all the nooks and crannies and, in case of the lamb, the slashes. Place the meat in a snug-fitting roasting tray, top with any leftover marinade and cover loosely with tinfoil. Bake the meat in the preheated oven until sweet and tender. This will take an hour and a half for the pork ribs and the lamb (but if you like your lamb pink, it will only need an hour), and an hour and 20 minutes for the spatchcocked chicken.

Now you're going to finish your meat on a medium hot barbecue. Place it carefully on the bars of the barbecue and sear it well on one side, then turn it over. While it's cooking, use your reserved rosemary sprigs to baste the meat with the sticky juices from the bottom of the roasting tray. Keep turning and brushing the meat until you've built up a lovely sticky, charred crust, then take it off the barbie and rest it on a serving dish for a few minutes. Meanwhile, pop your roasting tray on the barbie or over a gas hob and let the juices reduce a bit.

Cut the pork into individual ribs, carve the leg of lamb into slices or tear the chicken into pieces, and serve with a bowl of the lovely marinade juices from the roasting tray and some barbecued vegetables (see page 86).

serves 4 to 6

1 x 1.8kg free-range or organic chicken, spatchcocked (see page 268 for how to do this)
or
1 x 3kg leg of lamb, on the bone, slashed evenly 0.5cm deep
or
2kg pork rib racks

for the marinade
1 heaped teaspoon cumin seeds
2 tablespoons fennel seeds
5 cloves
sea salt and freshly ground black pepper
a bunch of fresh thyme or lemon thyme, leaves picked
a bunch of fresh rosemary, leaves picked and chopped, a few whole sprigs reserved
zest and juice of 1 orange
1 bulb of garlic, broken into cloves and peeled
4 heaped teaspoons sweet smoked paprika
6 tablespoons balsamic vinegar
150ml organic tomato ketchup
8 tablespoons olive oil
10 bay leaves

barbecue

85

# My favourite barbecued veggies

A barbecue is not just for searing and chargrilling meat – you should think of it as another heat source available to you, like your oven or your hob. A sort of extension of your kitchen into your garden! If you want to get some really different results out of your barbecue, a great idea is to wrap some interesting vegetables in a double-thickness tinfoil parcel, adding some water or wine, a bit of butter or olive oil, and a little salt and pepper. The parcel can then be steamed over the barbie or baked, depending on how moist the veggies are.

## Barbecue-steamed stuffed onion

Put a small red onion on a chopping board and cut it halfway down into four, without cutting all the way through. Push a few sprigs of rosemary and a knob of butter into the centre. Double-wrap in tinfoil and, when the barbecue has cooled down a little, place the packet directly on to the coals. Leave for 15 minutes, then carefully remove the foil and peel off the outer layer of onion, as it'll probably be charred because of its sugar content. You'll have a perfectly good onion underneath, so tuck in!

## Barbecue-steamed green leaves

Rip up some spinach, rocket, Swiss chard and watercress. Fold a double piece of tinfoil in half and seal up the two sides to make a little bag. Drop in your leaves, and drizzle in some olive oil and lemon juice. Season with sea salt and seal the last edge tightly. Wait until the coals have cooled down a bit, then steam the bag on the barbecue for 5 minutes.

## Barbecue-steamed fennel

Fold a double piece of tinfoil in half and seal up the two sides to make a little bag. Cut a fennel bulb in half and then into slices and add these to your tinfoil envelope. Squeeze in the juice of ½ a lemon, leaving the lemon half in the bag. Add ½ a sliced fresh red chilli and a good drizzle of olive oil, then season with sea salt and freshly ground black pepper. If you want, you could add a few bits of fresh rosemary. Seal the last edge tightly and place on the bars over a medium hot barbie until cooked. This should take about 25 minutes.

## Sweet potatoes with cumin, lime and chilli

In a pestle and mortar, bash up a few dried chillies, a teaspoon of ground cumin and a dessertspoon of sea salt. Give your sweet potatoes a scrub under the tap, prick them about ten times with a knife, then, while they're still wet, dust them with the spicy mix. Roll them individually in foil and submerge them under the hot ash. If you want to put them among the coals, double-wrap them in foil so the skin doesn't burn. Stab with a knife to check if cooked after 20 minutes. Serve with a squeeze of lime.

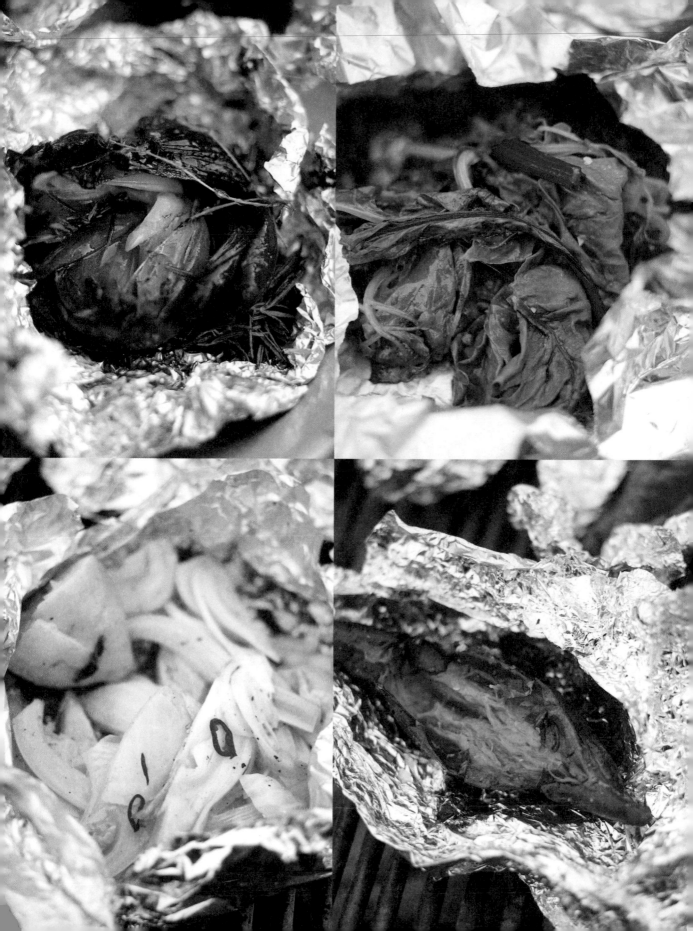

# How to . . .

## . . . make a simple barbecue

It's so easy and cheap to make your own barbecue – you really should have a go. All you need to do is put a couple of bricks on the ground with a solid, 8cm-deep roasting tray on top of them. I've had a go at doing this in parks or even on our outside table. Scrunch up some paper and place it in the tray, with some dry kindling wood. Pile some coal in and around the wood, to give you a kind of pyramid shape. Light the paper and kindling and watch carefully to make sure the flames don't go out. When the fire has burned down and the coals are white hot and ashy, place a metal cake rack on top of them. Easy. For a Korean vibe, have a selection of lovely thin little pieces of marinated fish and meat ready, with skewers, dips and seasonings alongside, so everyone can cook for themselves.

## . . . light your barbecue

There are three ways you can do this:

**The conventional way** is to use rolled-up bits of paper, dry kindling, twigs and coal (as described above), in that order, to form a tepee shape. Build the coals up around the outside. This will ensure good air circulation and therefore good burning.

**The easiest way** is to use a Grenadier electric firelighter (www.grenadier.co.uk). I have one of these for lighting barbecues, or for getting a nice fire going at home in the winter. These bits of kit are great because you don't have to find dry wood or kindling or scrunch up bits of paper to get the fire started. But, most important of all, there is absolutely no need to use any chemical firelighters or liquid fuels. It will even light wet wood and coals in just a few minutes! Please don't use those little firelighter blocks you can buy in bags – they give off really dreadful fumes that will end up flavouring your food. Horrible.

**The cheat's way** (which I saw used in Japan!) is to place a piece of chicken wire or a cake rack over a portable gas hob. Put about six or seven pieces of coal on top of it with a few more on top to make a little pyramid and turn the heat up to full whack. By burning the coals directly on the flames like this, you'll kick-start them.

When they're half-glowing, carefully lift the wire or rack (making sure that any kids are out of the way) and take the coals over to your barbecue. You can do this by using tongs to put the coals into a large pot. Add more coals in and around the glowing ones.

## . . . keep your barbecue under control

The most common food disaster that happens in gardens every summer is the old classic – barbecued food that's raw in the middle but cremated on the outside. It's easy to stop this happening because it's simply about controlling the heat. All you have to do is stack your coals high on one side of the barbecue – this will give you immediate, searing heat – and decline them slowly towards the other side until you have a single layer of coals. It's a bit like having a high and low setting, just like you have on your hob. Use this simple tip and your barbecue skills will improve straight away! Remember, you're in control – there's no excuse for letting things burn.

You don't want flames leaping up when you cook over a barbecue – they will only discolour and burn your food. Keep them down by using a water spritzer. Just spray any flames as soon as they start.

## . . . barbecue safely

When writing this chapter I thought I'd do a bit of research about how people in the UK these days get on with lighting fires and barbecues, and I was so amazed by what I came across that I thought I'd share it with you here. It's quite shocking. Read on . . .

4.6 million people have used white or methylated spirits to light their barbecue; 1.7 million have used petrol; 1.2 million have used aerosols, which are highly combustible and can explode if exposed to a naked flame; and over 600,000 have used perfume.

Please never use any of these things – I can't stress enough how dangerous they are near a naked flame. No wonder there are about 1,000 highly uncontrollable barbecue fires each year in Britain. You also need to ensure that your barbecue is stable, secure and in a safe place away from kids. This is definitely something to bear in mind, as one of my mate's kids pulled a barbecue on top of her and broke her leg – thank goodness it wasn't lit at the time.

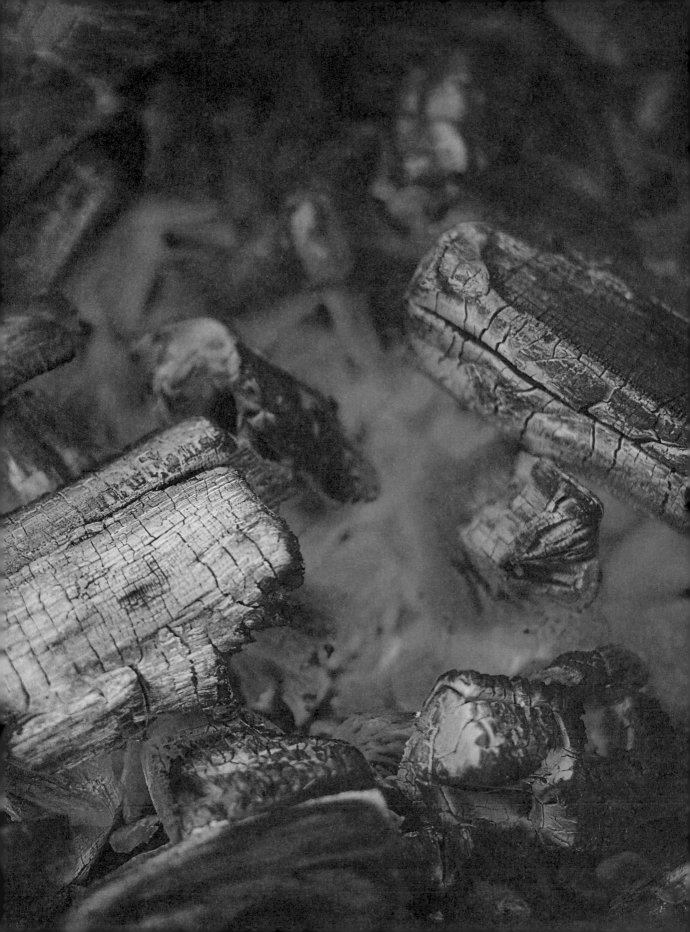

# cabbage
## family

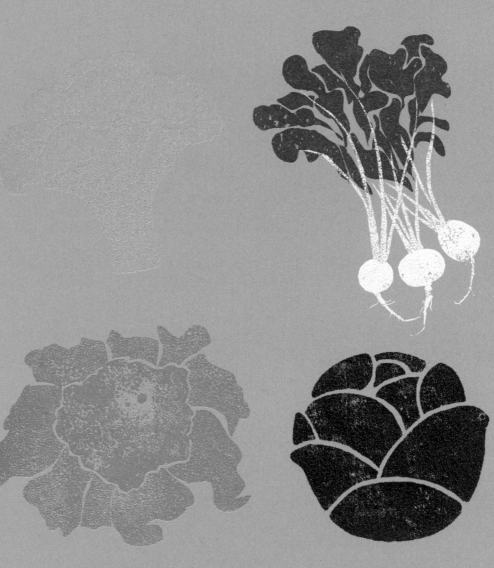

The cabbage family is mainly made up of different varieties of cabbage, broccoli and cauliflower, but also includes such diverse things as kohlrabi and turnips. The proper name for this group of vegetables is 'brassicas'. The great thing about growing them is that you'll have some varieties available for most of the year. The flavour from home-grown ones is incredible, so you're in for a treat!

Crossbreeding within the brassica family has taken place over many thousands of years, and there are now all sorts of varieties around the world, from the army of oriental cabbages and leaves, like pak choi, to the European varieties, some of which I'm lucky enough to have in my garden, like lime-green cauliflower, purple cauliflower, all the different colours of kale, and one of my favourites, cavolo nero (Italian black cabbage). As the vegetables in the brassica family have evolved over time, some parts of their structure have been exaggerated, so they've grown big swollen roots or leaves. To help you understand what the brassica family includes, I think the simplest way to get your head round it is to split them up into four main categories: roots, stems, flowers and leaves. Here are some examples.

## Roots

Swedes and turnips are swollen roots that grow at ground level. My favourite thing to do with the good old swede is to mash it with half the amount of carrot and some butter and flavour it with nutmeg, salt and pepper. You may not be a turnip lover, but I like to parboil them, slice them and fry them with some thyme or rosemary tips, smashed garlic and a splash of vinegar.

## Stems

Kohlrabi is a stem that can be either white or purple. Basically it can be treated like a potato – you can parboil it and then roast it with rosemary, oil and smashed garlic, or you can boil and purée it with some good oil or cream. Delicious. It can also be eaten raw.

## Flowers

You may not think of broccoli, or the good old cauli, as actually being flowers, but that is what they are. As well as the more usual green broccoli, you can also get purple sprouting and white sprouting broccoli and romanesco cauliflower. There are so many ways of cooking these brassica flowers, yet in this country the standard treatment is to boil them in salted water and serve them with a knob of butter. But it doesn't have to be this boring! They're actually great with big flavours like olives, tomatoes and garlic. Cauliflowers, in particular, really love chilli and spices – you only need to look at an Indian menu to see what I'm talking about. So the next time you're thinking of cooking cauliflower cheese again, try something different!

## Leaves

Lovely brassica leaves include kale, red cabbage, spring cabbage, Brussels sprouts and cavolo nero. Kale is great blanched in boiling water and tossed with olive oil and a little lemon juice. Red cabbage is classic with grated apples, a splash of vinegar and a little smoky bacon. With spring cabbage the lovely inner leaves only need lightly boiling and tossing in a little butter with some salt and pepper. Cavolo nero is incredible boiled with garlic, then drained and whizzed up in a food processor. It's great spread on crostini or served with gnocchi or as a ravioli filling.

# Curried cauliflower fritters

This is a really unusual but delicious way to eat cauliflower. The Japanese are brilliant at making lovely crispy batter for their tempura, so while I was over there recently I wanted to discover their secret. It turns out there are lots of different techniques, such as using cornflour instead of plain flour, or ice-cold sparkling water instead of tap water. In this recipe I'm going to use beer, though, as it gives such a nice colour and goes well with the spices. However, the best advice I was given is to fry the fritters in small batches and eat them straight away, so they're crunchy and hot.

PS This batter recipe can be used for all sorts of things, like fish fillets or thin chicken strips or any finely cut vegetable. You can leave the spices out if you prefer it plain.

First make your batter. Smash up the cumin and mustard seeds, chillies and peppercorns in a pestle and mortar until you have a powder. Put the flour into a mixing bowl and stir in the ground spices and the turmeric. Pour in most of the beer and whisk gently. Check the consistency – you want it to be the thickness of double cream. If it's too thick, whisk in the rest of the beer. Don't worry too much about having little lumps in the batter, as they'll just become nice crunchy bits when you start frying. Season with sea salt and put to one side.

Trim the bottom off the stalk and break the cauliflower into bite-sized florets. Slice up the stalk into 2cm pieces – this way it will all cook at the same rate. Wash the cauliflower, drain it and pat dry with kitchen paper. Place the cauliflower pieces in a bowl and dust with a little flour.

Pour the oil into a deep saucepan – you want it to be about 10 to 12cm deep – and heat it to 180°C. If you don't have a thermometer don't worry, just drop a piece of potato into the oil. When it floats to the surface and starts to sizzle, the oil will be at the right temperature so remove the potato from the pan.

Shake any excess flour off the cauliflower. One by one, dip the pieces into the beer batter, then carefully place them in the hot oil, moving them away from you as you do so. Make sure you stand back so you don't get splashed. It's best to fry them in batches so you don't overcrowd the pan (but serve them as soon as each batch is ready). Each time a batch of cauliflower is nearly ready, add some battered parsley leaves to the pan and fry for 40 seconds (you want to serve them scattered over the fritters). Fry the pieces gently, turning them a couple of times with a slotted spoon. When they're browned and crisp, lift them out of the oil, allowing any excess to drip back into the pan, and drain on kitchen paper. Dust with sea salt and squeeze over a little lemon juice.

serves 6

1 cauliflower
flour, for dusting
vegetable oil
optional: a small piece of
  potato, peeled
a small bunch of fresh flat-
  leaf parsley, leaves picked
sea salt
1 lemon

*for the batter*
1 teaspoon cumin seeds
2 teaspoons black
  mustard seeds
2–3 dried red chillies
1 teaspoon black
  peppercorns
200g self-raising flour
½ teaspoon turmeric
350ml cold beer
sea salt

cabbage family

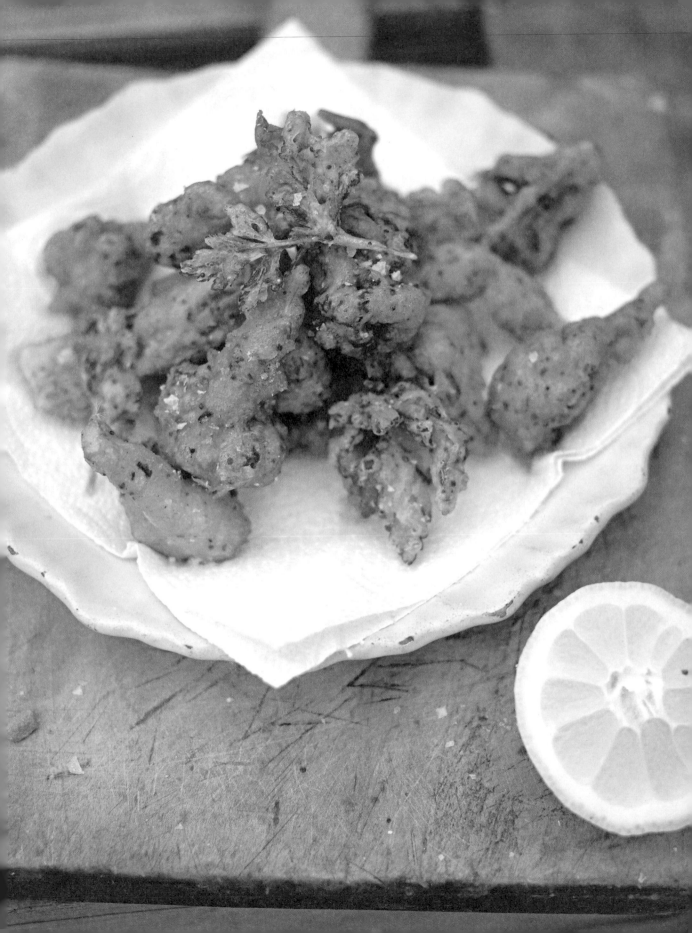

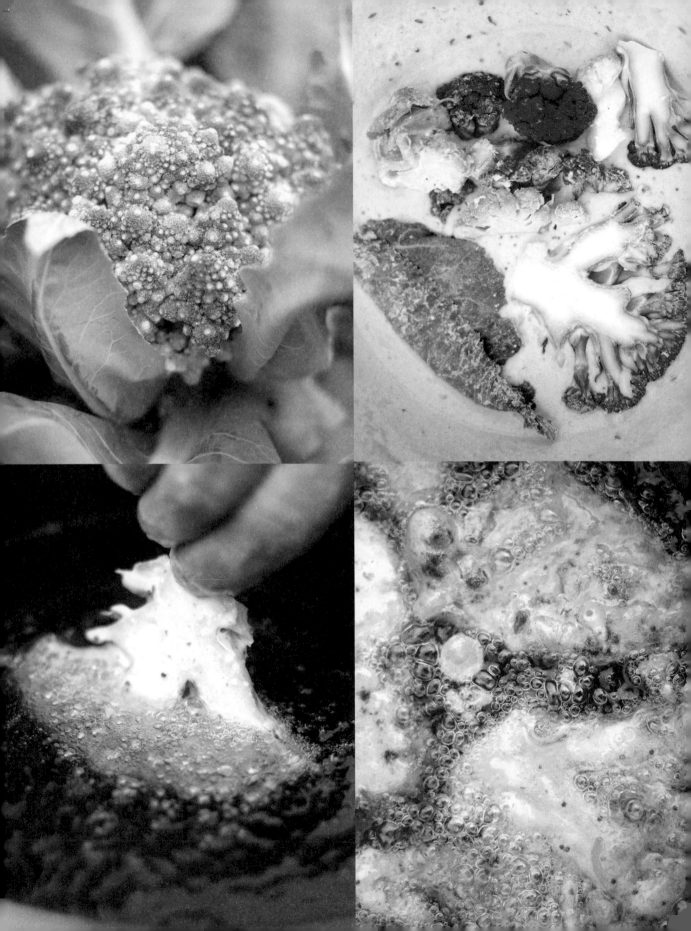

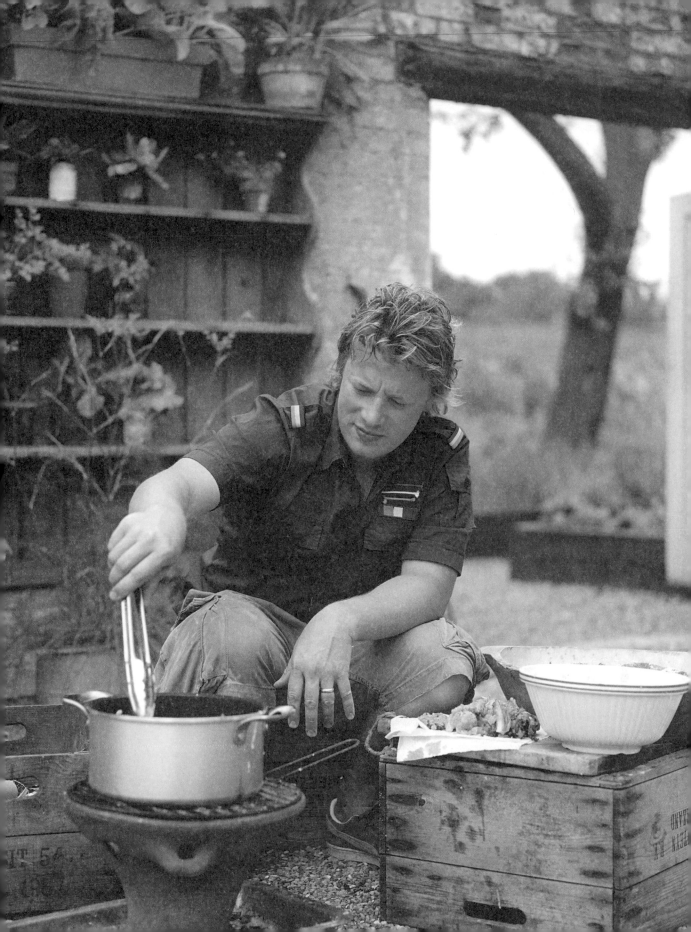

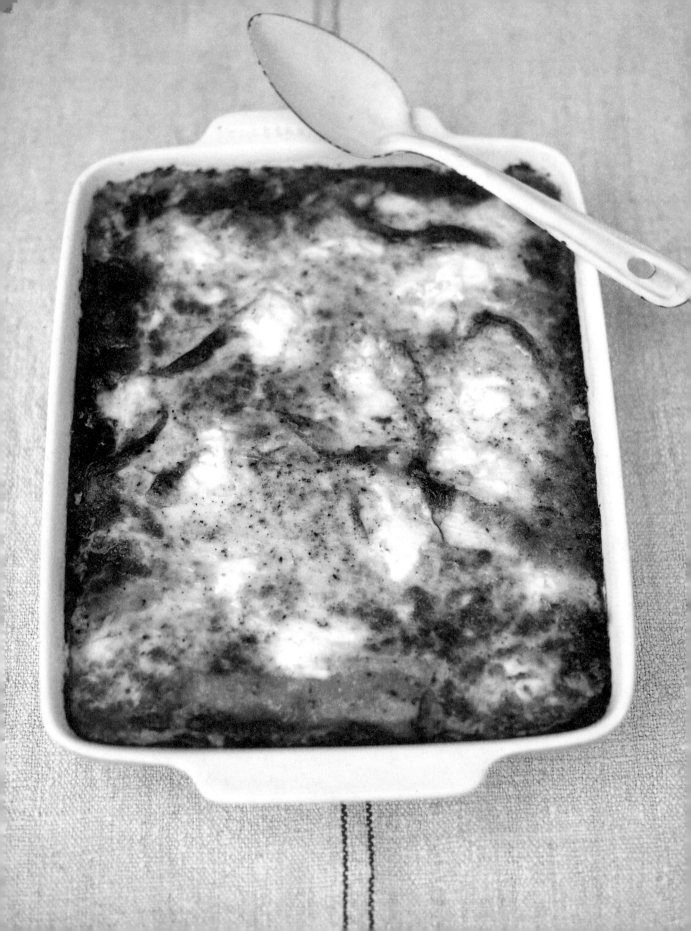

# Incredible baked cauliflower and broccoli cannelloni

This is a twist on the classic Italian dish of orecchiette with broccoli, anchovies and garlic – I've added cauliflower and made it an oven-baked dish. The flavours are amazing.

Preheat the oven to 190°C/375°F/gas 5. Bring a large saucepan of salted water to the boil and drop in the chopped broccoli and cauliflower. Boil for 5 to 6 minutes, until cooked, then drain in a colander, reserving the cooking water.

Heat a wide saucepan, pour in a couple of good glugs of olive oil and add the garlic. Fry for a few seconds, then add the thyme leaves, anchovies, anchovy oil and chillies and continue frying for a few seconds more before adding the cooked broccoli and cauliflower with around 4 tablespoons of the reserved cooking water. Stir everything together, put a lid on the pan leaving a little gap, and cook slowly for 15 to 20 minutes, stirring regularly – overcooking the veg not only intensifies their flavour but gives you the texture that you need for this recipe. Remove the lid for the last 5 minutes to let the moisture evaporate, then use a potato masher to crush the veg. Take the saucepan off the heat, taste the vegetables and season carefully with salt and pepper. Spread the mixture on a baking tray to cool. Meanwhile, get yourself another baking dish or roasting tray (the right size for fitting the cannelloni tubes snugly side by side – I test this by actually laying the tubes into the dish, then remove them and put to one side) and pour in the passata with a pinch of salt and a swig of red wine vinegar.

Now, to make a really quick and easy white sauce, mix the crème fraîche with half the Parmesan, a sprinkling of salt and pepper and a little of the reserved cooking water to thin it down.

Spoon your cooled broccoli and cauliflower mixture into a large sandwich bag and cut off the corner. Twist the top of the bag and squeeze it to pipe the filling into the cannelloni tubes. (If you prefer, use a teaspoon to push the mixture into the cannelloni or use a piping bag if you have one.) Fill the tubes up – don't be stingy! – and place them in a single layer on top of the passata. Lay the basil leaves over the cannelloni and spoon your white sauce evenly over the top. Season with black pepper, sprinkle over the remaining Parmesan and tear over the mozzarella. Drizzle with extra virgin olive oil and bake in the preheated oven for 30 to 40 minutes, or until golden and bubbling on top.

Dress the rocket leaves with a squeeze of lemon juice and about three times as much extra virgin olive oil. Serve the cannelloni with the rocket and some good crusty bread.

**serves 4 to 6**

sea salt and freshly
  ground black pepper
500g broccoli, washed,
  florets and stalks chopped
500g romanesco or white
  cauliflower, washed,
  florets and stalks chopped
olive oil
7 cloves of garlic, peeled
  and finely sliced
a small bunch of fresh
  thyme, leaves picked
1 x 25g tin of best-quality
  anchovies in oil, drained
  and chopped, oil reserved
2–3 small dried chillies,
  crumbled
500ml good-quality passata
good-quality red wine
  vinegar
500ml crème fraîche
200g Parmesan cheese,
  finely grated
16 cannelloni tubes
a small bunch of fresh
  basil, leaves picked
200g good-quality
  mozzarella cheese
extra virgin olive oil
4 large handfuls of rocket
  leaves, washed and dried
1 lemon

cabbage family

97

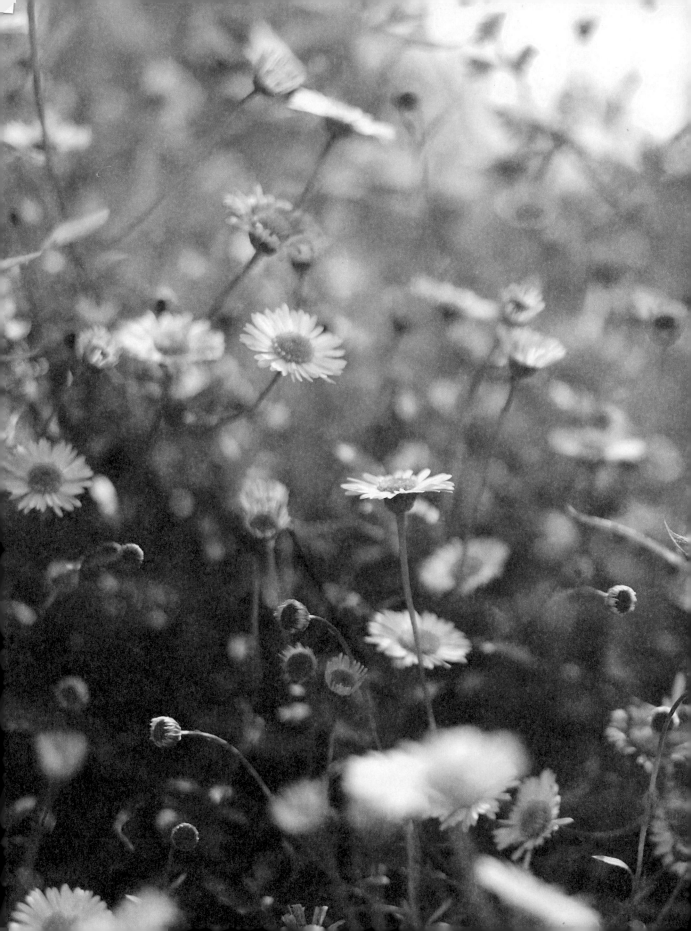

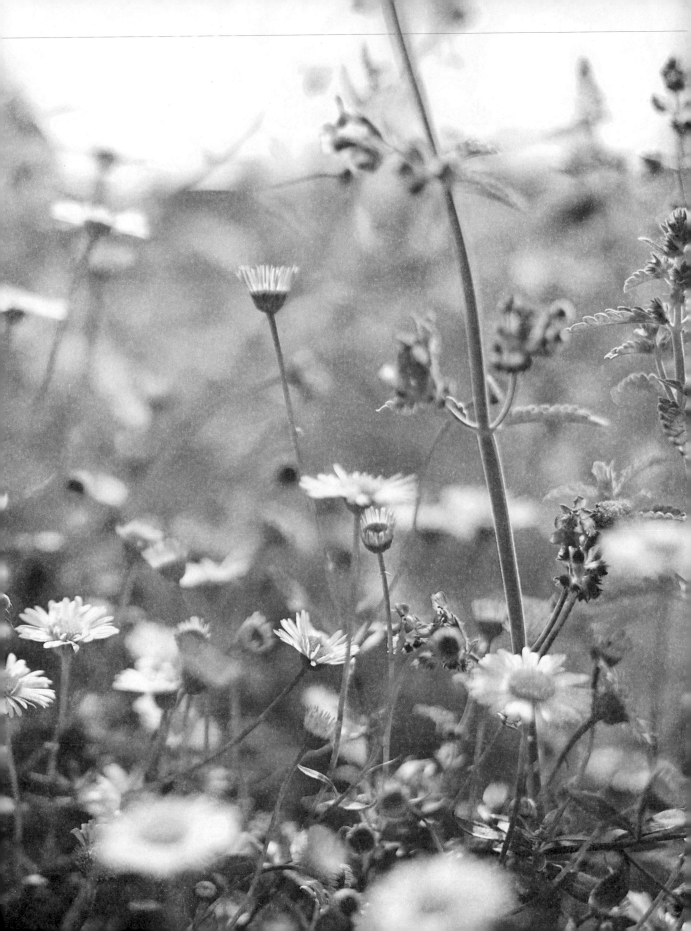

# English hot-pot of amazing summer greens and flaked gammon

I love this old-school English dish because it's good value, simple to make and tastes absolutely delicious. All you have to do is spend 5 minutes getting everything prepared and then you can let your oven or hob do the work for you! If you can get your gammon with the bone in it, your broth will be tastier.

Put your gammon into a large deep pot, cover with water and place over a medium heat. As soon as the water comes to the boil, drain the gammon and discard the water – this will get rid of any excess salt in the meat. Tie the bay, thyme and parsley stalks together in a little bunch.

Put the gammon back into the pot with the herb bunch and peppercorns. Cover with enough water to submerge the gammon. Bring to the boil, then reduce the heat and simmer very gently for around 1½ hours. Add the carrots, fennel, shallots, celery, potatoes and turnips to the pot, season and bring back to the boil. Simmer for about 45 minutes until cooked.

Remove the gammon and vegetables from the pot using a long pair of tongs or a slotted spoon and keep to one side in a large deep warm dish while you cook the greens. Add the shredded greens and broccoli to the pot and bring the stock back to the boil. Cook for 5 minutes until tender.

Check the seasoning of the boiling stock, then remove the greens and broccoli to the warm dish. Pull the meat apart using two forks, then take the bowl to the table, divide the meat and vegetables between your serving bowls and ladle over plenty of broth. Scatter over the reserved fennel tops, parsley leaves and celery leaves and drizzle over some good extra virgin olive oil. Lovely with a little bit of English mustard on the side.

serves 6 to 8

2kg smoked middle cut of gammon, with the knuckle
a sprig of bay leaves
a small bunch of fresh thyme
a few sprigs of fresh flat-leaf parsley, leaves picked, stalks reserved
a few peppercorns
6 medium carrots, scrubbed, tops left on (if in good condition)
1 large fennel, cut into 6 pieces, herby tops reserved
6 shallots or 1 large red onion, peeled and cut into 6 pieces
1 celery heart, quartered, yellow leaves picked and reserved
400g new potatoes (or bigger potatoes cut into small pieces), lightly scrubbed
6 small turnips, peeled
sea salt and freshly ground black pepper
4 generous handfuls of summer greens (use spinach, chard, kale or a mixture), roughly shredded
a good handful of purple sprouting broccoli, stalks trimmed
extra virgin olive oil

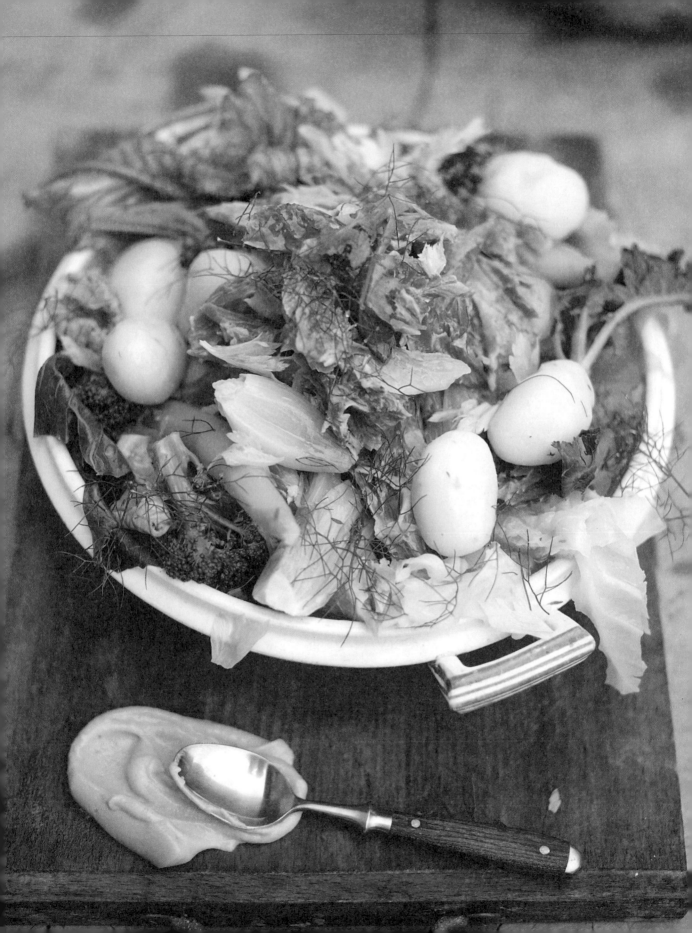

# How I grow the cabbage family

## Soil
Brassicas can grow well in most soil types, but they don't really like acidic ground. They need a bright spot in the garden.

## Planting
Sowing times vary quite a lot depending on the variety and type of brassica, so please check the seed packet. As a general rule, though, summer brassicas are usually sown in the early spring; autumn and winter cropping varieties should be sown from spring to early summer and spring cropping varieties can be sown from midsummer into autumn to grow over the winter.

Although you can sow straight outside, I sow my brassica seeds into module trays filled with organic sowing compost and keep them indoors to start off with. This way I don't waste any seed, I know exactly how many plants I've got and the baby seedlings are easier to keep safe, away from slugs, bugs and bad weather conditions. To sow, all you need to do is fill each module with your potting compost, make a hole with your finger or the end of a little stick, 1 to 2cm deep, and pop in a couple of seeds. Cover them with a little soil and water gently.

Seedlings are ready for planting outside when they're about 6 to 9cm tall. I tend to plant leafy brassicas about 30 to 60cm apart, staggered alternately down two adjoining rows. Root brassicas can be closer, 15 to 30cm. The final size these vegetables will grow to is often determined by the planting distance, as they will tend to fill their allotted space then stop. Baby brassicas, like baby cabbage or caulis, are usually bred to be planted much closer together than their bigger brothers. The one thing they all have in common is that they like to be planted firmly so they can take root properly and not get blown over in the wind. So remember to pat the soil down really well around the seedlings when you're planting.

## Harvesting and storing
Cabbages and Brussels reach a certain size and then stop growing, so pick them when they look big enough. They can also be pulled out of the ground, roots and all, and hung upside down in a cool place, like an unheated shed – they'll keep reasonably fresh like this for a month or two. Swedes should be picked when they reach the size of a grapefruit; turnips when the size of squash balls. If left too long they may turn woody and tough. The heads of caulis, broccoli and calabrese should be picked when they are firm, with no open flowerbuds, and eaten as soon as possible. Leafy types like kale and greens can be picked a few leaves at a time.

## My growing tips
- A big pest of brassicas is cabbage root fly, because the maggots burrow into the ground near the stem and chew through the plant's roots. As I'm growing my veg at home organically, I can't spray to get rid of this pest. Instead I use a little plastic thing called a 'brassica collar' which protects the plants.

- Watch out for caterpillars, in particular those of the cabbage white butterfly, as they can chomp through the leaves and devastate a cabbage in a matter of days. The easiest, and most environmentally friendly, way to stop them is to cover your plants with fine netting or garden fleece as soon as you see the pretty white butterflies in your garden. The netting will stop them laying eggs on your precious brassicas and it means you don't have to spray pesticides all over plants you want to eat!

- If you're not too squeamish, you can simply pick the caterpillars off the leaves – they are usually well hidden, so look underneath the leaves as well. Chuck the caterpillars into a wild bit of the garden or over your fence – or, even better, boil them up and sauté them in a little garlic and butter (a joke!).

- Don't grow brassicas in the same bit of ground year after year. If you do, you'll risk a build-up of soil-borne pests and diseases.

- Fold big leaves over the developing heads of cauliflower. This protects them from scorching in strong summer sun or being damaged by frost in winter.

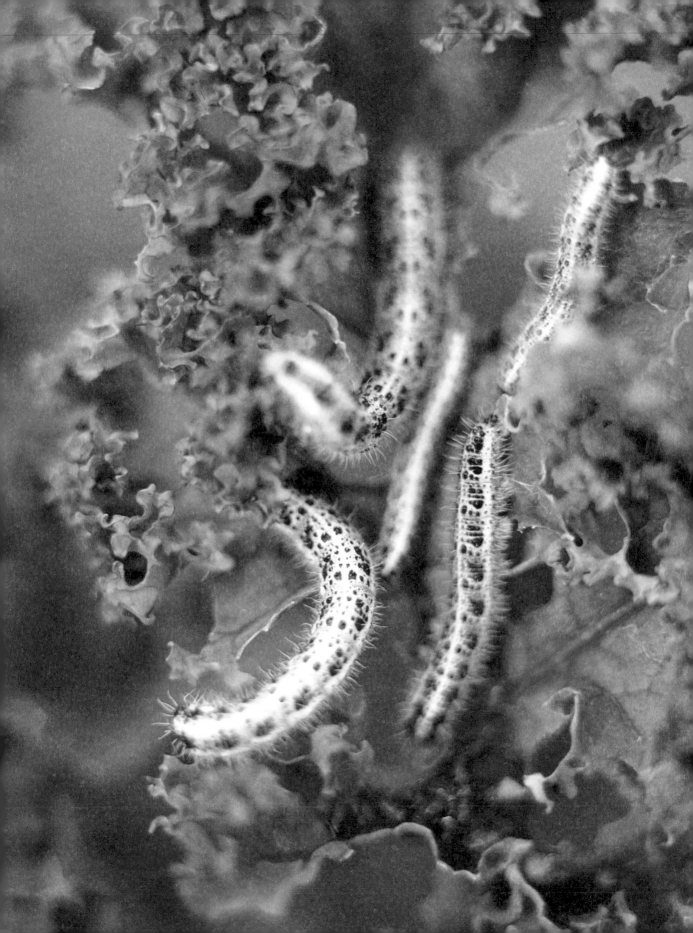

# carrots and beets

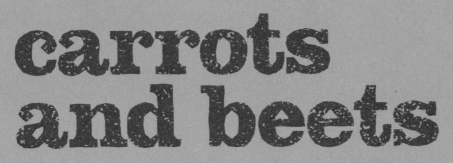

You might not expect to see carrots and beets in a chapter together but to me they're kind of inseparable. They're similar to sow, they're low-maintenance, you can eat the delicious young fragrant leaves from both vegetables when they're small (try them in salads or stir-fries) and the actual root itself is the vegetable that we eat. However, though most people eat carrots on a regular basis, beets don't seem to be on their radar in the same way. Personally, I think they should be!

As far as excitement and general use in your kitchen is concerned, carrots and beets both deliver. I like to cook them in a similar way – they are delicious either boiled and dressed with good olive oil or butter, a squeeze of lemon juice and a pinch of salt and pepper, or shaved raw into ribbons (using a speed peeler) to give a crunch and flavour to any everyday salad. However, my favourite thing to do is boil them for 10 minutes, toss them with some good olive oil, salt, pepper, a little swig of red or white wine vinegar, woody herbs like thyme and rosemary and some smashed garlic, and roast the little monkeys at 180°C/350°F/gas 4 until they're lightly golden, with intense flavour. Come on Eileen, now we're talking! Flavourwise, carrots and beets are both sweet, which is why even though they're vegetables they work really well in cakes – you may be familiar with carrot cake, but try baking one with beetroot instead. Delicious!

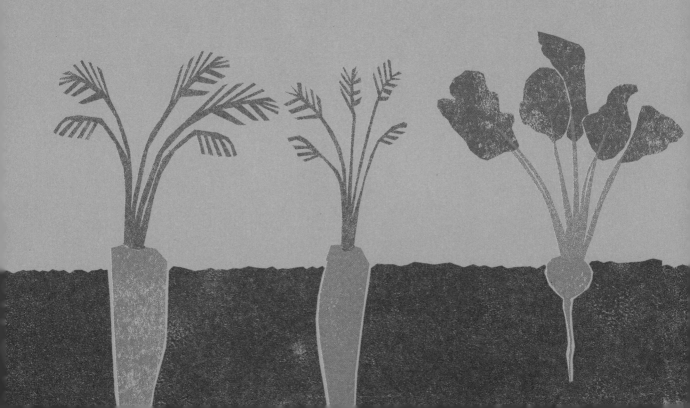

Now, we've all grown up with carrots that are orange. But did you know that historically they weren't orange – they were more purple in colour? Originating from the Middle East, they've been eaten for thousands of years. But it wasn't until patriotic Dutch growers began to cultivate orange carrots in the sixteenth century, to respect their royal House of Orange colours, that they became so popular. There are so many other colours, and shapes, on offer though – check out what's available at good supermarkets or from online seed companies (see page 395 for the ones I've used). Look for yellow, pink, white, red, even purple and black ones – amazing! Go and have a look round, or make your life even easier and grow some interesting varieties yourself (maybe not the orange ones, otherwise it will look like you've bought them from the shop!). Be a bit more exciting – try other colours and interplant them in flowerbeds if you're short of space.

I've even grown some in buckets, bags and pots over the last year. Carrots won't let you down.

Beets are definitely the underdog of these two vegetables and probably more famous for being pickled and sold in jars. As with carrots, you can get beets in a whole variety of colours – from white and yellow, to a vivid candy-striped variety. And as I said above, they can be cooked in the same way as carrots. Just imagine putting a damn good roast on the table, or a fantastic steak with crispy potatoes, and then bringing out something unexpected like roast beetroot – that's how you get your friends talking and how you can introduce them to new favourites! You can turn beets into soup, boil and dress them, roast, steam or stir-fry them, or use them in salads. So don't read this and then do nothing about it – make beets a part of your life!

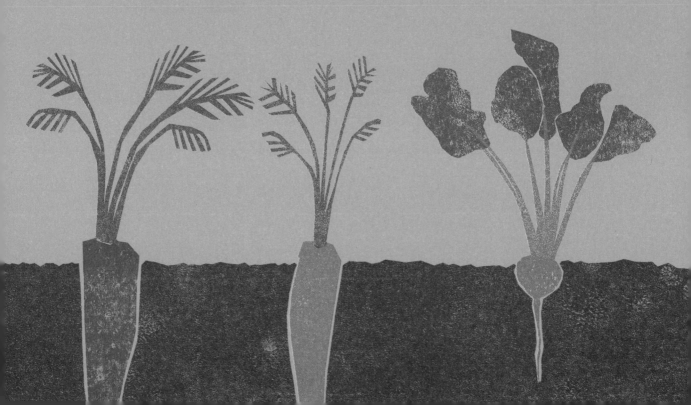

# Indian carrot salad

This is a beautiful fresh Indian-style salad with a zingy crispness that goes wonderfully with spicy lamb. The dressed carrots can be served on their own with some added apple or celery for extra sweetness and crunch.

Heat a large frying pan and fry your ground lamb until all the fat comes out of it. Add the garam masala and a good pinch of salt and give it a stir. Keep frying until the meat is lovely and crispy. Shave the carrots into long thin strips with a speed peeler or a mandolin slicer and keep them to one side.

Heat a small frying pan over a moderate heat and toast the cumin seeds for 30 seconds – they will start to smell nutty and gorgeous. You're not trying to cook the seeds here, you're just waking their flavours up a bit. Put them into a pestle and mortar and grind them up. Put the pan back on the heat and toast the sesame seeds until golden. Transfer them to a plate.

Slice your peeled shallots or onion wafer thin. As with all salads that contain onion, you don't want to be coming across great big chunks! If you don't feel confident about your knife skills, use the coarse side of a box grater instead. This will almost mush your onions to a purée, but at least you won't come across any big bits.

To make your dressing, put the lemon zest and juice into a bowl and add the shallots or onion, grated ginger, ground cumin and a pinch of salt. Whisk everything together with about 5 tablespoons of extra virgin olive oil. Pour the dressing over the carrots, add the coriander and mint leaves, and mix it all together using your fingers. It's important that you have a little taste to check whether the dressing needs more lemon juice, oil or seasoning.

Divide the crispy lamb mince between four plates and put the dressed salad on top. Sprinkle with the toasted sesame seeds. Served with naan bread, some yoghurt and lemon halves, this makes a great snack!

**serves 4**

600g good-quality
  coarsely ground lamb
2 teaspoons garam masala
sea salt
500g carrots (mixed colours
  if possible), peeled
1 tablespoon sesame seeds
a small bunch of fresh
  coriander, leaves picked
a small bunch of fresh
  mint, leaves picked

*for the dressing*
1 teaspoon cumin seeds
3 shallots or 1 small
  red onion, peeled
zest and juice of 1 lemon
1 heaped teaspoon
  freshly grated ginger
extra virgin olive oil

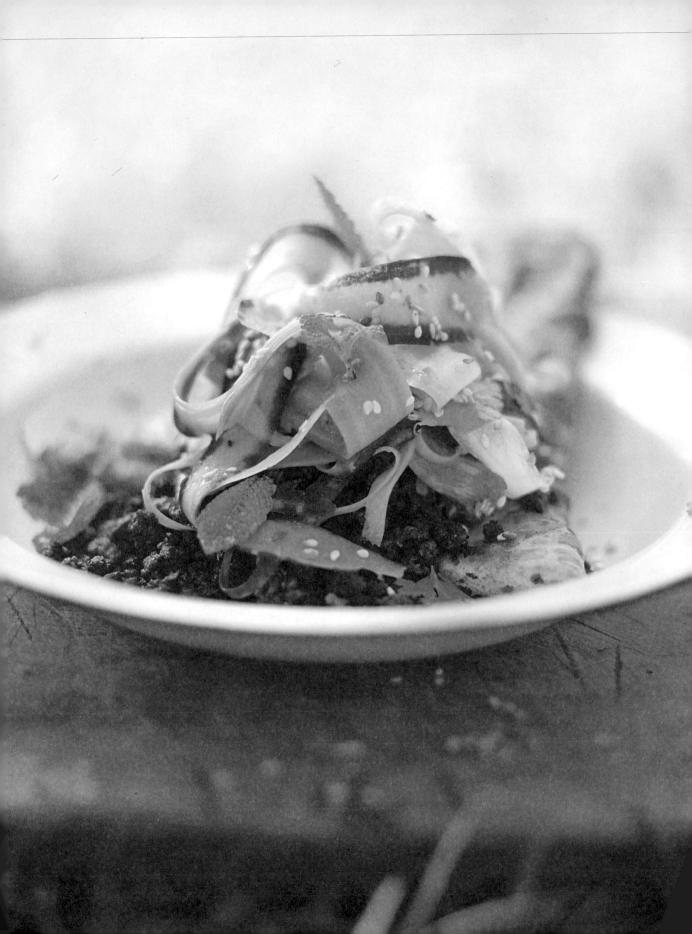

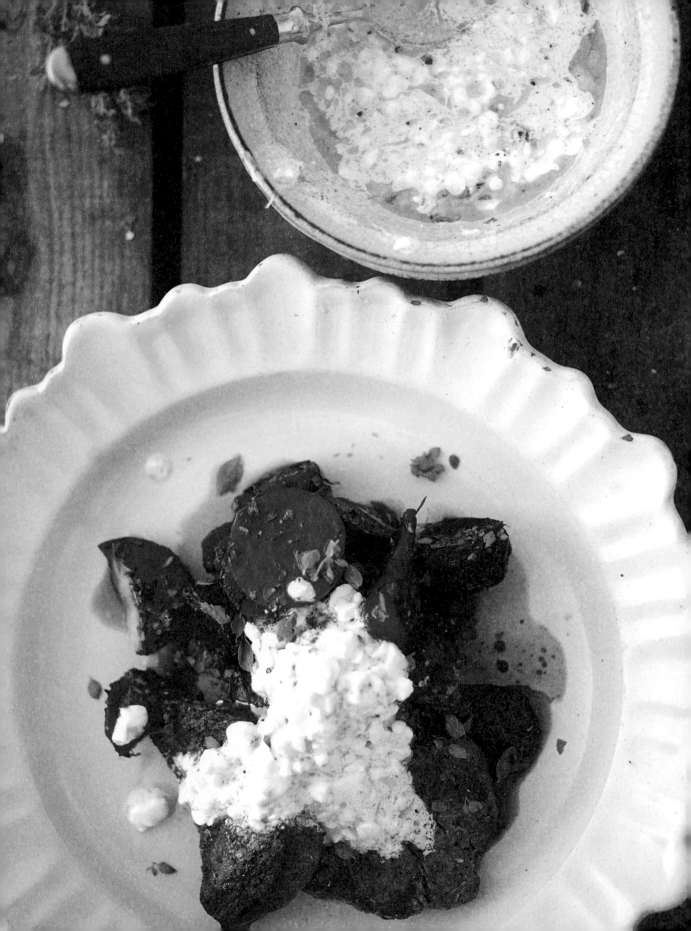

# Smoked beets with grilled steak and a cottage cheese dressing

I came across this method of smoke-cooking beetroots slowly on the barbecue or in the hot ashes of a fire when I was in America. My recipe uses small beetroots, which are easier to peel and don't take as long to cook, and rosemary sprigs to protect the beets from the direct heat of the coals. Alternatively, you can roast the beetroots in the oven at 200°C/400°F/gas 6 for 1½ hours – they'll still taste lovely, but you won't get the wonderful smoky flavour.

First light your barbecue or fire. Lay the beetroots on a double layer of foil – about 30cm (60cm unfolded) – and sprinkle the rosemary leaves on top. Roll up the foil, folding in the edges and twisting the ends together. Stab the foil a few times all over with a knife to allow the smoke to get inside and flavour the beetroots. Lift the rack of your barbecue and carefully insert your foil package among the coals, making sure you place some coals on top too. Leave it to cook for 30 to 40 minutes, or until the beetroots are tender, then remove the package and allow it to cool down. Unwrap it and remove the beetroots, discarding the rosemary sprigs.

Once cooled slightly, peel the beetroots and discard the charred skin. Cut the beets into irregular chunks and place in a bowl. Add the vinegar, 3 tablespoons of extra virgin olive oil, plenty of salt and pepper and half the parsley and tarragon. Toss, have a taste and adjust the seasoning if necessary.

Put the cottage cheese into a bowl and add the juice and finely grated zest from half your lemon. Stir in 2 glugs of extra virgin olive oil, the thyme leaves and some salt and pepper and gently fold it all together, so the oil and lemon marble through the cottage cheese. Taste the dressing and squeeze in a bit more lemon juice if you like.

Lightly rub a little dressing on to your 4 steaks. Place them on the barbecue and cook to your liking, turning them every minute, then remove them to a plate and allow to rest.

To serve, divide the dressed beets between two plates. Top each plate with 2 steaks and a spoonful of cottage cheese dressing. Scatter over the remaining herbs and enjoy!

serves 2

8 small beetroots,
 tops trimmed
a small bunch of fresh
 rosemary, leaves picked
1 tablespoon red
 wine vinegar
extra virgin olive oil
sea salt and freshly
 ground black pepper
a small bunch of fresh flat-
 leaf parsley, leaves picked
 and roughly chopped
a small bunch of fresh
 tarragon or basil,
 leaves picked and
 roughly chopped
4 x 100g fillet steaks

*for the cottage cheese
 dressing*
4 heaped tablespoons
 cottage cheese
1 lemon, halved
extra virgin olive oil
a few sprigs of fresh
 thyme, leaves picked

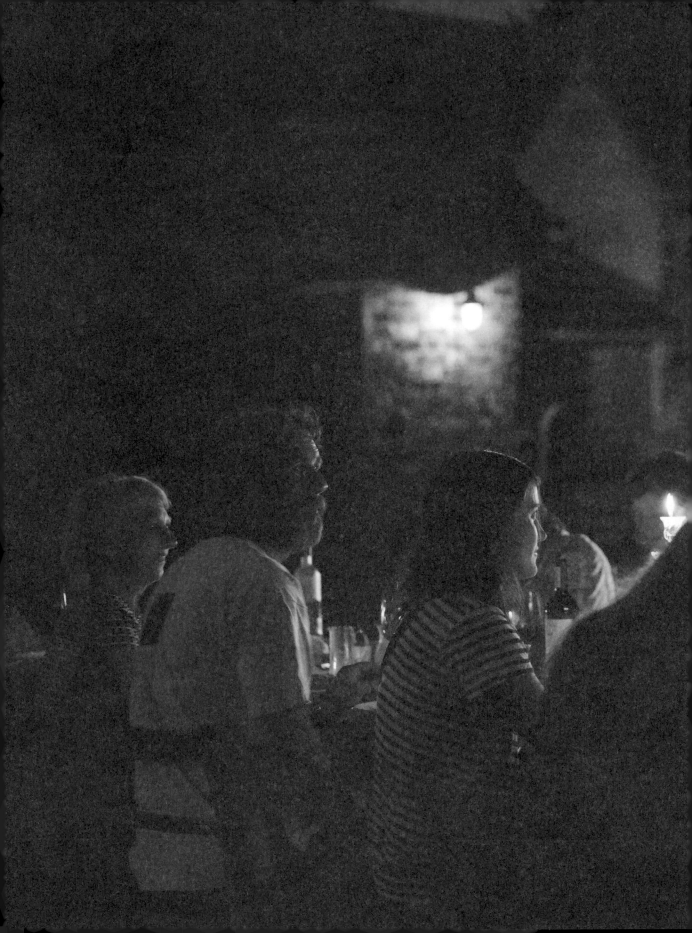

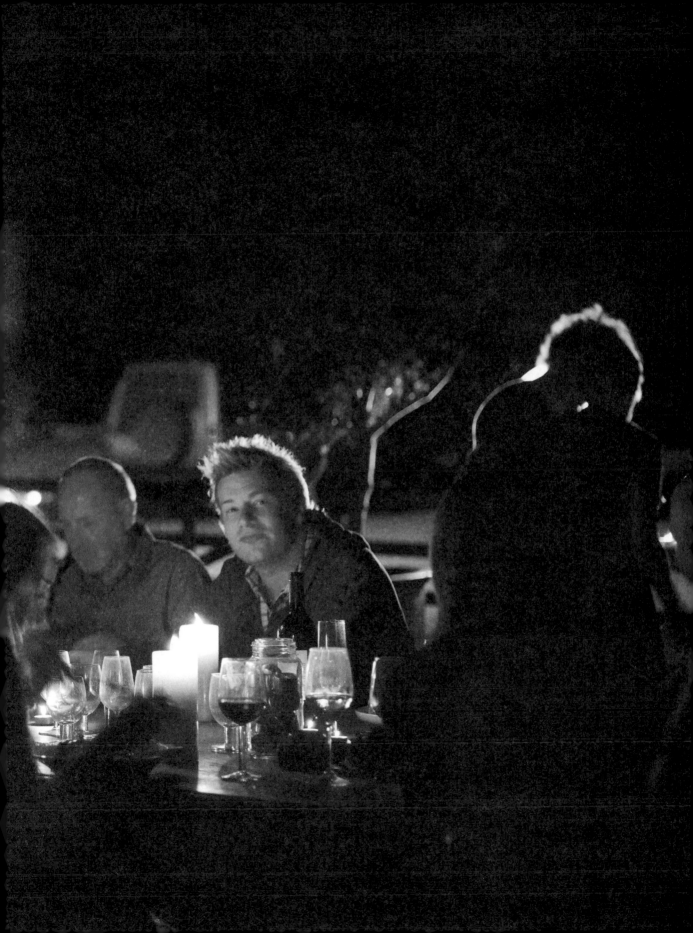

# Roasted carrots and beets with the juiciest pork chops

Carrots and beets are particularly good when roasted as it brings out their natural sugars. The best advice I can give you is about flavouring them. A few smashed garlic cloves, a woody herb like rosemary, thyme, sage or bay, and a splash of vinegar, or squeezed lemon or orange juice, can accentuate their natural flavour.

Preheat the oven to 220°C/425°F/gas 7. Put your carrots into a large pot and your beets into another, and add enough water to cover them. Season with salt and bring to the boil. Cook for 15 to 20 minutes until just tender, then drain and place in separate bowls. Peel your beets, and cut any larger carrots and beets in half or into quarters. Smaller ones can stay whole.

Now add your flavourings while the veg are still hot. Toss the carrots with half the smashed garlic and a glug of olive oil, then lightly season. Add the orange juice and the thyme leaves and toss again. Mix the beets with the rest of the garlic, the rosemary, balsamic vinegar and salt and pepper. You can now put the veg either into separate ovenproof dishes, or together on a large roasting tray with the carrots in one half of the tray and the beets in the other. Place in the middle of the preheated oven and roast for around half an hour or until golden.

While the carrots and beets are cooking, lay the chops on a board and score through the skin and the streaky-looking part of the meat. This will give you lovely crackling. Look at the picture – you'll see what I mean. Firmly press a sage leaf on to the eye meat on both sides of each chop. Season with salt and pepper.

When the vegetables start to colour, heat a large ovenproof frying pan or small roasting tray on the hob, add a good glug of olive oil and put in the chops. As soon as you've got nice colour on one side, turn the chops over and place the tray in the oven for 10 minutes, or until the chops are crisp on the outside and just cooked through and juicy in the middle. Remove the chops to a warmed plate. Pour most of the fat away from the tray and add a squeeze of lemon juice to it. Stir and scrape the lovely sticky bits off the bottom and drizzle all over the chops. Remove the carrots and beets from the oven – they should be nice and sticky by now. Serve them with the chops and a glass of wine.

**serves 4**

750g carrots, mixed colours
  if available, peeled
750g beets, different sizes
  and colours if available
sea salt and freshly
  ground black pepper
1 bulb of garlic, broken
  apart, half the cloves
  smashed, half left whole
extra virgin olive oil
juice of 1 orange
a few sprigs of fresh
  thyme, leaves picked
a few sprigs of fresh
  rosemary, leaves picked
5 tablespoons balsamic
  vinegar
4 thick organic pork
  loin chops, skin on
8 fresh sage leaves
1 lemon

carrots and beets

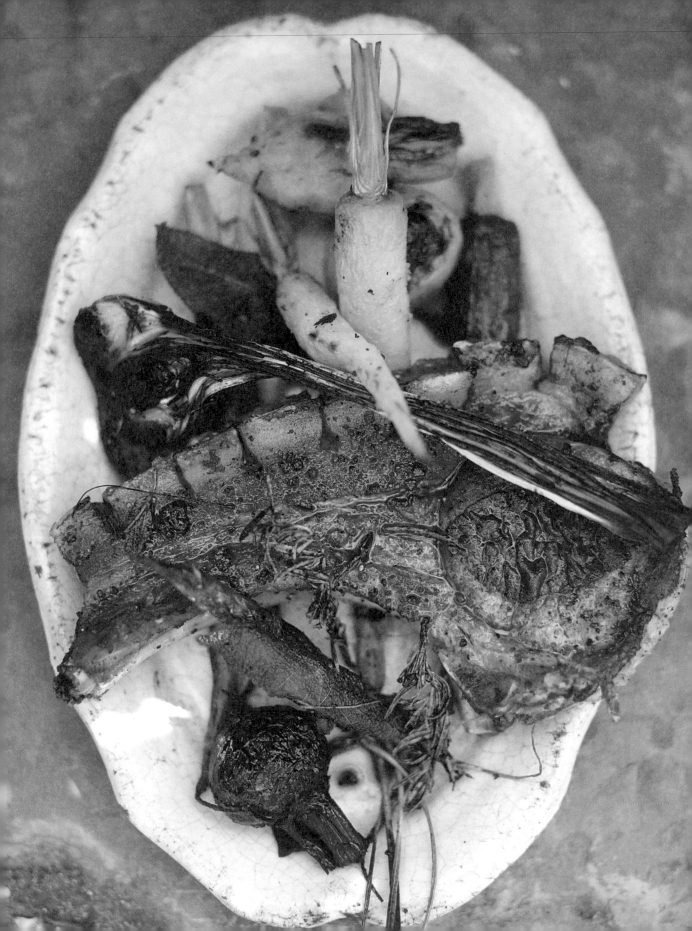

# How I grow carrots and beets

## Soil

Carrots and beets are usually sown straight into the ground. Carrots are a little fussier than beets – they prefer light, fertile soil rather than a dense clay (there's no need to add manure over winter). If clay is what you have in your garden, don't despair, because they can be grown in big pots or troughs filled with good light potting compost. They need a light soil, because if they hit a hard bit they'll simply split in two to grow round the lump, and you'll end up with some pretty funny-shaped carrots! Beets aren't as fussy as carrots, so any good garden soil will do.

## Planting

By choosing different varieties of carrot and beet, and sowing 'little and often', every three or four weeks from February to August, you can have crops from late spring right through to winter. With careful storage you could have them all year round.

To sow carrots, level off the soil and make furrows about 1 to 2cm deep, 15 to 20cm apart. Sprinkle the seeds lightly and evenly into the furrow. Then cover them over with soil and water them gently. Beets are usually sown straight into the soil, just like carrots, but I often start my seeds in pots or module trays indoors, and plant them outside when they're slightly bigger. I sow two or three seeds per module and when they're big enough I plant each little group out together without disturbing the roots. This way I can space them out more easily, and it's more economical on seed.

## Harvesting and storing

Two months after planting, you can start eating your carrots and beets. Left longer most varieties simply get bigger, until the weather starts cooling in autumn. If you want to eat baby beets or carrots, simply pull them out of the ground earlier.

To store any type of root vegetable, like carrots or beets, turnips, swede or Jerusalem artichokes, even potatoes, you can do something called 'clamping'. In the old days, before we had fridges and freezers, this is the method that everyone would have used to store their root veg. All you need to do is get yourself a wooden crate or a thick polystyrene box and pour in a layer of moist sand. Brush it over with your hands to get it even. Remove any excess soil from your veg, then twist any green stalks off them and place the vegetables next to each other, but not touching, in one layer on the sand. Cover them with more sand and then repeat the process, layering vegetables and sand to the top of the crate. Store the crate in a cold shed or garage, or outside under cover. Clamping the veg like this will keep them really well for four to five months without losing too much nutritional value and flavour.

## My growing tips

- I love growing carrots from mixed colour seed packs because then you'll always get a surprise when you pull them up.

- As your carrot and beet seedlings grow you may need to thin them out a little. All you need to do is pull up some of the little plants, leaving a good strong one every 5 to 8cm. This will allow the ones that are left behind more room to grow. After thinning, make sure you mound the earth back up around the remaining plants and give them a little sprinkle of water, as their roots will have been disturbed. The baby carrots and beets that you pull up are lovely to cook with, so enjoy them!

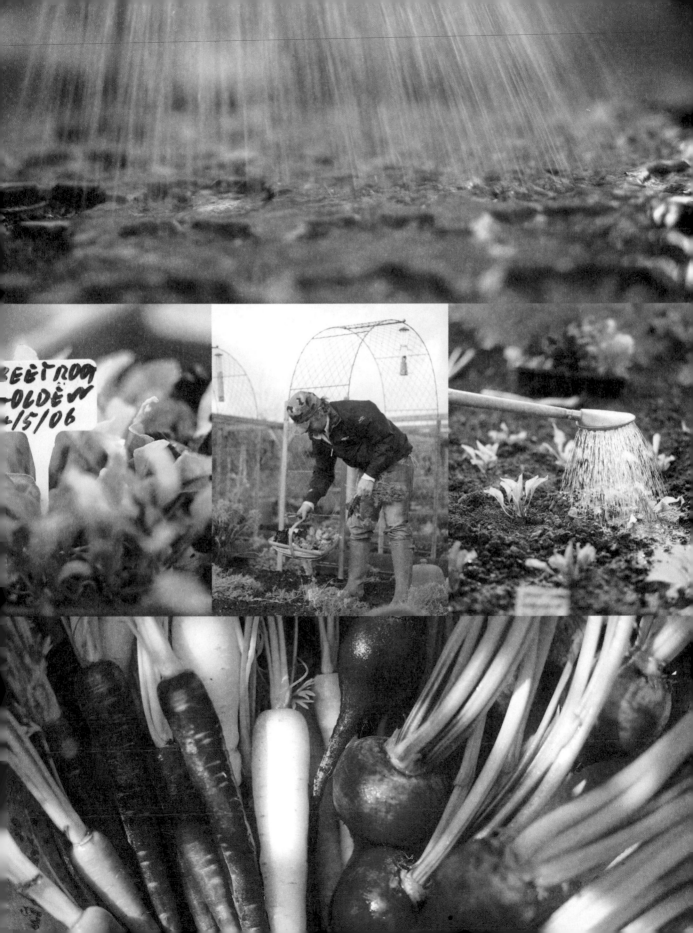

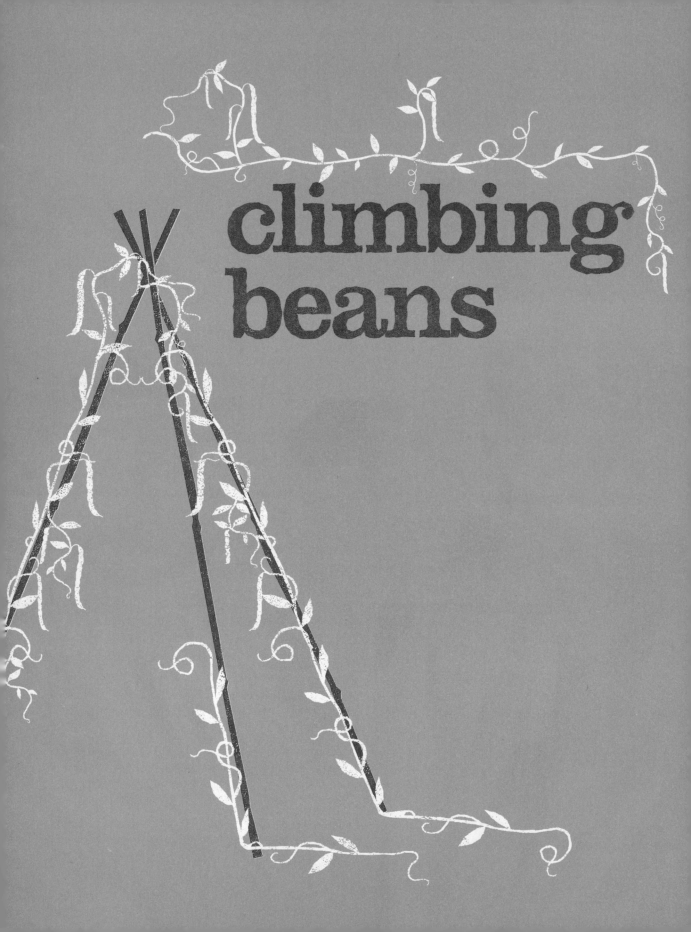

# climbing beans

In August 2006 we were supposed to be in the middle of our glorious British summer and enjoying the sunshine, but instead it just seemed to pour with rain. A lot! Yet we shouldn't ever complain, because the garden loves a mixture of sun and rain – it makes everything go a bit berserk and things grow much quicker. Especially beans – you'll see a massive difference in their growth after just ten to fourteen days if you've had a nice bit of rain. The pods can go from being tiny flower buds to almost fully grown in this very short space of time – just amazing.

Climbing beans naturally grow around anything they touch. Given a supporting framework, like canes or trellises, they will climb up houses, against walls, over arches – you name it. In fact, in some countries you'll see beans of all types planted alongside and underneath other crops like sunflowers and sweetcorn – not only does this make good use of the available space but it gives the grower much more yield from his land.

The whole climbing bean family is completely diverse – some types are loved for the beans inside the pods, others for the actual bean pods, some for both! The best thing is that beans go well with almost everything: alongside meat and fish; tossed warm or cold into salads; or added to soups and pasta dishes. Some can be served on toast, as well as being the hero of their own dishes. There's absolutely nothing wrong with simply boiling or steaming beans and dressing them with a knob of butter or a splash of extra virgin olive oil, as they'll be delicious like this. However, don't think this is the only way you can cook them. Beans are such fantastic carriers of flavours that they are brilliant when wok-fried, stewed or braised with spices. They are also full of protein, so a perfect choice for vegetarians.

# Beef carpaccio with marinated bean salad

Carpaccio is very thinly sliced raw meat. I like mine Italian style, with the meat sliced a little more thickly. This makes it a bit more rustic and you can really taste the quality of the meat. I also like to sear the meat very quickly before slicing it up, as this gives you a contrasting encrusted edge of flavour. It's lovely with this marinated bean salad – you can simply use green beans, or a mixture of different ones.

You don't need loads of meat for this, just a couple of slices per person, which should allow you to spend a little more on a good-quality piece of beef.

Bring a large pot of salted water to the boil. Drop in the beans and cook for about 5 minutes. When perfectly done, drain them in a colander.

To make the marinade, mix the shallot or onion in a bowl with the herbs, mustard, vinegar and 4 tablespoons of extra virgin olive oil. Season with salt and pepper to taste, then add the hot cooked beans and toss. Put to one side to allow the beans to cool down and take on all the fantastic flavours.

Place the beef fillet on a chopping board and season it all over with salt and pepper. Run the thyme sprigs under hot water for a few seconds – this will help to release their fragrant oils. Strip the leaves from the stalks and chop them up roughly. Sprinkle the thyme over the fillet, then roll the meat around the chopping board so that any excess seasoning and herbs stick to it.

Get a heavy frying pan very hot and add a splash of oil, followed by the beef fillet. Fry for 1 minute only, turning it every few seconds to sear and encrust all the lovely flavourings on to it. Take the meat out of the frying pan and put it on a plate to rest for a minute. (Once seared, you can serve straight away or you can keep the meat covered on a plate until needed. I prefer not to keep it in the fridge.)

Using a sharp knife, now slice the seared fillet this thick: ┝━━┥ Lay each slice on a board and flatten as much as you can by pressing down on them with the side of a chopping knife – it works a treat. Lay two or three slices out flat on each plate. Season again lightly and place a pile of beans on top, spooning over some of the marinade. Sprinkle over any leftover herb leaves and drizzle with some good extra virgin olive oil.

serves 4

sea salt and freshly
  ground black pepper
250g green or mixed beans,
  topped but not tailed
1 x 500g piece of beef fillet
a few sprigs of fresh thyme
olive oil

*for the marinade*
2 small shallots or ½ a
  small red onion, peeled
  and very finely chopped
a handful of fresh soft
  herbs (chervil, parsley,
  yellow inner celery,
  tarragon), leaves
  picked and chopped
1 teaspoon Dijon mustard
1½ tablespoons white
  wine vinegar
extra virgin olive oil

climbing beans

118

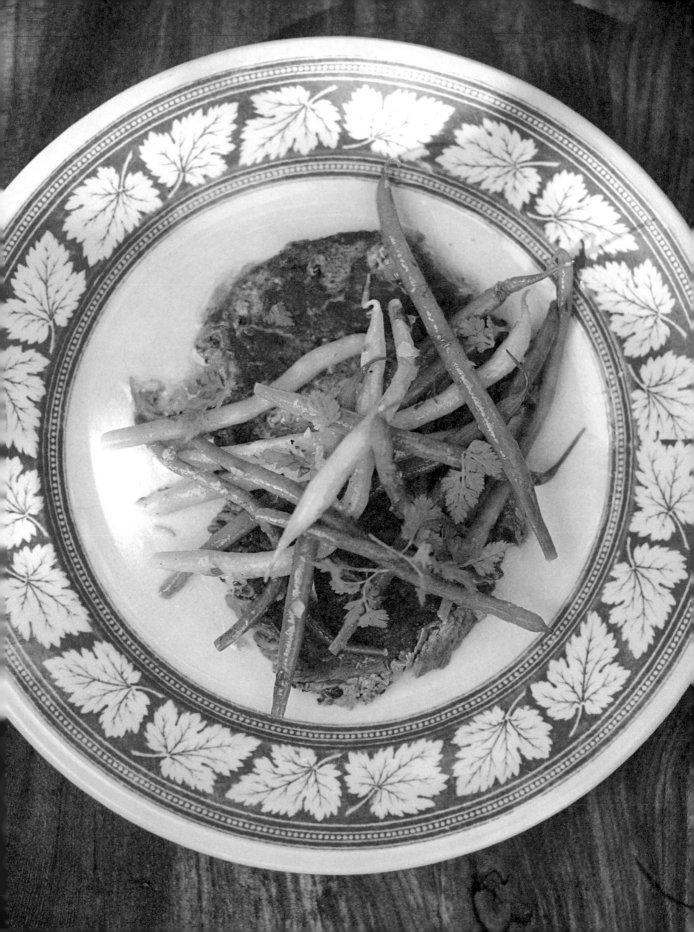

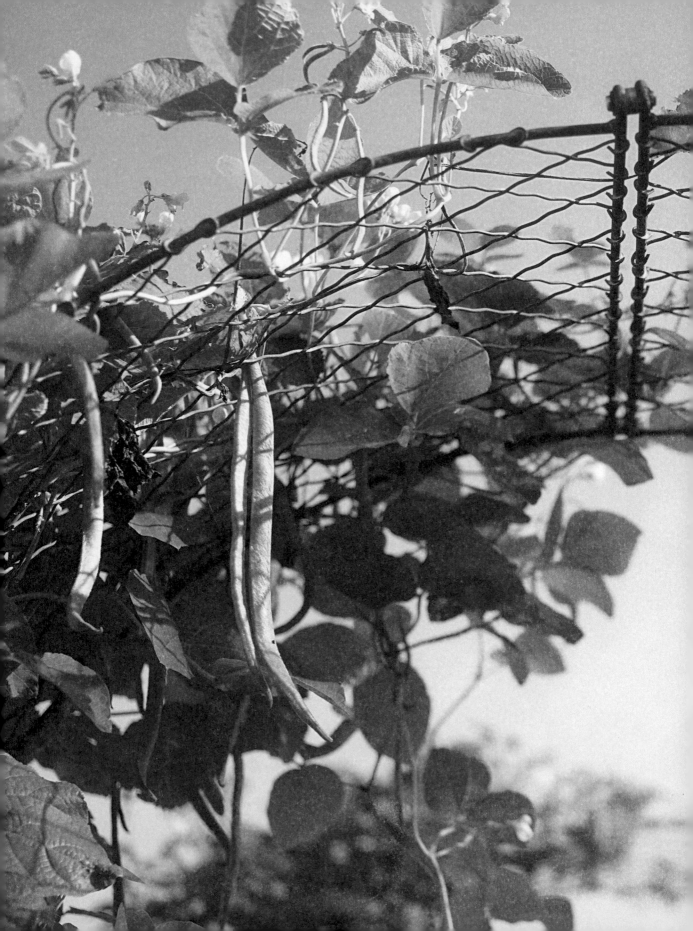

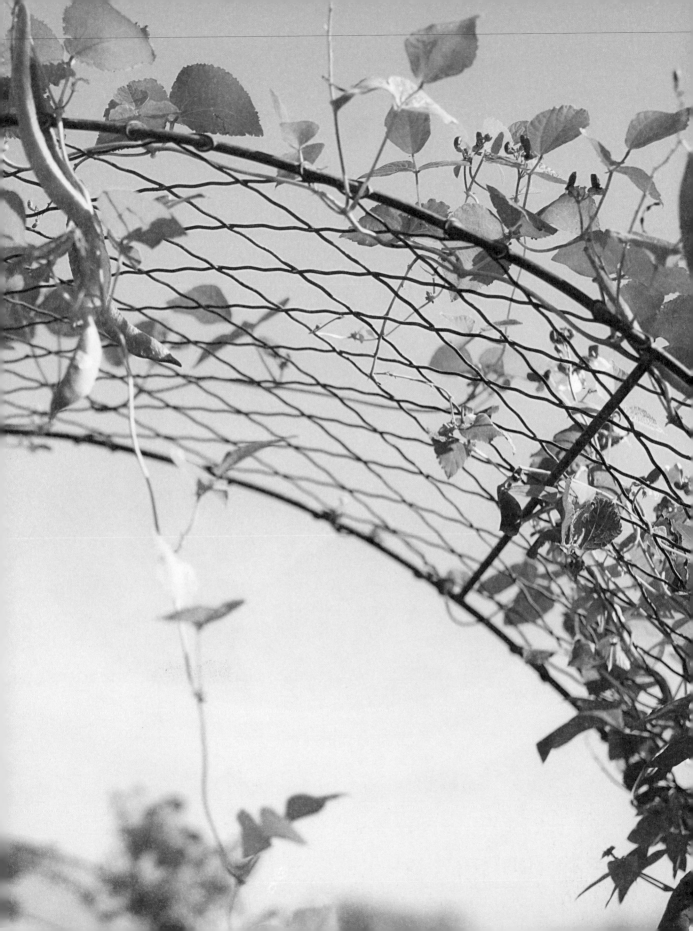

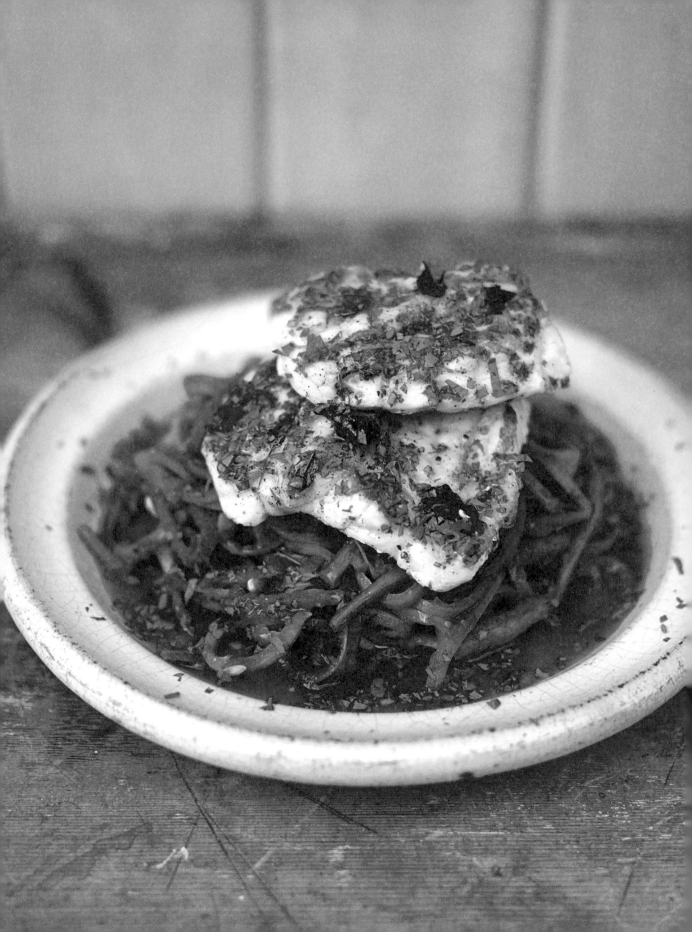

# Grilled butterflied monkfish with a sweet runner bean stew

I absolutely love to cook runner beans this way. They take on fantastic flavour and go so well, when eaten hot, with roasted fish or white meat. They're also really good served cold as an antipasto. Please give them a try. To finish off this dish I'm going to use a great flavour enhancer called gremolata. The classic combination is garlic, lemon zest and flat-leaf parsley, all chopped together really finely. It can be sprinkled over stews, broths, soups or pasta dishes at the last minute. It really brings a dish to life. You get the fragrance and sharpness of the lemon and the hum of the garlic.

Feed the runner beans through a bean cutter. If you don't have one, just run your speed peeler down each side of the bean to get rid of the stringy bits and then cut them into 1cm pieces at an angle.

Your runner bean stew can be cooked in advance or started just before you cook the fish. Heat a large saucepan, big enough to hold all the ingredients, and add 2 tablespoons of olive oil plus the oil from the jar of anchovies. Chop 4 of the garlic cloves and fry them gently with the anchovies and dried chilli until it all goes soft and the anchovies break down into a mush. Pour in the crushed tomatoes or passata and add the beans and the rosemary sprigs. Season and bring to the boil. Place a lid on the pan and simmer gently for 12 to 15 minutes or until the beans are nicely cooked. If the sauce gets a little dry, add a splash of water and give the beans a stir.

Lay the monkfish pieces on a chopping board and slice them horizontally *almost* in half, so they open out like a book. Try to get them so you have an even thickness on both sides. Score the fish lightly and put to one side.

To make the gremolata, finely chop the remaining clove of garlic with a pinch of salt. Next, finely chop the parsley and finely zest the lemon. Mix these with the garlic, give it all one last chop and put aside to sprinkle over at the end.

Heat a very large griddle pan or frying pan (or use two smaller ones). Season the fish well with salt and pepper and rub lightly with olive oil. Cook the fish for 2 minutes each side or until just cooked through (don't be tempted to overcook it).

Take the beans off the heat, taste and season them once again if necessary. Remove the rosemary sprigs and squeeze in the juice from the lemon. Place a pile of beans on each plate and top with a piece of fish. Drizzle with oil and sprinkle over the basil leaves and gremolata. Or you could serve the whole lot on a big platter in the middle of the table – family service style!

serves 4

600g runner beans, trimmed
olive oil
1 x 100g jar of good anchovy fillets, in oil
5 cloves of garlic, peeled
1 dried red chilli, crumbled
700g jar of passata or 2 x 400g tins of tomatoes, crushed
2 sprigs of fresh rosemary
sea salt and freshly ground black pepper
4 x 200g thick pieces of monkfish, skinned and trimmed properly – ask your fishmonger
a bunch of fresh flat-leaf parsley
1 lemon
extra virgin olive oil
a small bunch of fresh green or purple basil, leaves picked

climbing beans

# Humble home-cooked beans

My first thought when I saw these beans on a menu in Italy was 'Beans on toast?' But then I tasted them. I felt pretty humbled that such a simple dish had been made to taste so gorgeous. Once you've learned how to season and cook them in the right way, you can apply the method to cannellini beans, butter beans, borlotti beans, haricots verts, lentils, even chickpeas. If you've grown your own beans, good on ya! Fresh ones will take about 45 minutes to cook, but you're more likely to get dried beans as they're cheap, and very reliable to cook. However, they will need soaking for at least 12 hours.

Drain your soaked beans, then give them a good wash. Place them in a deep pot and cover them with cold water. Throw in your garlic, herb sprigs, bay leaves, celery stick, potato and tomatoes. Place the beans on the heat and slowly bring to the boil. Cover with a lid and simmer very gently for 45 minutes to an hour, depending on whether you're using fresh or dried, until soft and cooked nicely. Skim if necessary, topping up with boiling water from the kettle if you need to.

When the beans are cooked, drain them in a colander, reserving enough of the cooking water to cover them halfway up when put back in the pot. Remove the garlic, herbs, celery, potato and tomatoes from the beans. Squeeze the garlic cloves out of their skins and pinch the skin off the tomatoes. Put the garlic, tomatoes and potato on to a plate, mash them with a fork and stir back into the beans. Season well with salt and pepper, and pour in three generous glugs of extra virgin olive oil and a few splashes of vinegar. Stir in the parsley and serve on some toasted sourdough bread.

serves 4

300g dried borlotti
  or cannellini beans,
  soaked in cold water
  for at least 12 hours
3 cloves of garlic, unpeeled
a few sprigs of fresh thyme
a sprig of fresh rosemary
3 bay leaves
1 stick of celery, trimmed
1 small potato, peeled
  and halved
2 cherry tomatoes
extra virgin olive oil
red wine vinegar
a few sprigs of fresh
  flat-leaf parsley, chopped
4 slices of sourdough bread

climbing beans

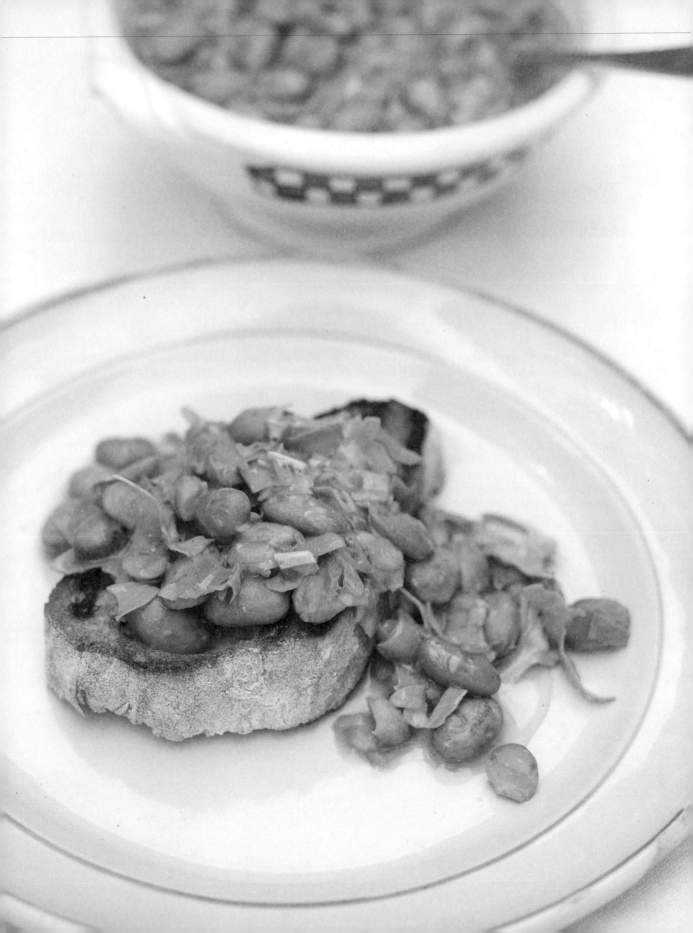

# Four ways to serve your humble home-cooked beans

Here are my four favourite ways to make humble home-cooked beans (see page 124) the hero of the dish. Each recipe is enough for one.

## Creamy beans with fresh crab and chilli

Mix some lovely cold, picked **crabmeat** with a little chopped **fresh chilli** and some picked **fennel tops**. Spoon the warm home-cooked beans on to a plate and top with the crab mixture.

## Crispy red mullet with beans

Get yourself 1 or 2 **red mullet fillets**. Season them with **sea salt and freshly ground black pepper** and fry in a glug of **olive oil** on a medium heat for a couple of minutes on each side. Chop a handful of **rocket** and stir it into your warm home-cooked beans with a little **lemon zest** and some **extra virgin olive oil**. Spoon the beans on to a plate, top with the perfectly cooked red mullet fillets and sprinkle over some **smoked paprika**.

## Warm salad of beans and bread

Toast 2 slices of good-quality **bread** and tear them into rough chunks. Place in a bowl with a handful of chopped **tomatoes**, some **sea salt and freshly ground black pepper**, a drizzle of **extra virgin olive oil** and a swig of good **balsamic vinegar**. Spoon some of your warm home-cooked beans on to a plate, followed by the bread and tomato mixture. Serve topped with a slice or two of **prosciutto** and some **baby basil leaves**.

## Beans with scallops and pancetta

Take up to 3 **scallops** and wrap a slice of **pancetta** round each one. Thread them on to a skewer or a sturdy sprig of fresh rosemary and fry them on each side in a little **olive oil** until golden. Spoon your delicious warm home-cooked beans on to your plate and top with the scallops. Serve with a squeeze of **lemon**, a drizzle of **extra virgin olive oil** and any juices from the pan. Brilliant!

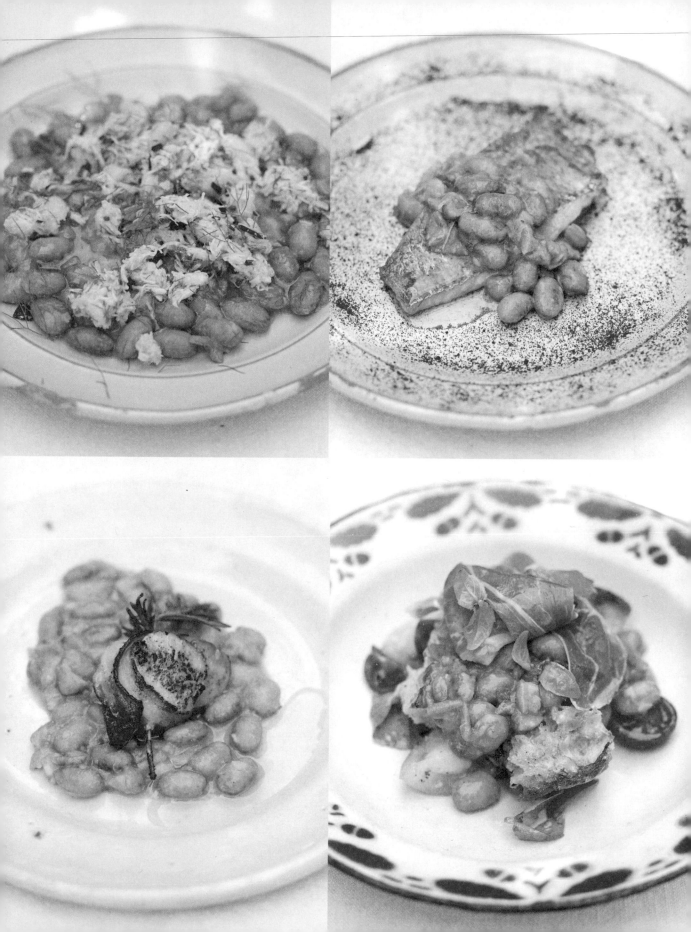

# How I grow climbing beans

## Soil

The best type of soil for growing beans is a good free-draining soil to which manure has been added over the winter. This can either be dug in or left on the surface as a mulch for the earthworms to dig in for you. The ideal spot for planting should be sunny and partly sheltered.

## Planting

I usually sow my beans indoors in April or May and I use organic, biodegradable grow-tubes, which you can buy from any good garden shop (or try making your own out of loo-roll tubes or by rolling a piece of card up and stapling it together), or small, deep pots – even plastic yoghurt pots will do the job, but you need to remember to prick a few holes in the bottom of them first. Fill almost to the top with good organic sowing compost and press gently to firm it down. Add a little more if needed and press down again. Make a hole about 3 to 5cm deep in the soil and drop in two seeds per pot and fill the holes back up with a little more compost. Water thoroughly and place on a sunny windowsill or in a warm, light, frost-free place for three to four weeks.

When your plants are 15 to 20cm high, you can plant them outside in your garden. All climbing types of bean need some structural support (over a wire arch, for instance), using little twigs or thin canes to help them start climbing. My favourite way is to build a trellis shaped like a tepee, using bamboo canes. To do this, push eight long canes into the ground so that they form a circle. Bring them in together at the top and secure them with string or wire.

Make a hole big enough to take one bean plant near the base of each cane. If you're using biodegradable grow-tubes, you can put the whole tube containing the plant into the soil. Otherwise, lift the plants out of their pots and plant one next to each stick. Wind the first few bean-shoot tendrils around the bottom of each bamboo cane – this will help to guide the plants as they grow (there's no need to secure them). From this point on, the plants will grip the canes for themselves. Don't forget to water them well.

## My growing tips

- Don't worry if you think your beans look a bit boring in the garden – they're not the most exciting plant in terms of how they look, but, like strawberries, they will give you a lovely surprise when you go along one day to check on their progress. Under the leaves you will come across a little treasure trove of beans all growing away, and the best thing is that they're hidden from the birds pecking away at them. Nature is a clever thing.

- Most plants in the bean family are called 'feeder crops'. This means they grab nitrogen from the air and concentrate it in their roots. They use what they need for their own growth, then release the rest of it into the soil, improving its fertility for future crops. As nitrogen is a major nutrient for plants, growing beans is a good organically friendly way of enriching the soil without using chemical fertilizers.

- Beans absolutely hate drought, and you'll notice their growth rate slowing down and the pods drying up if they go for a while without any rain. Make sure you give them a good soaking of water every few days if you haven't had many showers.

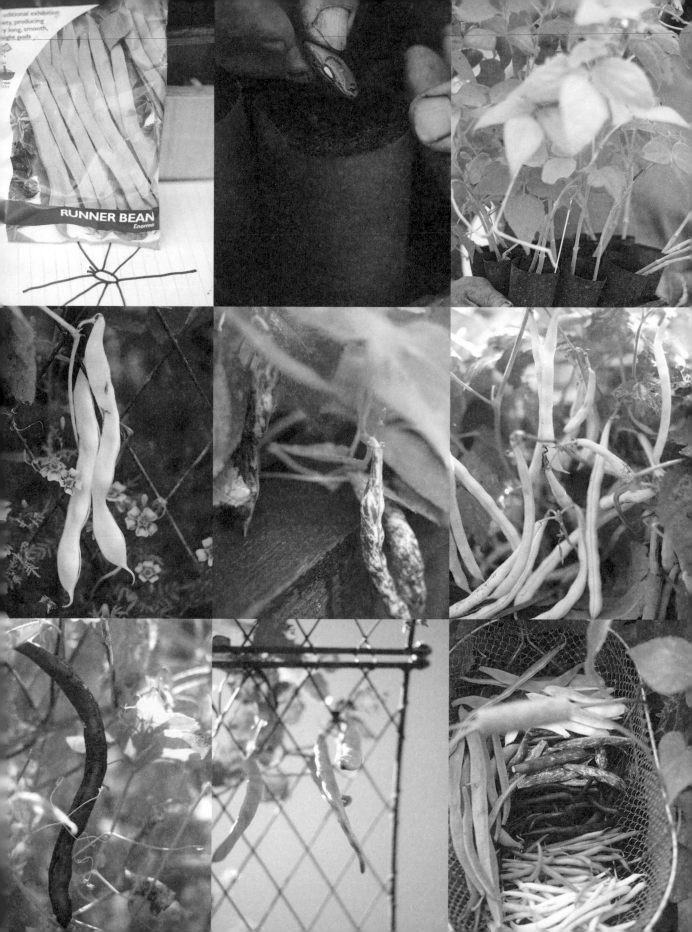

Courgettes are part of the squash, marrow and cucumber family. In Britain they're available everywhere now, but I don't think they're loved as much as, say, the good old garden pea. I might be wrong, but I would think it's to do with not many people knowing how to cook them properly. Most of those I've spoken to about courgettes feel unemotional about them and wouldn't miss them if they went without. If boiling them is all that's done with them, I can understand why!

We've only had courgettes available in Britain for the last fifty years, so this really makes them a super-modern vegetable. These same fifty years have seen some of the darkest cooking moments in British history. By this I mean that during this time people have stopped cooking so much at home and fast food and microwave meals have taken over. So this is not going to help the courgette's case for being a great little vegetable that everyone should be cooking! But have no fear. We shall get you to be a courgette expert without any problems.

When they're small and crunchy, you can finely slice or shave courgettes raw into salads, but they do like to be dressed with lemon juice, olive oil, salt, pepper and soft herbs. They also benefit from spices, like fresh chilli. And they're delicious paired with Parmesan cheese. So, the next time you're making a mixed salad of spinach and watercress, chopped tomatoes and avocado, get yourself a baby courgette, shave it with a speed peeler, dress it up and toss it into the salad – you'll be amazed how delicious it will be. Courgettes are lovely when grilled on the barbecue or in a griddle pan – simply slice them up about 0.5cm thick and grill them dry. Once they've got some char marks on them, dress them with some olive oil and lemon juice. They are also great when they're roasted until lightly golden and slightly blistered. Simply leave small courgettes whole or halve them lengthways, then toss them in oil with a swig of red wine vinegar, add some smashed garlic and drizzle with olive oil before roasting.

Perfect flavour partners for courgettes are thyme and mint. Have a go at roughly slicing up courgettes any way you like so you have some different shapes going on (removing and discarding any fluffy insides from larger ones), then put them in a high-sided pot with a little finely chopped mint or thyme, olive oil, salt and pepper and slowly fry on a low heat for 20 to 25 minutes, stirring every so often. The sweetness and intensity of flavour will blow your mind! Finish with a squeeze of lemon juice and some more chopped mint. Serve with anything.

I would definitely encourage you to have a go at growing your own courgettes because one of the biggest benefits is that you get the flowers along with the courgettes themselves. They have a sweet, pollen-like taste and are a fantastic receptacle for filling with seasoned meats or cheeses, especially ricotta with soft herbs. You can bake or roast them, even batter and deep fry them. Or you can simply tear them up and throw them at the last minute into salads, soups, stews, risottos, or pasta dishes.

# courgettes

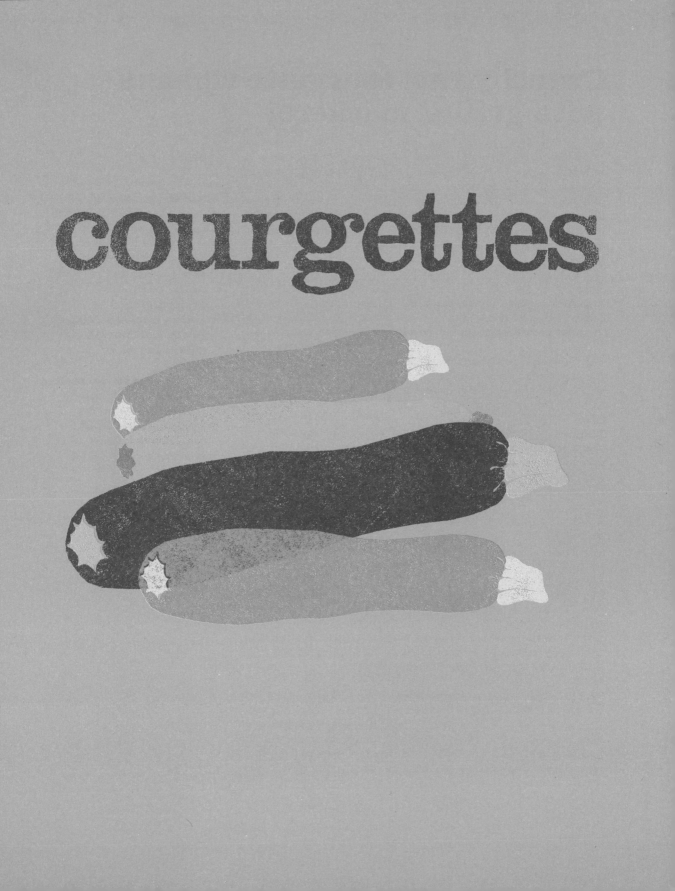

# Crunchy raw courgette ribbons with grilled mackerel

These zingy, crunchy courgettes are delicious and contrast so well with a meaty fish like mackerel. They'd also go equally well with pork chops or tuna steaks. Mackerel is an incredibly underrated fish – it's packed with omega-3 oils, so it's really good for you. Only buy it when it's really fresh, though. If in doubt, use your nose! It should smell like the seaside, not fishy. In this recipe I'm cooking it on the barbecue, but it's fine to use a griddle pan or put it under a screaming hot grill instead.

First light your barbie and get yourself a nice bed of glowing hot coals. Brush the bars clean using a wire brush so the fish doesn't stick to them. If you're not using the barbie, preheat your grill to its maximum or heat up your griddle pan.

Put the lemon zest into a large bowl and add the lemon juice, together with three times as much good extra virgin olive oil. Add the chopped chilli and season the dressing to taste with salt and pepper.

To finely slice your courgettes into beautiful thin ribbons, you need either great knife skills or, more realistically, an everyday speed peeler. Slice or peel them straight into the bowl with the dressing in it. Don't toss together, though, until the fish is cooked.

Using a knife, score the skin of each fish about 0.5cm deep on both sides. Rub the fish with olive oil and season inside and out with a little salt. Pop a rosemary sprig into the cavity of each fish.

Lay the fish on the hot bars of the barbecue, in your griddle pan or under a hot grill and let them cook for a couple of minutes on each side or until they're crisp and golden, with lovely charred marks. Then give them a further minute on their belly to make sure they're done. They're cooked when the flesh can be removed from the bone easily.

Add the rocket and half the basil leaves to your courgettes. Tear in any courgette flowers that you might have. Toss delicately, using the tips of your fingers, making sure you dress every little ribbon of courgette. Serve the courgettes next to the grilled mackerel, with a wedge of lemon, the rest of the basil leaves sprinkled over and a drizzle of extra virgin olive oil.

serves 4

zest of 1 lemon, juice of ½
extra virgin olive oil
1 fresh red chilli, deseeded and finely chopped
sea salt and freshly ground black pepper
6 small green and yellow courgettes or 12 pattypans
4 x 200g mackerel, scaled, gutted and cleaned, gills removed
olive oil
4 sprigs of fresh rosemary
2 big handfuls of rocket, washed and spun dry
a small bunch of fresh basil, leaves picked
lemon wedges, to serve

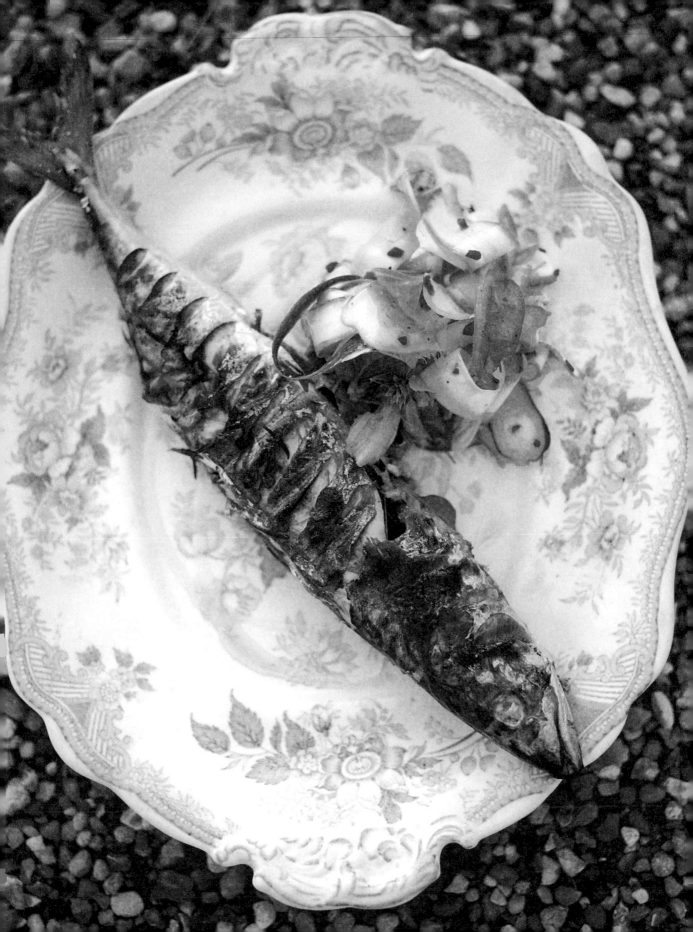

# Beautiful courgette carbonara

Carbonara is a classic pasta sauce made with cream, bacon and Parmesan and is absolutely delicious. Try to buy the best ingredients you can, as that's what really helps to make this dish amazing. I'm using a flowering variegated variety of thyme but normal thyme is fine to use. When it comes to the type of pasta, you can serve carbonara with spaghetti or linguine, but I've been told by Italian mammas (who I don't argue with!) that penne is the original, so that's what I'm using in this recipe. Before you start cooking, it's important to get yourself a very large pan, or use a high-sided roasting tray so you can give the pasta a good toss.

Put a large pan of salted water on to boil. Halve and then quarter any larger courgettes lengthways. Cut out and discard any fluffy middle bits, and slice the courgettes at an angle into pieces roughly the same size and shape as the penne. Smaller courgettes can simply be sliced finely. Your water will now be boiling, so add the penne to the pan and cook according to the packet instructions.

To make your creamy carbonara sauce, put the egg yolks into a bowl, add the cream and half the Parmesan, and mix together with a fork. Season lightly and put to one side.

Heat a very large frying pan (a 35cm one is a good start – every house should have one!), add a good splash of olive oil and fry the pancetta or bacon until dark brown and crisp. Add the courgette slices and 2 big pinches of black pepper, not just to season but to give it a bit of a kick. Sprinkle in the thyme leaves, give everything a stir, so the courgettes become coated with all the lovely bacon-flavoured oil, and fry until they start to turn lightly golden and have softened slightly.

It's very important to get this next bit right or your carbonara could end up ruined. You need to work quickly. When the pasta is cooked, drain it, reserving a little of the cooking water. Immediately, toss the pasta in the pan with the courgettes, bacon and lovely flavours, then *remove from the heat* and add a ladleful of the reserved cooking water and your creamy sauce. Stir together quickly. (No more cooking now, otherwise you'll scramble the eggs.)

Get everyone around the table, ready to eat straight away. While you're tossing the pasta and sauce, sprinkle in the rest of the Parmesan and a little more of the cooking water if needed, to give you a silky and shiny sauce. Taste quickly for seasoning. If you've managed to get any courgette flowers, tear them over the top, then serve and eat immediately, as the sauce can become thick and stodgy if left too long.

serves 4

sea salt and freshly
  ground black pepper
6 medium green and
  yellow courgettes
500g penne
4 large free-range or
  organic egg yolks
100ml double cream
2 good handfuls of freshly
  grated Parmesan cheese
olive oil
12 thick slices of pancetta
  or smoked streaky bacon,
  cut into chunky lardons
a small bunch of fresh
  thyme, leaves picked
  and chopped, flowers
  reserved (if you can get
  hold of flowering thyme)
optional: a few courgette
  flowers

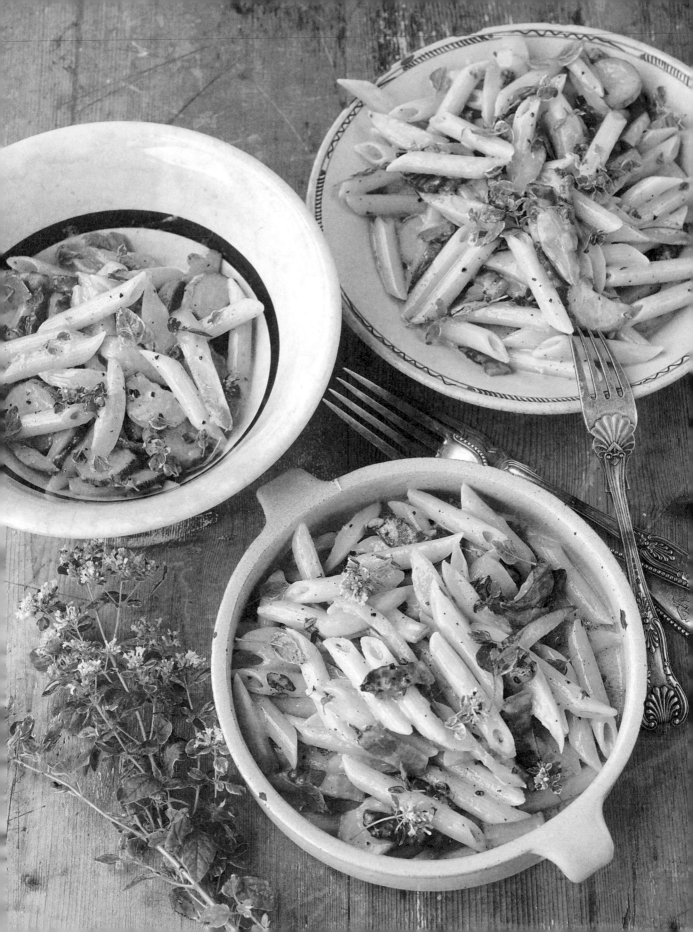

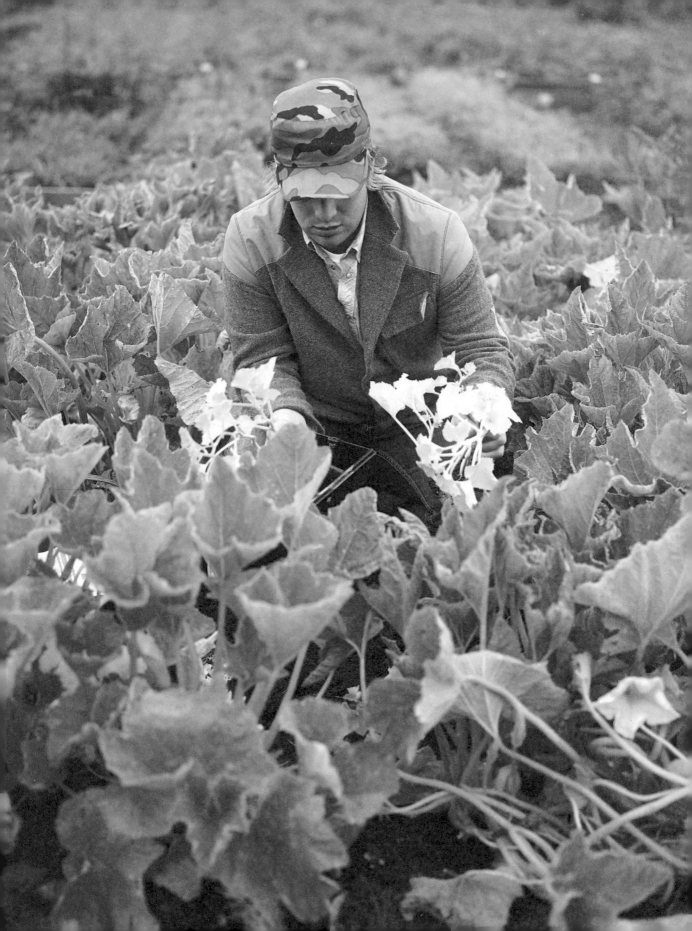

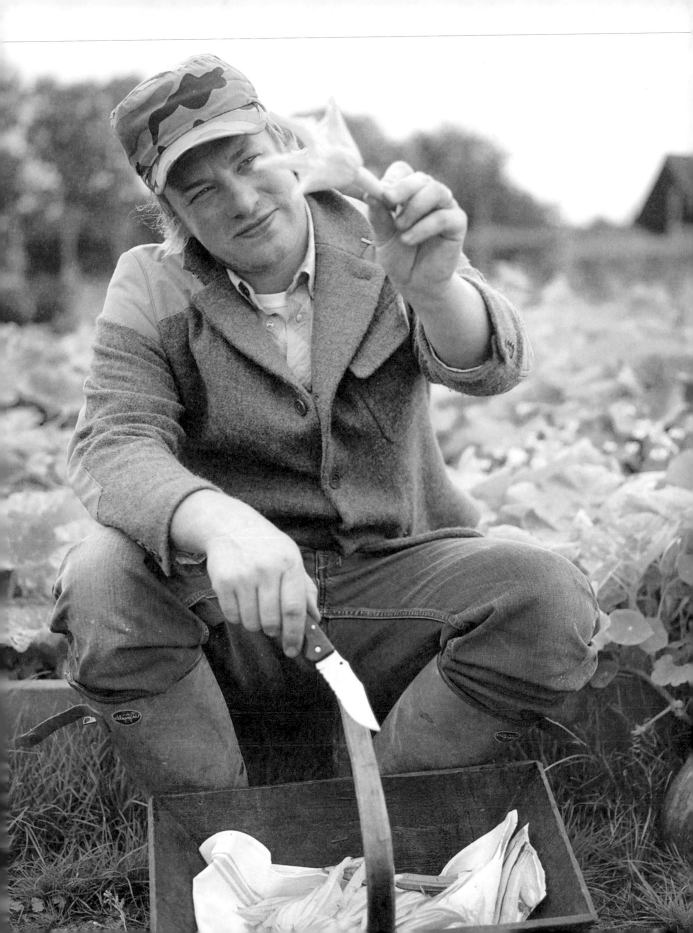

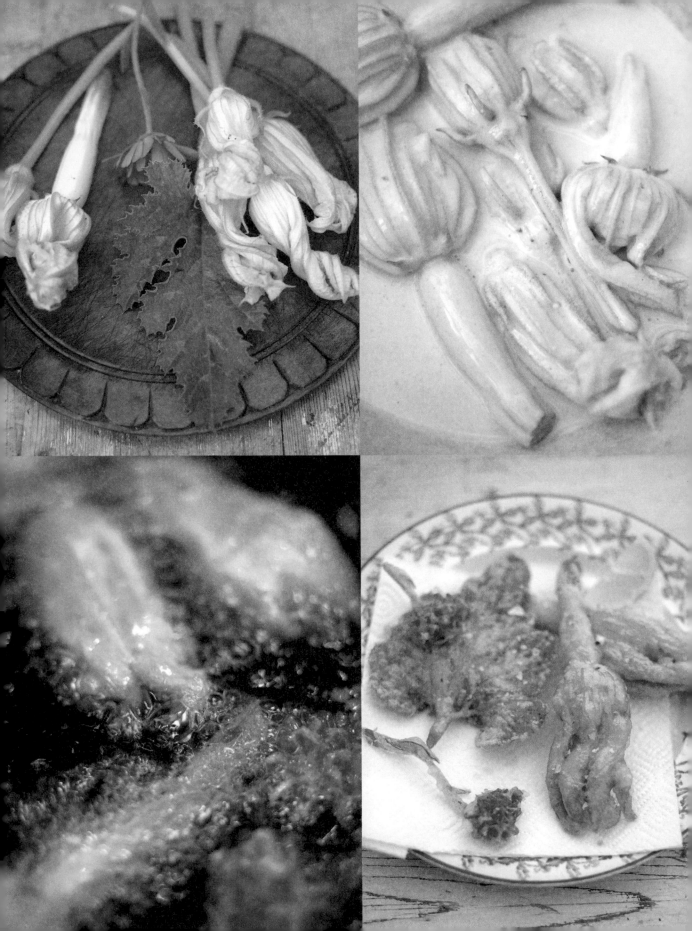

# Crispy courgette flowers stuffed with ricotta and mint

These stuffed courgette flowers look and taste amazing! Make sure they're eaten straight away, while they're still crisp and hot. If you can't get hold of any flowers you can still make the recipe using just the courgettes – it will be like an Italian tempura.

Beat the ricotta in a bowl with the nutmeg, the Parmesan, lemon zest and most of the chopped mint and chilli. Season carefully to taste.

To make a lovely light batter, put the flour into a mixing bowl with a good pinch of salt. Pour in the white wine and whisk until thick and smooth. At this point the consistency of the batter should be like double cream or, if you dip your finger in, it should stick to your finger and nicely coat it. If it's too thin, add a bit more flour; if it's too thick, add a little more wine.

Open the courgette flowers up gently, keeping them attached to the courgettes, and snip off the pointed stamen inside because these taste bitter. Give the flowers a gentle rinse if you like.

With a teaspoon, carefully fill each flower with the ricotta mixture. Or, as I prefer to do, spoon the ricotta into the corner of a sandwich bag. Snip 1cm off the corner and use this as a makeshift piping bag to gently squeeze the filling into each flower, until just full. Carefully press the flowers back together around the mixture to seal it in. Then put the flowers to one side. (Any leftover ricotta can be smeared on hot crostini as a snack!)

Now for the deep-frying bit. Get everyone out of the way if you can and make sure there are no kids around. Have tongs or a spider ready for lifting the flowers out of the oil, and a plate with a double layer of kitchen paper on it for draining. Pour the oil into a deep fat fryer or large deep saucepan so it's about 12cm deep. Heat it up to 180°C or, if using a saucepan, put in your piece of potato. As soon as the potato turns golden, floats to the surface and starts to sizzle, the oil is just about the right temperature. Remove the potato from the pan.

One by one, dip the courgettes with their ricotta-stuffed flowers into the batter, making sure they're completely covered, and gently let any excess drip off. Carefully release them, away from you, into the hot oil. Quickly batter another one or two flowers and any small courgette (or parsley) leaves if you have any – but don't crowd the pan too much otherwise they'll stick together. Fry until golden and crisp all over, then lift them out of the oil and drain on the kitchen paper. Remove to a plate or board and sprinkle with a good pinch of salt and the remaining chilli and mint. Serve with half a lemon to squeeze over. Bloody delicious. Eat them quick!

serves 4

200g good-quality crumbly ricotta cheese (not supermarket ricotta; best bought from a deli)
¼ of a nutmeg, finely grated, or a pinch of ground nutmeg
a small handful of freshly grated Parmesan cheese
grated zest of 1 lemon
a small bunch of fresh mint, leaves picked and finely chopped
1–2 fresh red chillies, halved, deseeded and very finely chopped
sea salt and freshly ground black pepper
200g self-raising flour, plus a little extra for dusting
350ml decent white wine or sparkling water
8 courgette flowers, with courgettes still attached
vegetable oil
optional: a small piece of potato, peeled
optional: a few sprigs of parsley
2 lemons, halved

# How I grow courgettes

## Soil

Courgettes like to grow in a good soil which has been mixed with some manure or organic planting compost. They also prefer a warm, sunny, open space. It's important that they don't get hit by any frost.

## Planting

Get yourself a packet of seeds from any garden centre or online seed supplier (see page 395). I find it's always best to start them off indoors in mid April to early May before planting outside. It's so easy – just fill a plastic tray (one that's divided into large 'pods') with your prepared soil, make a little hole in the soil of each pod, about 2cm deep, and drop in one or two seeds. Cover them up and place the tray somewhere warm, like a greenhouse or a sunny windowsill.

After about four weeks you can plant the courgettes outside in your prepared soil. Plant them about 80 to 100cm apart and surround each of them with a little circular ridge. This will help when it comes to watering – the water won't run away but will stay inside the ridge near the roots. You'll be absolutely amazed at how quickly they grow with some good manure – I know I was!

## Harvesting

Courgettes should be picked when they're small, as this is when they are at their most nutritious and tasty. They will begin to fruit immediately after they start flowering, which is usually four to five weeks after you plant them outside. Anything over 10cm long will be spongy, cotton-woolly and very seedy, so try to avoid growing, or buying, anything over that size. It's important that you don't cut all your courgettes at the same time. You need to leave a few female plants (with the flowers) and a few male ones too, otherwise they will stop producing.

## My growing tips

- If you leave a courgette on the vine for even slightly too long, it will ripen into something resembling a marrow, but it will be fibrous and lacking in flavour so you won't be able to do much with it.

- Courgettes love water, so make sure you keep an eye on them after it rains as they'll have a mad growing spurt!

- The more bumblebees there are round the flowers, the more courgettes you'll get. Gotta love those bees! Watch out for slugs, though – they love both courgettes and their flowers.

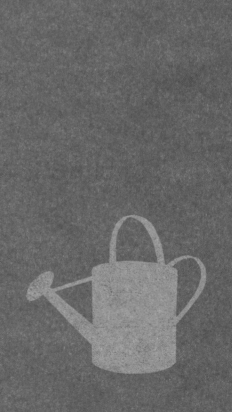

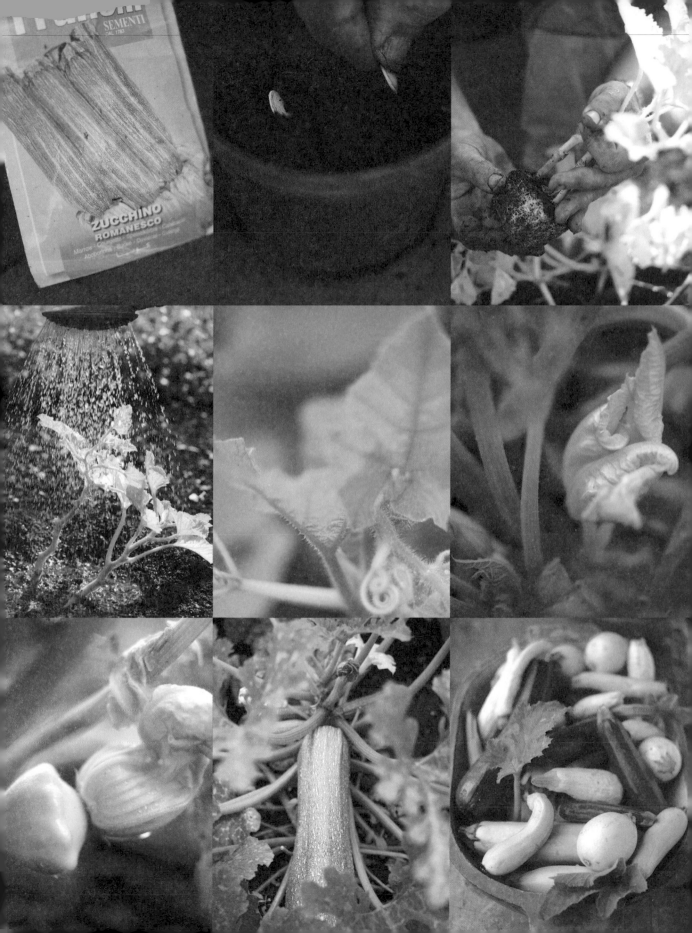

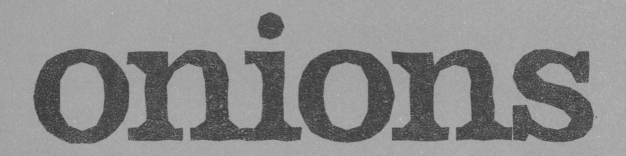

# onions

Onions are the most widely eaten vegetable in the world and can be used, usually chopped or sliced, in almost every type of food, but they are rarely eaten as the hero of a dish, or on their own. Certainly in the UK we use them in our cooking all the time, but more as a basic ingredient for things like soups, stews and risottos. In this chapter I want to celebrate the onion by giving you a really tasty onion soup, an unusual salad using pickled onions and an amazing way of baking them in balsamic vinegar, making them dark and sticky.

Not just onions but the whole allium family (garlic, shallots, leeks and chives) are fantastic vegetables in their own right, plus they're very good for you. Onions and garlic help fight off colds and can also lower cholesterol levels. Not only that but they have anti-inflammatory and antiseptic properties too. So let's all get eating them!

Like me, when you chop onions you probably end up crying. There are loads of old wives' tales about how you can stop this reaction but the only thing that works for me is to wear a scuba-diving mask that covers my eyes and nose, with a snorkel to finish the outfit off! The reason onions make us cry is because when you cut into them a chemical reaction happens and sulphur is released – it's this that gets into our eyes, making them sting. As long as you cover your eyes (with a mask or goggles!) you'll be all right. Cutting onions under running tap water, or completely under water, can also help, or you can try chilling them first or chopping them in a food processor. Some chefs even freeze their knives before cutting them! Have a go at all these and see what suits you best. Or failing that, just have a ruddy good cry!

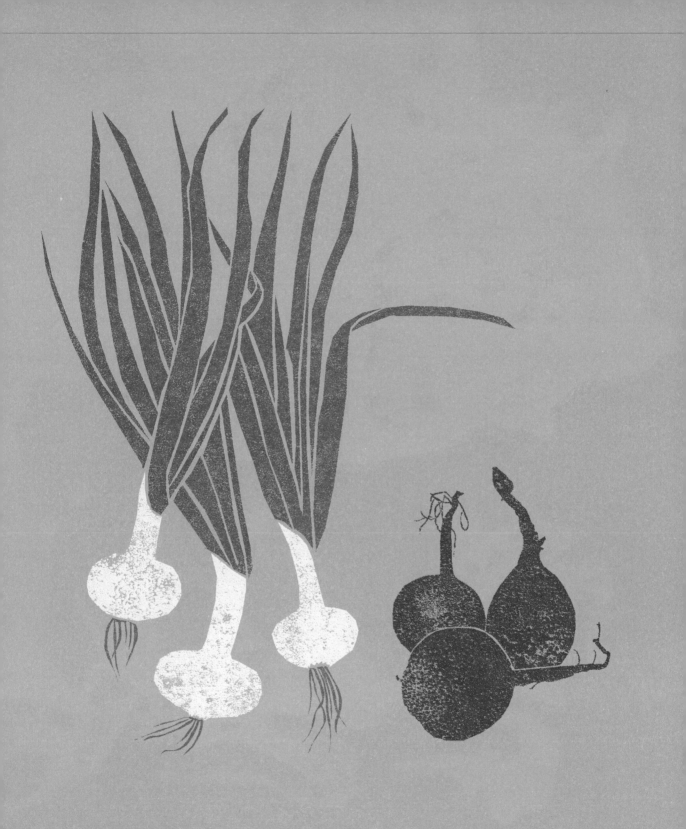

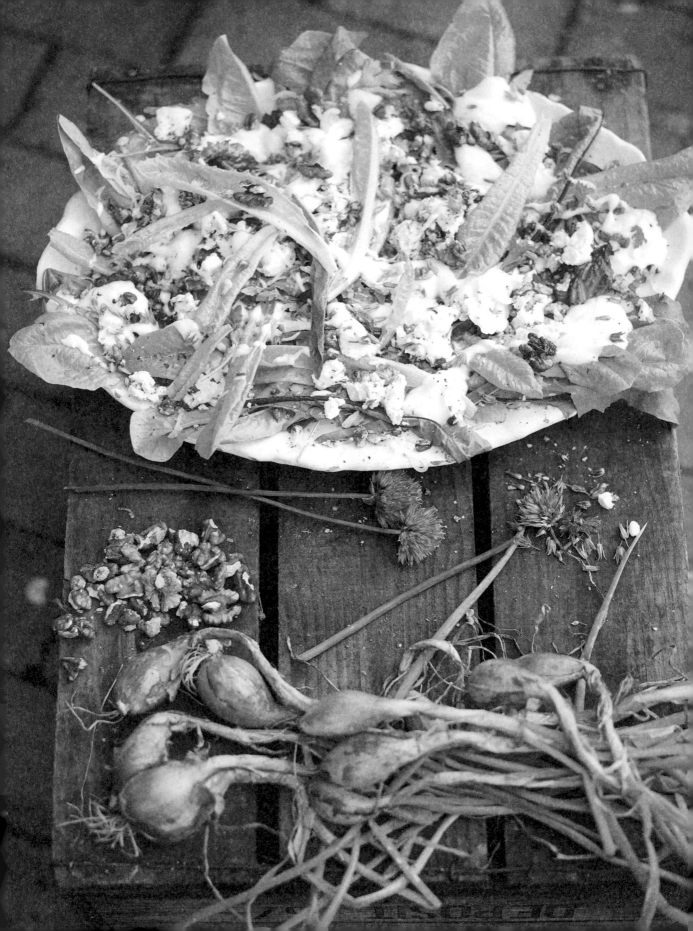

# Cheese and onion salad with creamy herb dressing

In this recipe, you basically pickle the onions very quickly. Usually pickling is a lengthy process, but if you get the onions really finely sliced, the salt and vinegar get to penetrate them straight away. The main rule when you're making a salad with any kind of onions in it is to make sure that they're sliced wafer-thin or chopped very small. There's nothing worse than salads with great big chunks of onion in them – clumsy, lazy, horrible!

Have a go at this recipe, even if you think you don't particularly like onions in salads, as they're quite mild. You can use sweet red onions instead of shallots if you like. And feel free to use any interesting mixed salad leaves.

Place the shallots in a small bowl with a generous pinch of salt and pour over just enough white wine vinegar to cover. You'll pour away the excess salt and vinegar once the onions are pickled, so don't worry if you think it's a bit much! Scrunch everything together with your hands and leave to marinate for at least 10 minutes.

To make the dressing, mix 4 tablespoons of olive oil with the crème fraîche and the red wine vinegar. Whisk everything together and season to taste.

Squeeze the shallots hard with your hands and drain. Place the salad leaves on a plate. From a height, sprinkle over the shallots and the crumbled Roquefort. Scatter over the crumbled walnuts – it's really nice if they're still a bit warm from being toasted. I like to drizzle over the dressing at the table. Finish by throwing over some torn-up chive or allium flowers, if you have them.

serves 4

8 small or 4 banana
  shallots, peeled
  and finely sliced
sea salt and freshly
  ground black pepper
white wine vinegar
1 romaine or cos lettuce,
  washed and spun dry,
  leaves separated
1 round lettuce, outer
  leaves removed,
  washed and spun dry,
  leaves separated
4 large handfuls of mixed
  salad leaves (such as
  rocket, oak leaf, and
  a little dandelion),
  washed and spun dry,
  leaves separated
100g Roquefort
  cheese, crumbled
a good handful of walnuts,
  toasted and crumbled
optional: a small handful
  of chive or allium flowers

for the creamy herb
  dressing
extra virgin olive oil
2 tablespoons crème fraîche
1 tablespoon red
  wine vinegar

onions

145

# English onion soup with sage and Cheddar

There's something so incredibly humble about onion soup. It's absolutely one of my favourites but unfortunately I only ever get to make it in the restaurant or for myself as the missus thinks she's allergic to onions. (She's not, because I whiz them up into loads of dishes without her knowing!)

If you have the opportunity, get hold of as many different types of onion for this soup as you can – you need about 1kg in total. Sweat them gently and you'll be amazed at all the flavours going on.

Put the butter, 2 glugs of olive oil, the sage and garlic into a thick-bottomed, non-stick pan. Stir everything round and add the onions, shallots and leeks. Season with salt and pepper. Place a lid on the pan, leaving it slightly ajar, and cook slowly for 50 minutes, without colouring the vegetables too much. Remove the lid for the last 20 minutes – your onions will become soft and golden. Stir occasionally so that nothing catches on the bottom. Having the patience to cook the onions slowly, slowly, gives you an incredible sweetness and an awesome flavour, so don't be tempted to speed this bit up.

When your onions and leeks are lovely and silky, add the stock. Bring to the boil, turn the heat down and simmer for 10 to 15 minutes. You can skim any fat off the surface if you like, but I prefer to leave it because it adds good flavour.

Preheat the oven or grill to maximum. Toast your bread on both sides. Correct the seasoning of the soup. When it's perfect, ladle it into individual heatproof serving bowls and place them on a baking tray. Tear toasted bread over each bowl to fit it like a lid. Feel free to push and dunk the bread into the soup a bit. Sprinkle with some grated Cheddar and drizzle over a little Worcestershire sauce.

Dress your reserved sage leaves with some olive oil and place one on top of each slice of bread. Put the baking tray into the preheated oven or under the grill to melt the cheese until bubbling and golden. Keep an eye on it and make sure it doesn't burn! When the cheese is bubbling, very carefully lift out the tray and carry it to the table. Enjoy.

serves 8

a good knob of butter
olive oil
a good handful of fresh sage leaves, 8 leaves reserved for serving
6 cloves of garlic, peeled and crushed
5 red onions, peeled and sliced
3 large white onions, peeled and sliced
3 banana shallots, peeled and sliced
300g leeks, trimmed, washed and sliced
sea salt and freshly ground black pepper
2 litres good-quality hot beef, chicken or vegetable stock
8 slices of good-quality stale bread, 2cm thick
200g freshly grated Cheddar cheese
Worcestershire sauce

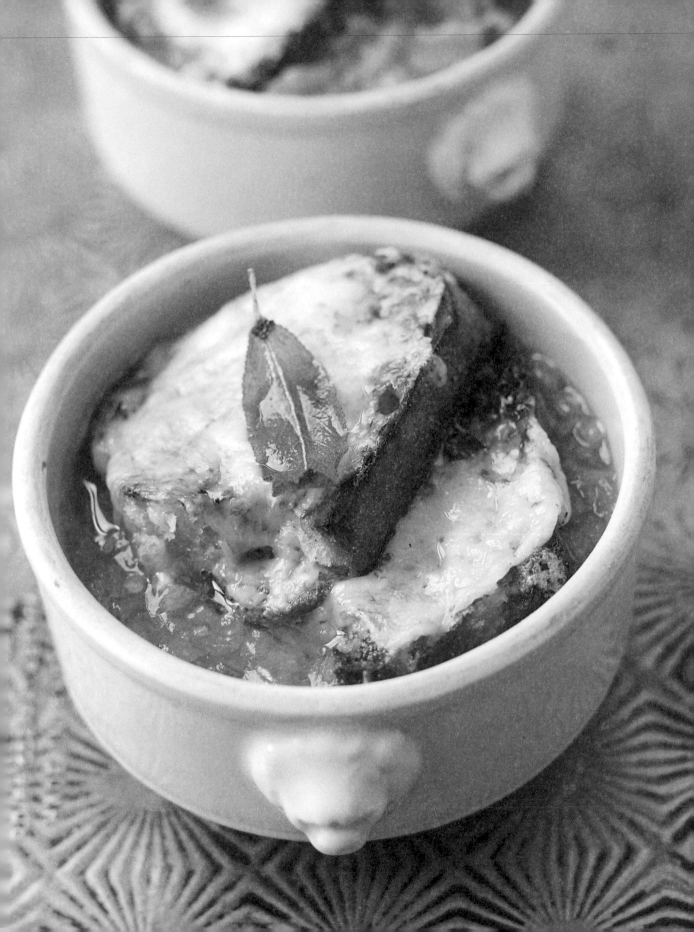

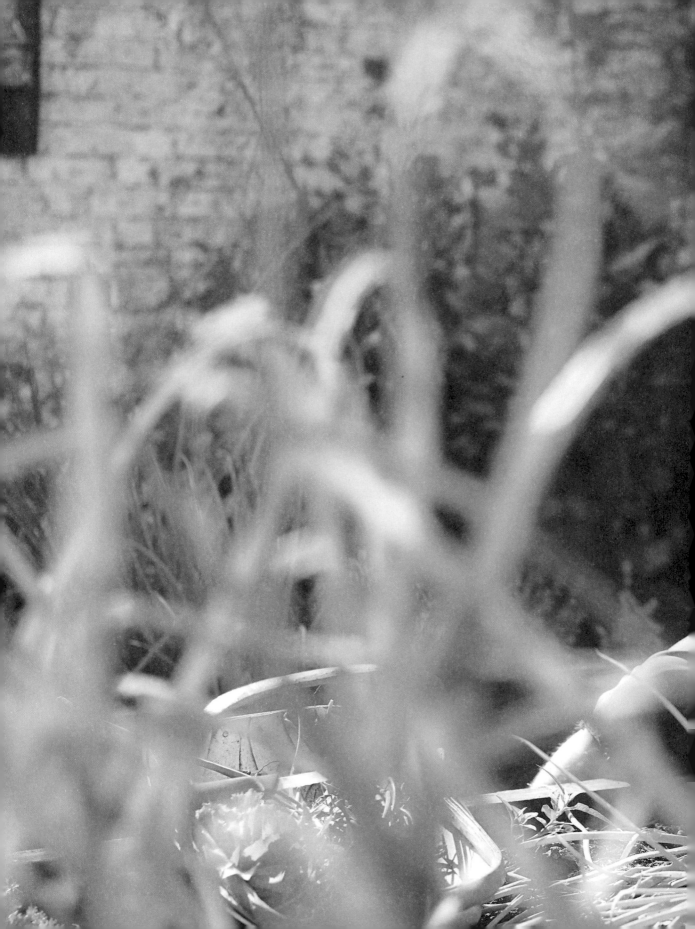

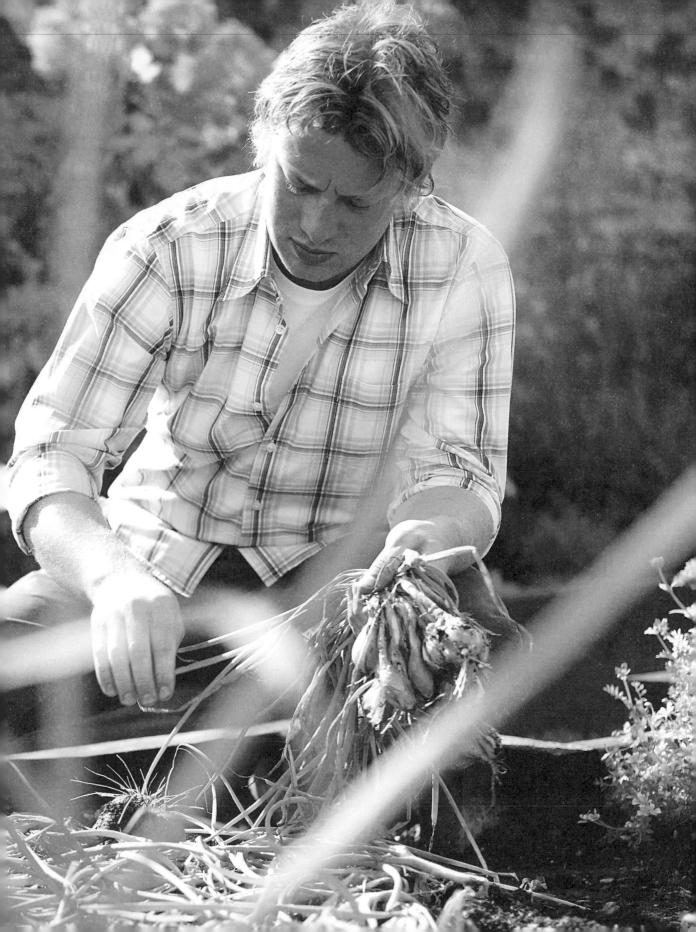

# Balsamic-baked onions and potatoes with roast pork

This dish has attitude – it uses a lot of balsamic vinegar but, trust me, it works really well! The onions and potatoes are baked in the vinegar, making them crispy, dark, sticky and sweet. I've chosen to serve them with roasted pork, but beef or lamb works just as well. I prefer red onions for their colour and sweetness.

Preheat the oven to 200°C/400°F/gas 6. Put the potatoes into a pan of boiling, salted water and cook for around 8 minutes, then drain and return to the pan. Chuff them up a bit by shaking the pan.

To prepare the meat, scatter a handful of finely chopped rosemary leaves over a large chopping board. Sprinkle over some salt and pepper and the ground fennel seeds. Roll the pork across the board, pressing down hard so all the flavourings stick to it.

Get a large roasting tray that your pork will fit snugly into, and place it on a hob over a medium high heat. Pour in a little olive oil and place the pork in, fat side down, sprinkled with any flavourings remaining on the board. After a few minutes, when the pork fat is lightly golden, turn it over and add the garlic cloves, onion, celery and bay leaves to the tray. Place on the bottom shelf of your preheated oven for an hour, basting it halfway through. (For the last 20 minutes of cooking, you may need to cover the pork with a bit of damp greaseproof paper to stop it colouring too much.)

Get another roasting tray, into which you can fit the potatoes in one layer, and heat it on the hob. When hot, pour a glug of olive oil into it and add the butter, rosemary and garlic. Add the potatoes and toss them in all the flavours. Add the onions and all the balsamic vinegar and season with salt and pepper. Cook for 5 minutes on the hob to reduce the balsamic vinegar a little. Place the tray on the top shelf and cook for around 50 minutes, until the potatoes and onions are dark, sticky and crispy – removing the tray to toss the onions and potatoes halfway through.

After an hour, the meat should be cooked. Prick it with a sharp knife – if the juices run clear, it's done; if not, pop it back in the oven for another 10 to 15 minutes, keeping the potatoes warm. Remove it from the oven and let it rest on a plate for 10 minutes. Pour away most of the fat from the tray and mash up the garlic and onion. Place the tray over the hob and add the white wine. Simmer until the liquid has reduced by half, scraping all the meaty, marmitey goodness off the bottom to make a tasty little sauce, and season if necessary. Pass through a sieve into a serving jug. Then slice the pork and serve it with your incredible baked onions and potatoes, drizzled with the pan juices. Great with some nice greens or a rocket salad.

**serves 6**

1.5kg medium-sized waxy potatoes (such as Charlotte), peeled and quartered lengthways
sea salt and freshly ground black pepper
olive oil
200g butter, cubed
a bunch of fresh rosemary, leaves picked and chopped
1 whole bulb of garlic, quartered or smashed
5 medium red onions, peeled and quartered
350ml cheap balsamic vinegar

*for the pork*
a small bunch of fresh rosemary, leaves picked and finely chopped
2 tablespoons freshly ground fennel seeds
1 x 1.5kg boneless rolled pork loin, preferably free-range or organic, skin off, fat scored in a criss-cross pattern
olive oil
6 cloves of garlic, crushed
1 medium red onion, peeled and quartered
2 sticks of celery, trimmed and chopped
4 bay leaves
2 wineglasses of white wine
extra virgin olive oil

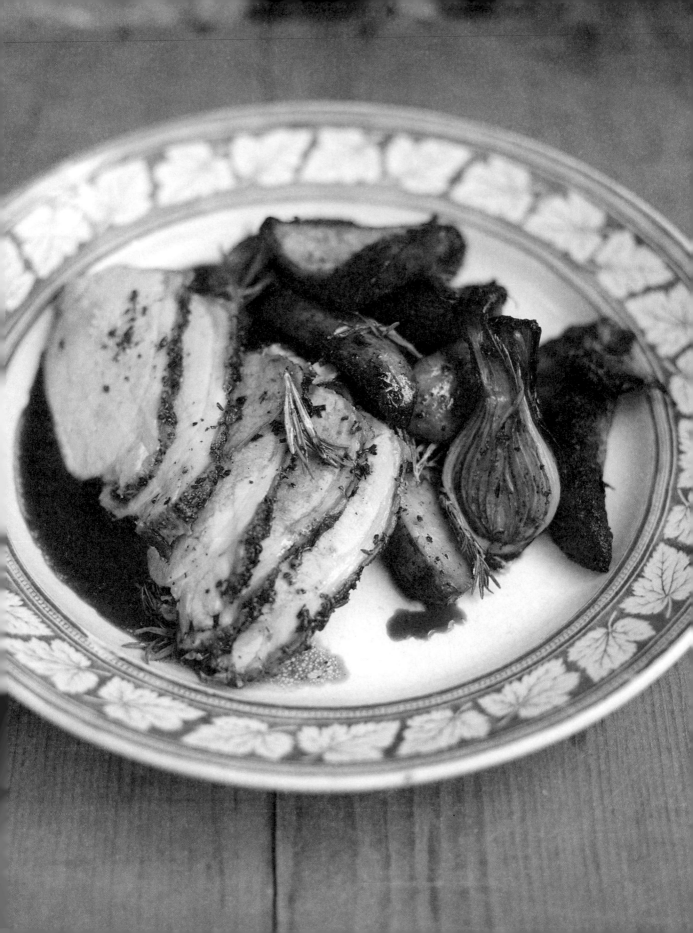

# How I grow onions

Onions are so cheap and easily available from supermarkets and farmers' markets these days, either fresh, frozen, pickled or dried, that you might be wondering why grow them yourself? Well, nutritionally there are loads of reasons for getting them fresh out of the ground, but I just think that a veg garden without onions or any of the allium family (this includes garlic and spring onions) seems a shame. Onion plants are real characters – sturdy and predictable but with so many cooking uses. Garden onions are juicy and they also have a crispness which you don't really get from onions that have been stored, so even though they're cheap to buy, I still think every beginner gardener should have a bash at growing some of these.

## Soil
You want to have free-draining and fertile soil (fed with some compost or manure the year before) and choose a spot that's open and sunny.

## Planting
Most of the onion family are sown or planted outside in March and early April, except for shallots, which can go in the ground from mid-February, and garlic, which prefers to be planted in late autumn.

Although you can plant from seed, my preferred option is to plant from 'sets' as it's so easy. These are little baby onions which you can pop straight into the ground. Simply rough up your soil, make a hole with your finger and plant your set so about half of it sticks out, pointy bit upwards. Pat the soil round it to firm it up a bit. You can plant single ones or, as I do, in threes leaving about 15 to 20cm between the clusters. How you space them will determine their size – single onions will end up being bigger as they've had more space to grow. With a little light and water you'll have full-size onions about four or five months later. Shallots and garlic are even cleverer. Plant a single shallot or garlic clove and they will slowly split and grow into as many as twelve new ones. Amazing!

## Harvesting and storing
I know my onions are ready in late July or August when their leaves have turned yellow and the plant has fallen over. I lift them out carefully with a fork, then separate the individual onions and leave them on a piece of paper or sacking to dry out naturally. If the weather is nice, I'll leave them in the sun. If it's anything like it was in August 2006, find somewhere light and airy indoors! Drying takes a couple of weeks, after which they'll get a protective, papery skin and, as long as they have no bruises or cuts, they'll keep right through the winter when bound with string and hung up.

## My growing tips
- Alliums are tough customers and don't need much looking after – they only really need watering if the weather is very dry.

- Snap off any flower stems that appear. If alliums are allowed to flower their roots don't swell up properly.

- It's very important to plant alliums in different parts of your garden every year so that there's less chance for diseases to build up in the soil and damage them.

- Birds like to pull up newly planted onions and shallots, so keep an eye out and pop them back in again if necessary.

- Alliums can be used as companion plants in the garden. As they have a strong smell they ward off unwanted bugs, so it's a good idea to plant them next to things like carrots, to repel the dreaded carrot fly, or even next to your roses to keep greenfly away. It's a great organic way of getting rid of pests.

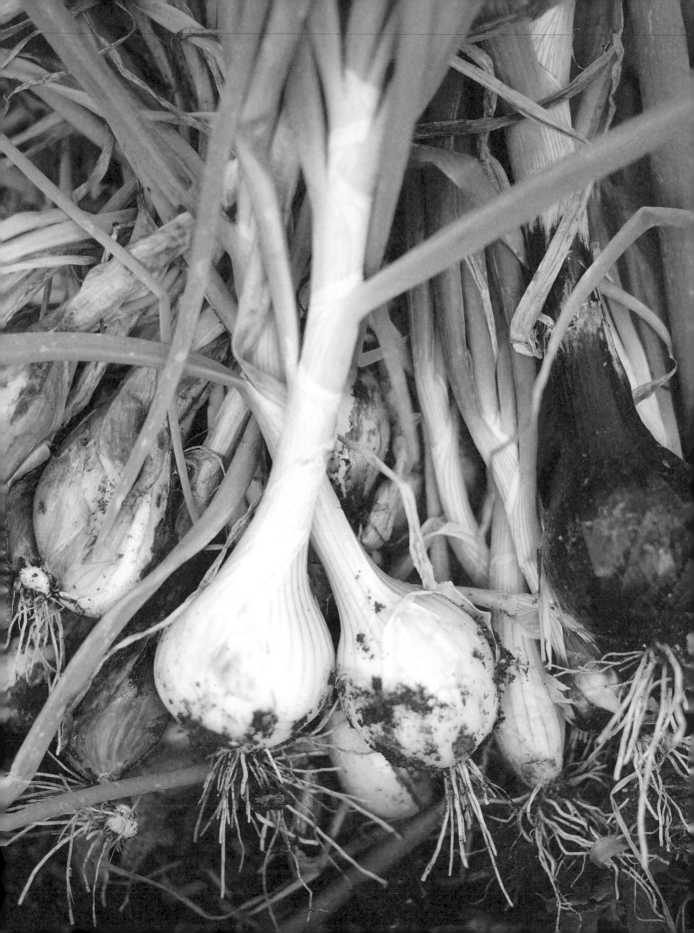

# peas and broad beans

I've loved having my own peas and broad beans in the garden this year. They're simple to grow, they look fantastic, it's exciting to watch them develop and they're a genius example of nature at work. Every time I break a pod open and see the lovely, velvety, cosy pouch with broad beans nestling safely inside, I get so excited! The other day I was picking some in the garden with Poppy and Daisy and we were checking out how amazing the natural packaging is in one of these pods. They're like a natural Jiffy bag – those envelopes with bubble wrap inside that keep things safe in the post.

Peas and broad beans belong to the legume family – of which there are about 1,000 varieties worldwide – and they're loaded with goodness. Legumes basically grow in pods and the main groups are peas, beans and lentils. People all over the world eat them as a major part of their diet because no other plant is so rich in protein or so cheaply grown. Next to cereal crops, legumes are one of the most widely grown and consumed human food sources – so peas and beans are pretty important little things! They're both lovely eaten raw, but remember, the fresher the better. Sprinkle them on top of stews, stir into pasta sauces or add to salads. They can be used across the board when slightly larger, and when very big they are better suited to being mashed and turned into fritters, for example. In Italy, plates of pecorino cheese are served with unpodded young broad beans to be enjoyed together as a nibble before dinner. Simplicity itself – genius. The trick is to eat your broad beans when they're small or medium-sized. It's never as much fun when they've grown big because you have to start peeling them and they go a bit 'floury' in texture.

When it comes to peas, don't let them get past their best. You don't want them too small, but you don't want them too big or old either, otherwise they'll be like little bullets, tough and woolly (great for making into mushy peas, though!).

You can eat the young shoots and leaves of peas and broad beans, and depending on the variety you can eat the pods as well, as you do with mangetout. The prize at the end of the growing season is when you find peas and beans that have hardened (like little beads). They can be dried and stored to see you through the winter or kept for seed. Dried peas became a staple food of European peasants during the Middle Ages because they were plentiful, easily stored, very nutritious and made a cheap meal.

Peas and broad beans are great plants to grow in your garden, not only because they give an incredible crop and have the most beautiful flowers but because they're what's called 'feeder crops' – this basically means that they provide the soil with much-needed nitrogen supplies. A bit like giving it a really good breakfast at the start of a long, hard day! If you grow your peas and beans in a different place each year, the goodness from the roots can feed the whole veg garden. It's called 'green manuring', and is definitely how nature intended us to improve our soil, not spraying or sprinkling it with loads of man-made fertilizers.

# Incredible smashed peas and broad beans on toast

England is famous for its mushy peas, so to celebrate this great little vegetable I've decided to do my own take on the whole mushy pea thing. This is the kind of food I love to cook and eat outdoors, especially when the sun's out. All my friends who have tasted this have absolutely loved it – so I know you will too.

Don't use frozen peas and broad beans for this because it sort of misses the point. Made with raw peas and sweet fresh broad beans, the whole thing will taste alive and just like summer. Think mown lawns and warm sunny evenings! Get them early enough in the season and they'll be even sweeter. Farmers' markets and good supermarkets are beginning to sell pea shoots – use them in the same way as salad leaves. They're great.

Pod the peas and broad beans, keeping them separate. Put any really small ones to one side to use in the salad.

This next bit is best done in a pestle and mortar, in batches if necessary. (You can pulse it in a food processor instead, but you won't end up with the lovely bashed and bruised flavour that makes this dish incredible.) Bash up half the mint leaves with the peas and a pinch of salt. Add the broad beans a few at a time and crush to a thick green paste.

Mash in a few tablespoons of extra virgin olive oil to make the paste really gorgeous and spreadable. Stir in the pecorino. If the mixture is a bit stiff, add a little more oil to loosen it. Add about three-quarters of the lemon juice – this will bring the whole story together. Have a taste and see what you think. You want the richness of the pecorino and the oil to balance nicely with the freshness of the peas, beans and mint. Season with more salt and some pepper if you need to.

Toast the bread on both sides, either on a barbecue or in a hot griddle pan. Rub each slice twice only (very important) with the cut side of the garlic and top with some smashed peas and half a ball of mozzarella.

Dress the pea shoots, the remaining mint leaves and the reserved small peas and beans with the rest of the lemon juice, olive oil, salt and pepper and scatter this salad over the crostini. Finish with a little more olive oil and a grating of pecorino. Very delicious!

PS Just to get you thinking, this paste tossed with tagliatelle . . . oooh! Dolloped over a piece of grilled white fish . . . double oooh!

serves 4

500g peas in their pods (about 150g shelled weight)
700g broad beans in their pods (about 250g shelled weight)
a small bunch of fresh mint, leaves picked
sea salt and freshly ground black pepper
extra virgin olive oil
50g finely grated fresh pecorino cheese, plus extra for serving
juice of 1 lemon
4 slices of sourdough bread
1 clove of garlic, unpeeled, cut in half
2 large balls of buffalo mozzarella cheese, torn in half
a handful of pea shoots

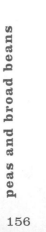

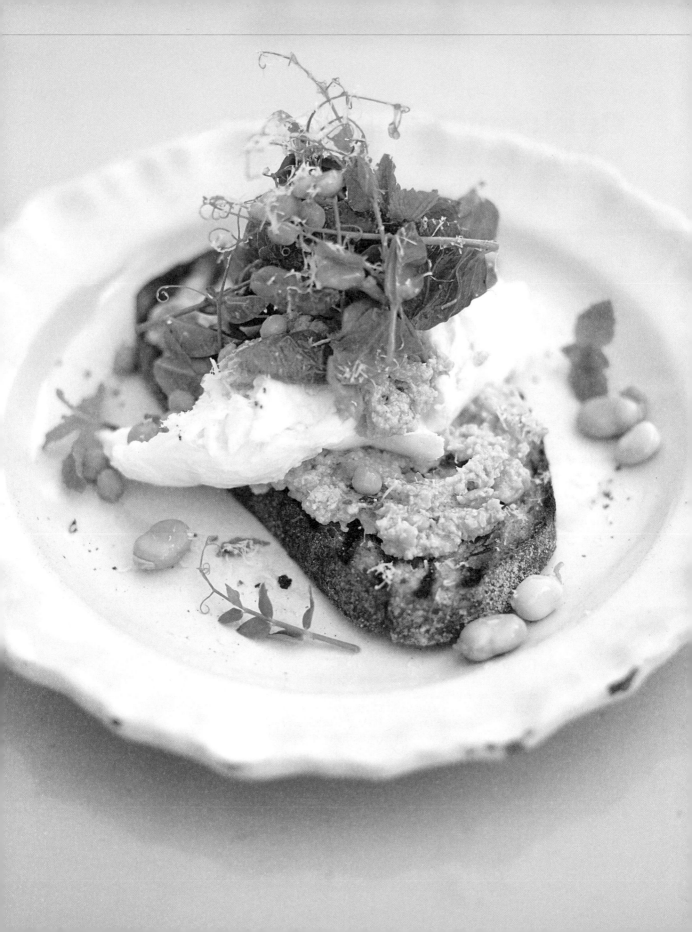

# Quick sausage meatballs with a tomato and basil sauce, spaghetti and sweet raw peas

This is a fantastic recipe that completely celebrates everything I love about peas. Even though they only make an appearance right at the end, it's a star performance. I like to serve a pile of unpodded peas in the middle of the table so that everyone gets to pod some over their own plate. It's also an incredibly fast recipe – you can be sitting down to eat within a minute of the pasta being done. The key to getting it right, though, is to buy really good-quality sausages.

Heat a large saucepan and add a few glugs of olive oil. Snip the sausages apart, then squeeze and pinch the meat out of the skins so that you get little meatball shapes – don't make them too big or they will take too long to cook. Try to get at least three balls out of each sausage. Don't worry about rolling them into perfect balls and making them look all fancy – rough and rustic is good! Put them into your pan. Keep frying and turning the meatballs until they're golden brown and cooked through.

Meanwhile, put the spaghetti into a large pan of salted boiling water and cook according to the packet instructions until al dente.

To make your tomato sauce, heat a separate pan and pour in some olive oil. Add the garlic and the chopped basil stalks and move them around the pan for a couple of minutes. Put some small basil leaves to one side for later, and sprinkle the rest into the pan. Add the tomatoes and season carefully to taste. Bring to a simmer, break up your tomatoes a bit more with a spoon and add a swig of balsamic vinegar – it's lovely for adding sweetness to the sauce.

Add the herbs to the pan of sausage meatballs, tossing everything in all the lovely flavours. Cook for around 30 seconds. When your spaghetti is cooked, drain it and divide the pasta and meatballs between four bowls. Spoon over the tomato sauce. Sprinkle over the reserved basil leaves and serve with a handful of fresh peas per person in the middle of the table, so that everyone can have a go at podding their own, and a little Parmesan for grating or shaving over the top.

**serves 4**

olive oil
8 good-quality pork
  sausages
500g spaghetti
sea salt
300g fresh peas, in
  their pods
a block of Parmesan
  cheese, to serve
a few sprigs of fresh
  marjoram, thyme or
  rosemary, leaves picked

*for the tomato sauce*
olive oil
2 cloves of garlic, peeled
  and finely sliced
a small bunch of fresh
  basil, leaves picked,
  stalks finely chopped
2 x 400g tins of good-
  quality plum tomatoes
sea salt and freshly
  ground black pepper
good-quality balsamic
  vinegar

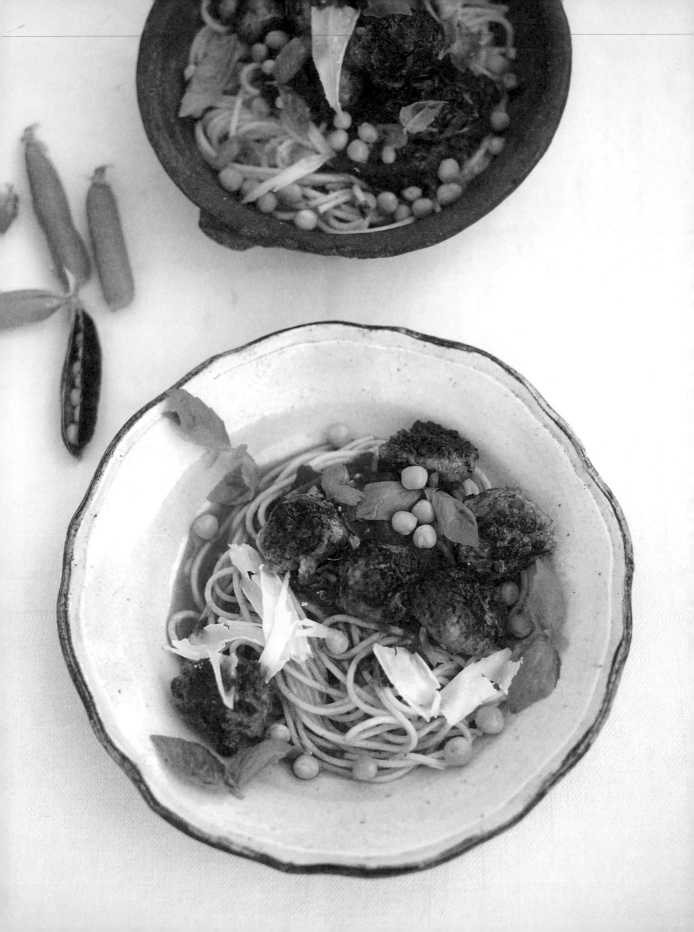

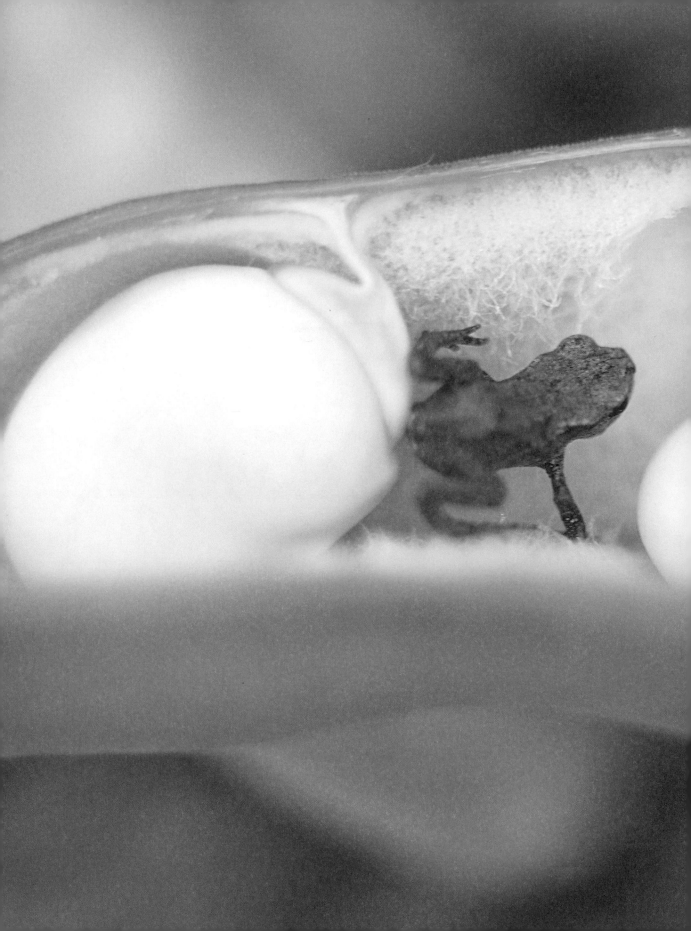

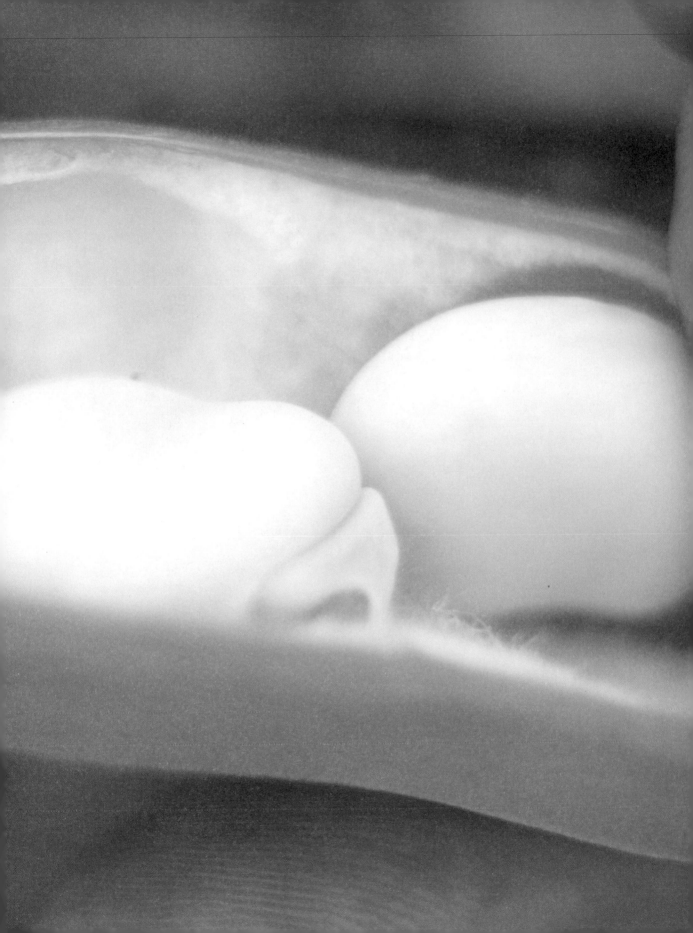

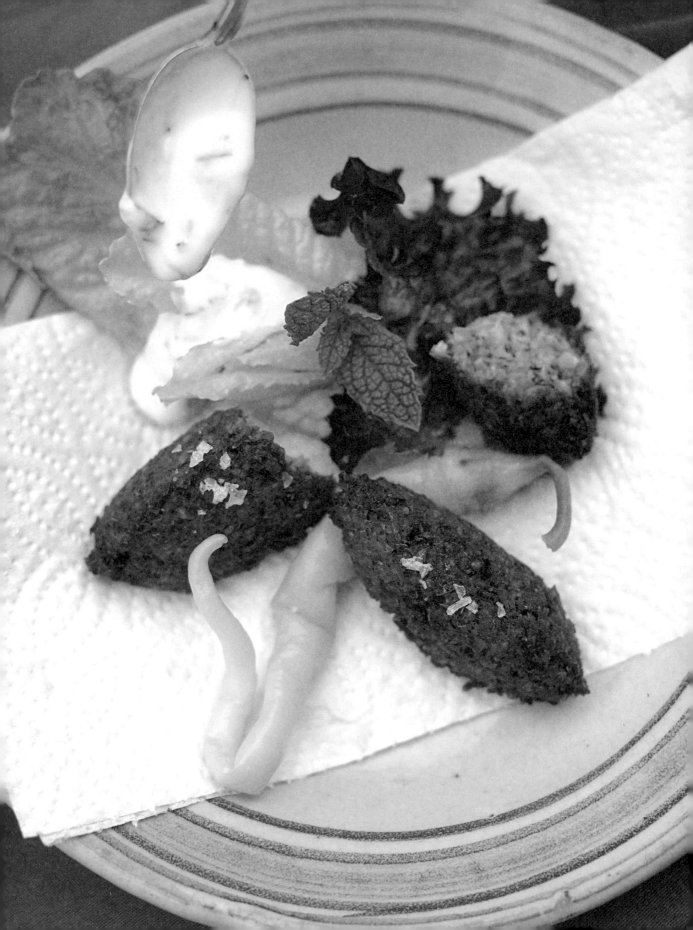

# Spicy broad bean fritters with lemon minted yoghurt

These fritters make a delicious snack. They not only taste awesome but they look amazing – dark and crunchy on the outside, bright green and soft inside! They're simple to make, and the spiciness just makes them work. This dish is best made with early season, fresh-as-a-daisy, pastel-green broad beans. Or you can use frozen broad beans – simply defrost them and pinch off the skins.

Boil any larger white-skinned broad beans for 30 seconds, then drain. When cool, pinch their skins off – they'll taste less bitter if you do this. Now whiz the coriander and half the mint in a food processor. Season with salt and pepper, then add the spices, chilli, broad beans and lemon zest and whiz until finely chopped (stopping once or twice to scrape the mixture off the sides). Sprinkle in the flour and pulse for a few seconds. Don't add any more flour or the mixture will become too dry.

Get a large saucepan and pour in the vegetable oil till it's 5 to 7cm deep. Be careful – keep kids and pets away, and make sure the handle isn't sticking out so you don't accidentally catch it and spill the hot oil. Heat the oil. To check whether it's hot enough for frying, drop in the piece of potato – as soon as it sizzles and floats to the top, you're in business. Remove the potato and discard it.

Cover a plate with a sheet of greaseproof paper. Scoop up a small amount of the broad bean mixture and either use your hands or two spoons to shape it into little rounds, then put them on to the plate. When they're all done, carefully lower one of them into the hot oil with a slotted spoon and fry until crispy brown. Remove with your slotted spoon and drain on a plate lined with kitchen paper. When you've got the hang of it, fry the rest of them – they should all fit into the pan at the same time but, if not, simply do batches.

For your lemon minted yoghurt, squeeze half the lemon juice into the yoghurt. Pick and chop the rest of your mint leaves and stir them in, adding salt and pepper to taste. Dress your salad leaves with a squeeze of lemon juice and some olive oil.

Sprinkle the fritters with salt and serve with the lemon minted yoghurt, the dressed salad leaves and some pickled chillies.

**makes 10**

1kg fresh broad beans, in their pods (about 300g podded weight) or 500g defrosted broad beans, skinned
6 sprigs of fresh coriander
a small bunch of fresh mint
sea salt and freshly ground black pepper
½ teaspoon cayenne pepper
1 level teaspoon ground cumin
½ a fresh red chilli, deseeded and finely sliced
zest and juice of 1 lemon
1 heaped teaspoon plain flour
1 litre vegetable oil
optional: a small piece of potato, peeled
4 tablespoons natural yoghurt
a few handfuls of mixed crunchy salad leaves, washed and spun dry
extra virgin olive oil
pickled chillies, to serve

# How I grow peas and broad beans

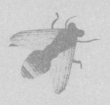

## Soil
Both peas and broad beans like a rich, well-drained soil. They perform badly if the soil is waterlogged or very acidic. Add compost or well-rotted manure to the soil the autumn before you sow. You can also reduce acidity by adding lime to the soil over the winter.

## Planting
Some varieties of peas and broad beans can be sown in autumn (mid-October to mid-November), while the soil still has some warmth in it, but I find it's best to sow them every three weeks from mid-February onwards so I get an ongoing crop. Broad beans don't like the heat of high summer, so make your last sowings by the end of April. Peas are more tolerant and can go in the ground up until mid-May. Both peas and broad beans can be started off early in pots and transplanted outside, but they are such hardy and robust seeds that it's much less effort to wait a couple of weeks for the weather to warm up a bit and sow them directly into the soil.

To sow peas, make small trenches in the soil (15cm wide, 4 to 5cm deep) with a 60cm gap between them. Sprinkle your seeds across the bottom of the trenches, cover with soil and water well.

To sow broad beans, make small trenches in the soil 3 to 5cm deep with a 25 to 30cm gap between them. Sow two seeds, with a 15cm gap between each pair, in the bottom of the trench, then cover with soil and water well.

## Harvesting
The picking season runs from late spring to summer and I think it's pretty obvious when your peas and broad beans are ready. Look at the lowest pods first, as they ripen from the bottom of the plant up. You're going to be the best judge, though – simply bust open their pods and common sense will tell you that if they're ridiculously small you should be patient. However, as the season doesn't last long, I think it's quite nice to use them while they're a manageable small size because you can make some exciting things with them.

Mangetout and sugar snap peas, which are eaten whole, should be picked every few days before they get too big. This also encourages more flowers to form, making new pods. With garden peas, keep checking and pick when they're nice and succulent.

## My growing tips
- It's important to water peas and beans during dry periods in the summer, especially when the flowers are forming and when the pods are swelling.

- Protect your beans and peas from birds with netting or by sticking a load of 60cm long twigs in the ground either side of your planting. This will stop birds sitting on the crops and eating them. Plus, the plants will appreciate something to grow up.

- Early sowings of peas will need protection from frost. You can use a cloche or garden fleece.

- Broad beans sometimes get blackfly, usually at the growing tip, where the sap is sweetest. To prevent it, pick out the top shoots once you have four or five offshoots of pods. Don't chuck the shoots away – they're bloody marvellous in salads (as are pea shoots)! Blackfly tend to be less of a problem with earlier sowings.

- If your garden is windy or exposed, consider growing dwarf varieties which can also be grown in large pots or growbags.

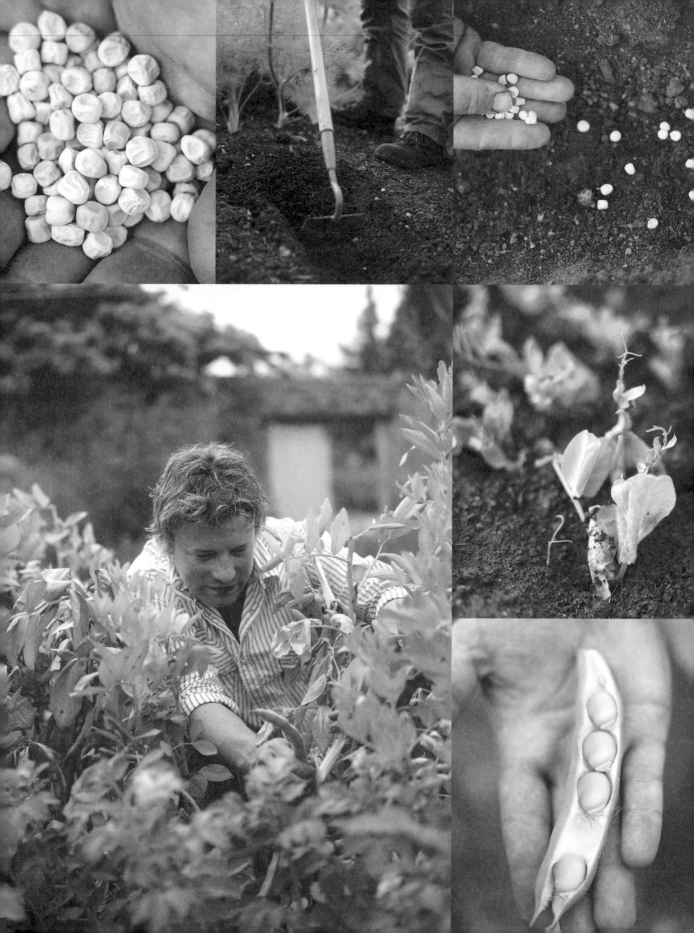

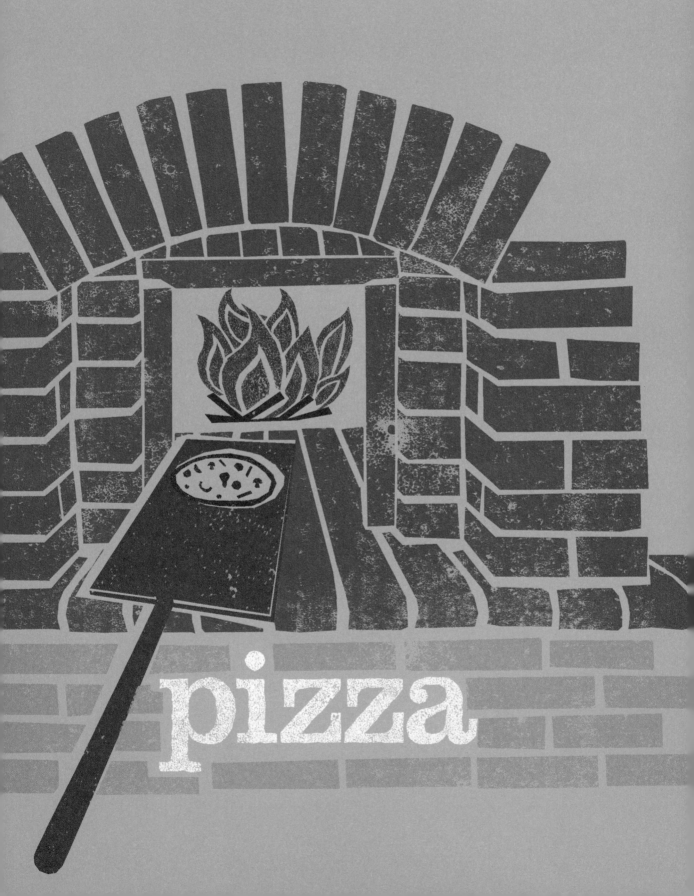

I decided to include this chapter in the book because I had a wood oven built in my garden last year, and I've been cooking some delicious pizzas in it. As these ovens reach very high cooking temperatures, they're perfect for cooking bread, and flatbreads like pizza. You may be thinking, 'But I don't own a wood oven.' It doesn't matter, though, because once I was happy that I'd mastered the perfect pizza in the wood oven, I worked on the recipes in this chapter so they give almost the same impressive results when cooked in my normal oven. Here's the trick ... buy yourself a pizza stone from a good cook shop or a thick piece of marble or granite from your local builders' merchant or stonemason. The great thing about these slabs is that you can measure up your oven and have a piece cut to size. Just preheat the pizza stone or slab in a very hot oven and your pizza bases will turn out really well when cooked on them – almost giving you wood oven results! You can also roast whole fish, big T-boned steaks and lamb chops on a pizza stone or slab. Treat yourself to one – you won't regret it!

I've also been using as many things as I can from the garden as topping ingredients for my pizzas. All summer I kept an eye on what was available to see whether I could get it on to a pizza! For example, Swiss chard can be simply cooked for a couple of minutes until it wilts and then chucked straight on – no messing! From all kinds of greens, to herbs, to thinly sliced potatoes, to one of my free-range eggs cracked over the top, I was amazed that I was able to use so many things from the garden. Not forgetting tomatoes, of course, for the all-important tomato sauce.

In the world of pizza there are two things that are incredibly important to get right. First and foremost is your dough and second is your tomato sauce. This chapter includes a basic recipe for the dough, which you can use in all the pizza recipes, as well as a recipe for a quick, easy and delicious tomato sauce (which you can use as the base for a whole load of other things too). See pages 182–3 for both recipes.

What I love most about pizzas is that they don't take much work to make and they're a great thing to put together if you've got a few mates coming round, or you just want to have some fun with the family. Particularly if you roll out the bases first and then put out bowls of all kinds of different ingredients so that everyone can make up their own topping. Pizzas are a really social, interactive, colourful type of food that most people enjoy eating, and at a pizza party everyone can inject their own personal tastes. My personal favourite is a plain Margherita pizza with a few added slices of coppa di Parma (cured shoulder of pork – you can buy this from good Italian delis), which crisp up really nicely, and, of course, loads of chilli. Not forgetting the cold beers ...

# Pizza bomba

Recently, I was in a restaurant on the island of Capri with my brother-in-law Salvatore, an Italian from Naples. When we were served these little balls of pizza on a big platter – 'bombas' he called them, which means 'little bombs' – I'd never seen him so excited in my life! It turned out that he used to eat these as a kid and they brought back lots of memories for him. As with ravioli parcels, you have to cook bombas gently to ensure that the inside flavourings are protected and that the outsides don't split open, so bear this in mind. You can cook them in batches if it helps – just don't rush things!

First, make your pizza dough. Dust your work surface with a little semolina or flour. Tear the knocked-back dough into 20 pieces about the size of a lime and dust them with a little semolina or flour. Roll each ball out into a 10cm circle about the thickness of a pound coin. You can now either keep these in the fridge, stacked and separated by olive-oil-rubbed and flour-dusted tinfoil, until you're ready to cook them, or you can make them into bombas and cook them straight away.

To make the bombas, place a dough circle on the palm of your hand, then cup your hand. Spoon in 1 tablespoon of tomato sauce, leaving the edges of the dough clear. Top with half a cherry tomato, a few of your larger basil leaves and a piece of mozzarella. Without spilling any of the filling, carefully pull the edges of the dough upwards and fold them over the top. Pinch and crimp the edges together to seal the join. Hug and cup the little ball in your hands to round it off, then dust with flour and place on a floured baking tray. Repeat until all your dough circles have been transformed into bombas, and don't worry if you're a little clumsy at first, you'll get better at making them as you go along.

Pour the oil into a sturdy, deep, appropriately sized saucepan, or a fryer if you have one, making sure it's about 10cm deep and doesn't reach all the way to the top of the pan (it'll bubble over otherwise!). Heat the oil until it reaches 180°C – you can test to see if it's hot enough by carefully putting in the piece of potato. When it sizzles and floats to the surface, the oil is ready, so remove the piece of potato and discard it.

Carefully put the little bombas into the hot oil using a slotted spoon and fry them for about 5 minutes – halfway through, turn them over. If they roll over and don't want to cook on the other side, use your slotted spoon to hold them under the oil until nice and golden all over. You can cook them in batches if your fryer isn't big enough to hold them all at once. Drain the bombas on kitchen paper and sprinkle with a pinch of salt. Heat the remaining tomato sauce and spoon on to a serving platter or individual plates. Place the bombas on top and sprinkle over the reserved basil leaves.

**makes 20**

½ x pizza dough recipe
  (see page 182)
flour, for dusting
300ml quickest tomato
  sauce (see page 183)
10 ripe cherry tomatoes,
  halved
a bunch of fresh basil,
  leaves picked, small
  leaves reserved
2 x 125g balls of buffalo
  mozzarella, each cut
  into 10 small pieces
vegetable oil
optional: a piece of
  potato, peeled

pizza

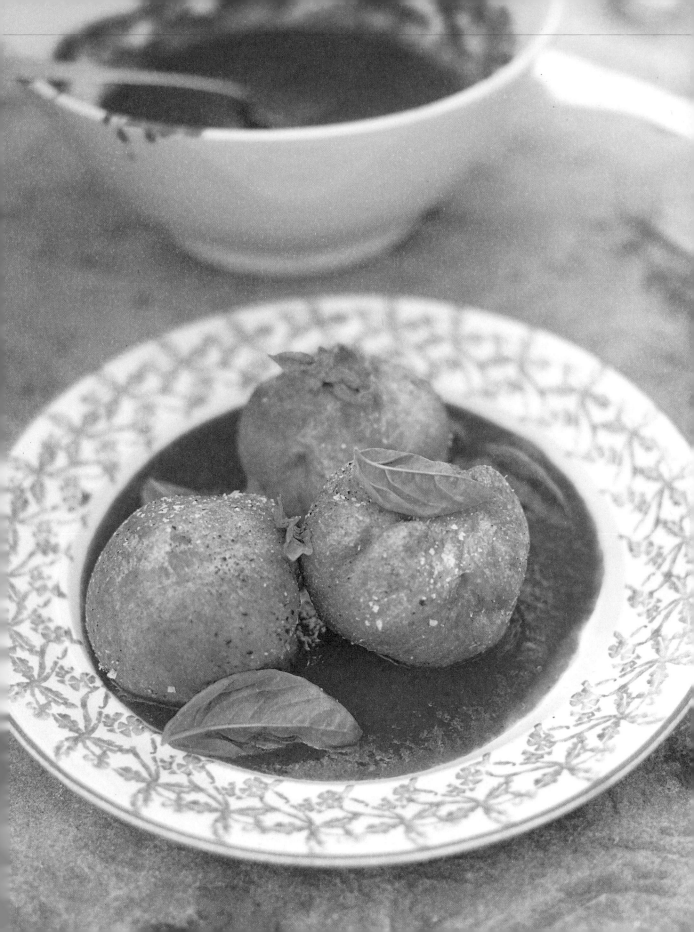

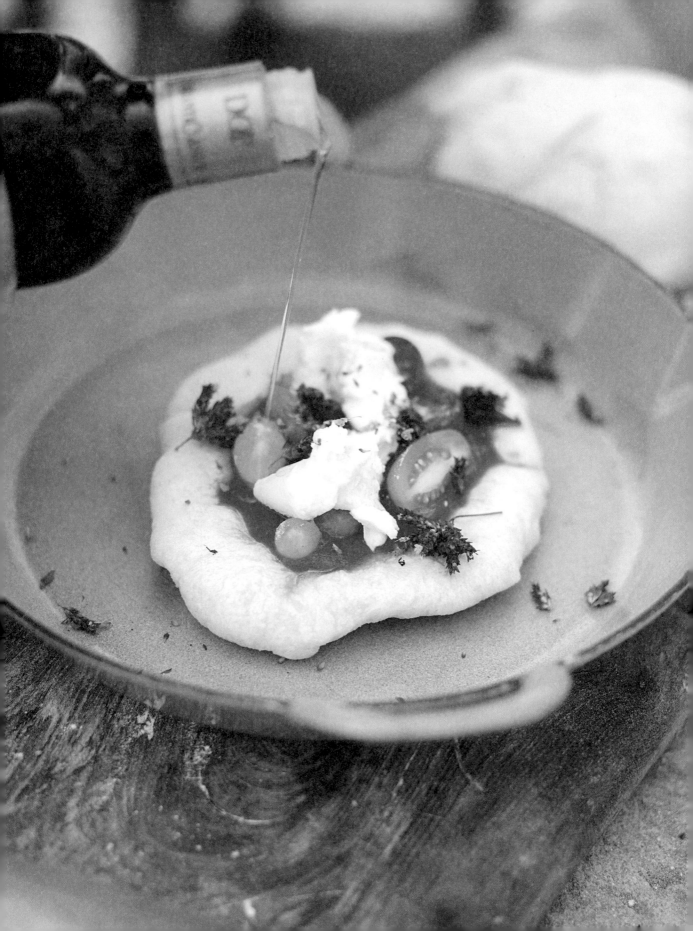

# Pizza fritta

This is the original pizza base recipe that all the others, all over the world, have come from! The base is fried in hot oil, giving it a kind of puffy, crispy, naan bread texture, which can be topped with simple combinations of ingredients. The pizza is then finished off under a hot grill. Really delicious, light and different.

First, make your pizza dough. Dust your work surface with a little semolina or flour. Tear the knocked-back dough into 10 pieces and roll each one out on a floured surface. You want to get them roughly circular, about 15cm across and about the thickness of a pound coin. You can now either keep them in the fridge, stacked and separated by olive-oil-rubbed and flour-dusted tinfoil, until you're ready to cook them, or you can cook them straight away.

Pour about 5cm of vegetable oil into a frying pan and place it on a high heat. You can test to see if it's hot enough by carefully putting in the piece of potato. When it sizzles and floats to the surface, the oil is ready so remove the potato and discard it. Carefully put in one of your pizzas, taking care to lay it in away from you so you don't splash yourself with hot oil. Fry for 30 seconds or so on each side, drain on kitchen paper, then remove from the oil with tongs and place on a baking tray. Do the same with all your pizzas. If, after a while, the oil starts to look a bit shallow, top it up and get it back to the right temperature first before frying any more.

Preheat your grill to its highest temperature. Once all the pizza bases are fried, smear each one with a spoonful of the tomato sauce, tear over some mozzarella, add a few cherry tomato halves and a sprinkling of oregano or a few leaves of basil. Season with salt and pepper, drizzle with extra virgin olive oil and grill for about 5 minutes, until the cheese is bubbling and golden.

makes 10

1 x pizza dough recipe
  (see page 182)
flour, for dusting
vegetable oil
optional: a piece of
  potato, peeled
400ml quickest tomato
  sauce (see page 183)
2 x 150g balls of
  buffalo mozzarella
20 cherry tomatoes, halved
a few pinches of dried
  oregano or 10 fresh
  basil leaves
sea salt and freshly
  ground black pepper
extra virgin olive oil

pizza

# Pizza Margherita . . . and so much more!

The real classic, simple pizza is put down to one man, Raffaele Esposito, of the Pizzeria Brandi in Naples. Over 100 years ago, when Queen Margherita was taking a tour of Italy, she saw many of the peasants eating this large flat bread and demanded to try one of these 'pizzas'. She loved it, so she ordered Raffaele to bake a selection of pizzas for her. He made a special one in the Queen's honour and topped it with tomatoes, mozzarella and fresh basil – to represent the colours of the Italian flag. It's still made all over the world. The great thing about a Margherita pizza is that when it comes out of the oven you can take it in lots of different directions by adding uncooked toppings to it. I love zingy rocket, shaved Parmesan and slices of uncured meat (as seen here) but things like picked crabmeat or prawns would be lovely too. Let your imagination go . . .

First, make your dough. Preheat the oven to full whack and place a large flat baking tray, pizza stone or granite slab in the oven to warm up. Remember that it will be very hot when you remove it later, so use triple-wrapped tea towels or a very thick oven glove. Be careful.

Tear the knocked-back dough into 6 pieces and roll each one out on a floured surface. You want to get them roughly circular, 30cm across, and about the thickness of a pound coin. You can now either keep them in the fridge, stacked and separated by olive-oil-rubbed and flour-dusted tinfoil, until you're ready to cook them, or you can put your tomato and cheese topping on and cook them straight away.

Place a pizza base on your pre-warmed flat baking tray, pizza stone or granite slab – the dough will start to bubble and cook immediately. Working quickly, spoon 3 to 4 tablespoons of tomato sauce into the middle and spread it out evenly, leaving the edge of the dough clear. Dot the pizza with mozzarella and sprinkle with some basil leaves. Season lightly with salt and pepper and drizzle with extra virgin olive oil.

Place the pizza in the preheated oven and cook for 8 to 10 minutes, or until the pizza base is golden, bubbly and crisp around the edges, and the tomato and cheese topping is melted and hot. Cook the rest of the pizzas the same way, adding the topping at the last minute just before they go into the oven (which needs to return to its preheated temperature first).

As each pizza comes out of the oven, place it on a plate or on a board and drape over three slices of prosciutto. Dress your rocket at the last minute with a squeeze of lemon juice, some olive oil and salt and pepper. Scatter the rocket over your hot pizza, grate over a little Parmesan and serve.

**makes 6 large pizzas**

1 x pizza dough recipe (see page 182)
flour, for dusting
300ml quickest tomato sauce (see page 183)
4 x 125g balls of good-quality mozzarella, torn into pieces
a bunch of fresh basil, leaves picked
sea salt and freshly ground black pepper
extra virgin olive oil
4 handfuls of rocket, washed and spun dry
1 lemon
18 slices of prosciutto
Parmesan cheese, to serve

pizza

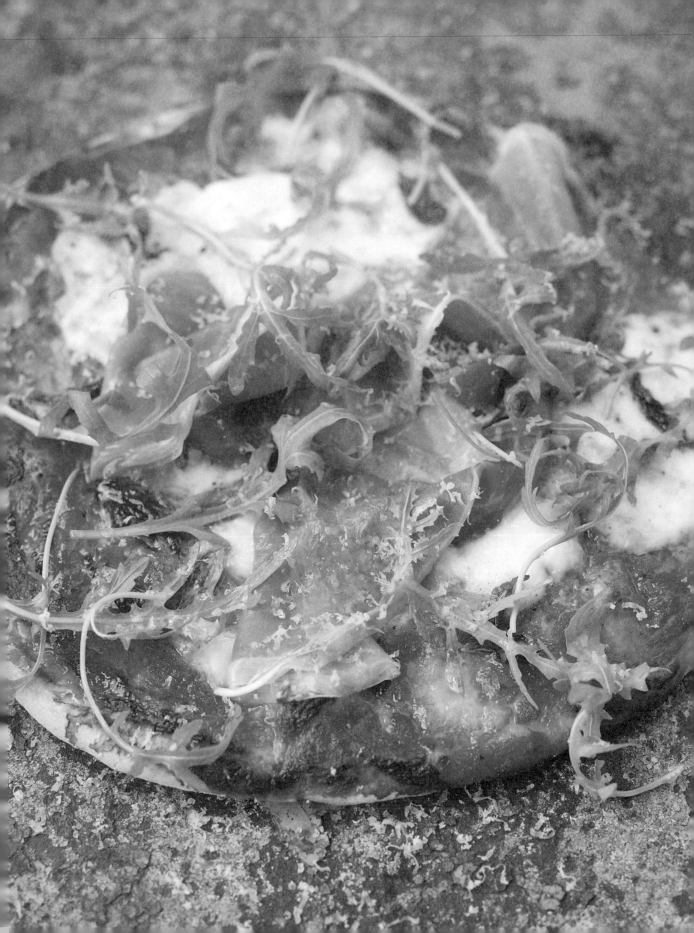

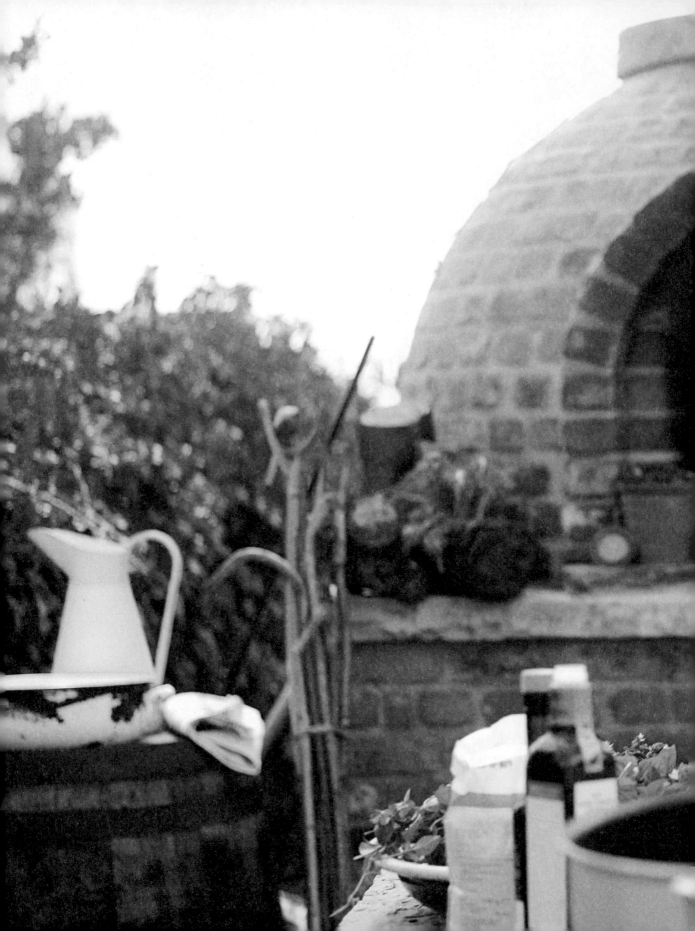

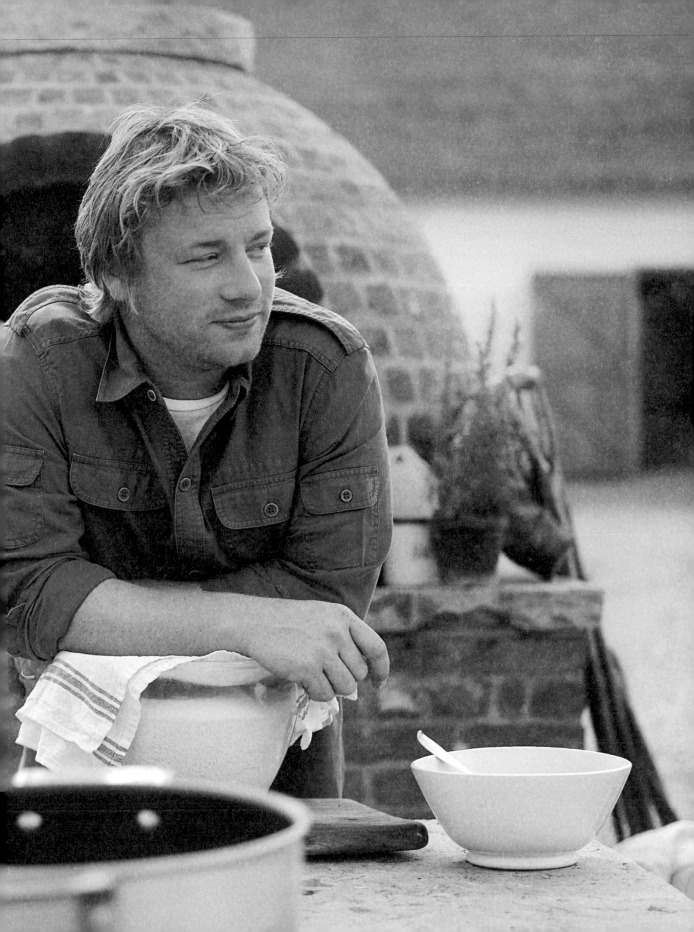

# Pizza quattro gusti

You can buy these pizzas in Rome, where they're made in massive rectangular trays and they look the business! They're great fast food and the best thing about them is that you can order whatever size you feel like eating, with as many different flavours as you like – 'quattro gusti' means four different flavours, 'otto gusti' is eight flavours. When you make this type of pizza feel free to use any flavour combinations you like. Don't worry about them merging into one another because I'll show you how to separate the quarters using strips of the dough. I think this is probably the biggest pizza I've ever made – great for a party! You'll need to get hold of a 30 x 40cm baking tray to make this.

PS For the seafood topping, if you can find agritti, which is a kind of Italian green that tastes a bit like seakale, do try it. It's also known as 'barba di frate' or monk's beard, and is available to buy from Seeds of Italy (see page 395).

Make your pizza dough. Preheat the oven to full whack, then dust your work surface with a little flour and roll out your knocked-back dough. You want to achieve a 30 x 40cm rectangle about 1.5cm thick.

Trim a 0.5cm strip off one long and one short side of the rectangle and lay these in the shape of a cross in the middle of your pizza, giving you four equal-sized rectangles within your big pizza. (See the picture on pages 178–9.) Pinch and shape the strips gently to form little crimped edges. Do the same to the four outside edges of your pizza, as this will help to keep your toppings nice and secure. Carefully place the pizza base in a large shallow-sided baking tray. (It's too large to cook on a pizza stone or granite slab, so we'll do it as they do in Rome.) Now you're ready to top it with your four flavours – you can make up your own, but the ones on the opposite page are my favourites . . .

Once you have assembled each quarter, place the pizza in the preheated oven and bake for 10 to 15 minutes until the dough is golden brown, the egg is just soft-baked and the clams are open. It's lovely to drizzle a little more extra virgin olive oil into the opened clams. What more can I say . . . tuck in!

**makes 1 enormous pizza**

½ x pizza dough recipe
  (see page 182)
flour, for dusting
100ml quickest tomato
  sauce (see page 183)
extra virgin olive oil
1 x 125g ball of mozzarella,
  torn into pieces
sea salt and freshly
  ground black pepper

*for the spicy salami topping*
**6 slices of salami • 2 pickled green chillies, finely chopped • a few sprigs of fresh flat-leaf parsley, leaves picked and torn**
Top one quarter of your pizza with 2 to 3 tablespoons of the tomato sauce and the slices of salami. Sprinkle with the chopped chilli and torn parsley leaves. Dot with half the mozzarella.

*for the seafood topping*
**2 cloves of garlic, peeled • 1 tablespoon white wine • a small handful of baby spinach or picked agritti, washed and spun dry • a few sprigs of fresh flat-leaf parsley, leaves picked and torn • 5 fresh clams, in their shells • 5 fresh or cooked prawns • a handful of fresh basil leaves • 3 cherry tomatoes, quartered • zest of ½ a lemon**
Smash up the 2 cloves of garlic with a pinch of salt in a pestle and mortar. Stir in a tablespoon of extra virgin olive oil and the white wine. Smooth this out over the second quarter of the pizza base. Top with the baby spinach or agritti and the torn parsley. Divide over the clams, prawns, basil leaves and cherry tomatoes. Finish with the lemon zest and a drizzle of extra virgin olive oil.

*for the Fiorentina topping*
**a few leaves of Swiss chard, washed, stalks removed and put to one side • juice of 1 lemon • 1 clove of garlic, peeled and chopped • 1 large free-range or organic egg**
Chop the Swiss chard stalks, drop them into boiling salted water and cook for 2 minutes. Add the leaves after a minute. Drain and squeeze dry, then put into a bowl. Drizzle with some extra virgin olive oil and the lemon juice and mix in the chopped garlic. Season and have a little taste – it's got to be just right, so add a little more oil or lemon juice if needed. Smooth 2 tablespoons of the tomato sauce over the third quarter of the pizza base. Lay the dressed chard on top, crack over the egg and dot with the rest of the mozzarella pieces.

*for the courgette topping*
**1 small yellow or green courgette, sliced lengthways with a speed peeler or into discs • 4 thin slices of pancetta • 75g taleggio cheese, roughly torn • ½ a fresh red chilli, thinly sliced • optional: a few courgette flowers**
Smooth 2 to 3 tablespoons of the tomato sauce over the last quarter of pizza. Divide over the sliced courgettes, and lay over the pancetta and the courgette flowers if you're using them. Top with the torn taleggio and sprinkle over the chilli.

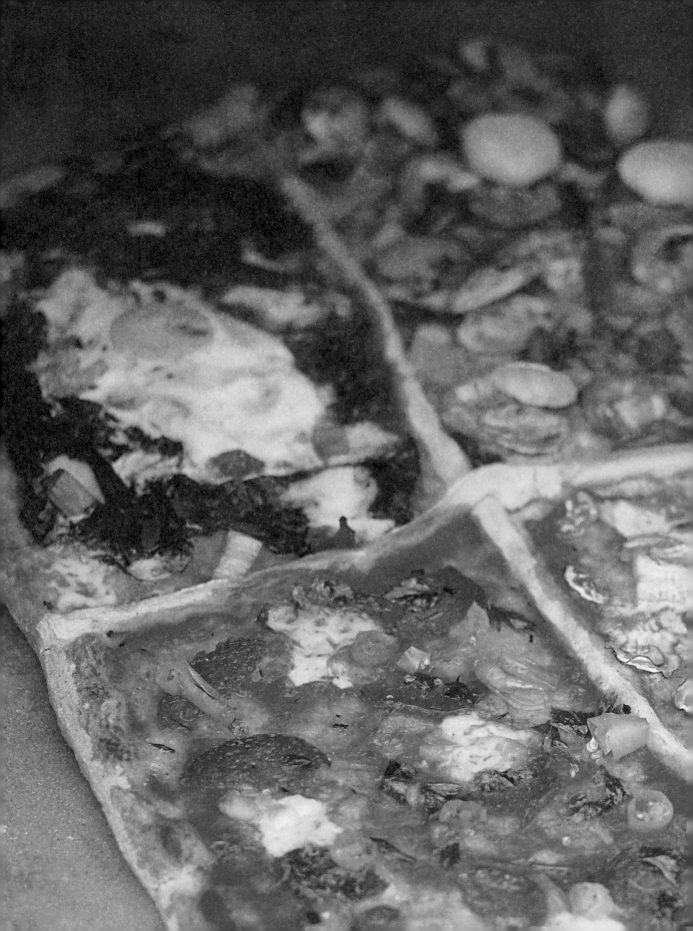

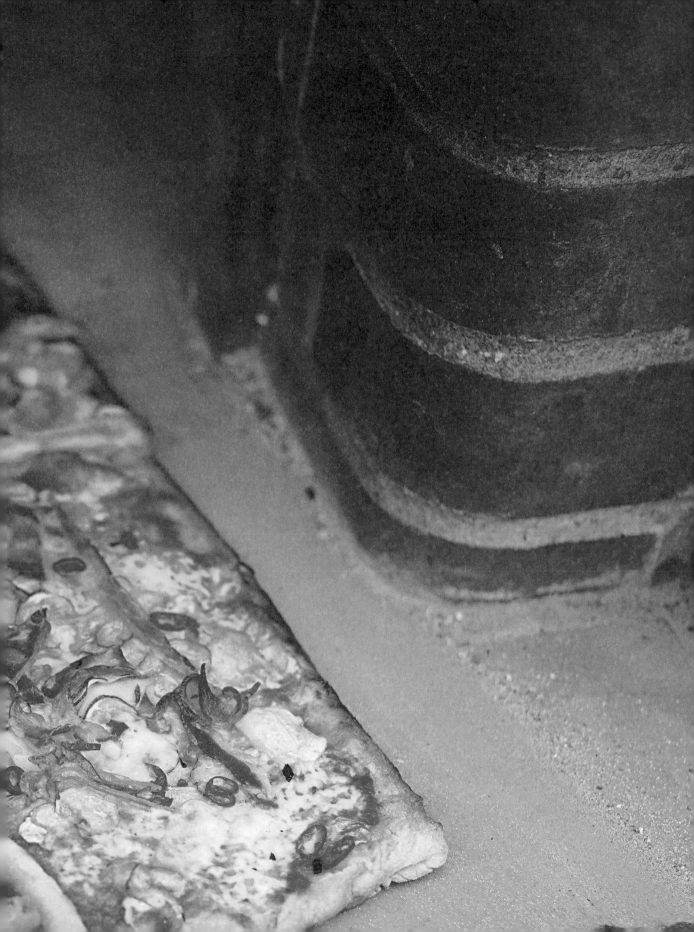

# Calzone

Calzone is a folded Italian pizza which, by the sheer nature of its shape, is far more portable than a normal pizza and looks a bit like a Cornish pasty. Although the flavourings can be the same as for pizza, Italians often fill their calzone with leftover veg from the night before, or with various things that need using up, mixed with lovely tomatoes and some melting mozzarella. Great served hot or cold.

First, make your pizza dough. Preheat the oven to full whack, then tear the knocked-back dough into four pieces and roll each one out on a floured surface. You want to get them roughly circular, about the thickness of a pound coin, and 30cm across. You can now either keep these in the fridge, stacked and separated with olive-oil-rubbed and flour-dusted tinfoil, until you're ready to cook them, or you can put your topping on and cook them straight away.

Pour a large glug of olive oil into a hot frying pan. Add the mushrooms and toss briefly in the hot oil before adding the sliced garlic and the thyme. Fry until the mushrooms are cooked and smell fantastic. Drop in the butter and toss the mushrooms in it to make them tasty and shiny. Season with a little salt and pepper.

Add the tomato sauce to the pan and stir. Cook for a few minutes, then add the spinach (in batches if you need to) and stir again. Simmer away the liquid until you're left with a thick, tasty mixture that's not too moist (otherwise it will burst through the dough when you're cooking the calzone).

Divide the mushroom and spinach mixture evenly between the four pizza bases and spread it out nicely. Top with pieces of mozzarella and season with salt and pepper. To make your calzone, carefully lift the far edge of the pizza dough and pull it over the top towards you – you basically need to fold it in half (imagine it looking like a big Cornish pasty!). Crimp the edges so none of the filling can spill out. Place the calzone side by side on a floured baking tray (use two if you need to), pizza stone or granite slab.

Cook for 10 to 15 minutes on the bottom of the preheated oven until the dough is puffed up and golden on top and the filling is hot.

**makes 4**

1 x pizza dough recipe
(see page 182)
flour, for dusting
olive oil
500g mixed mushrooms
(such as girolles,
shiitake, enoki and
chestnut), cleaned
and torn up
4 cloves of garlic, peeled
and finely sliced
4 sprigs of fresh thyme,
leaves picked
50g butter
sea salt and freshly
ground black pepper
200ml quickest tomato
sauce (see page 183)
300g spinach leaves,
washed and spun dry
2 x 125g balls of good-
quality mozzarella,
torn into pieces

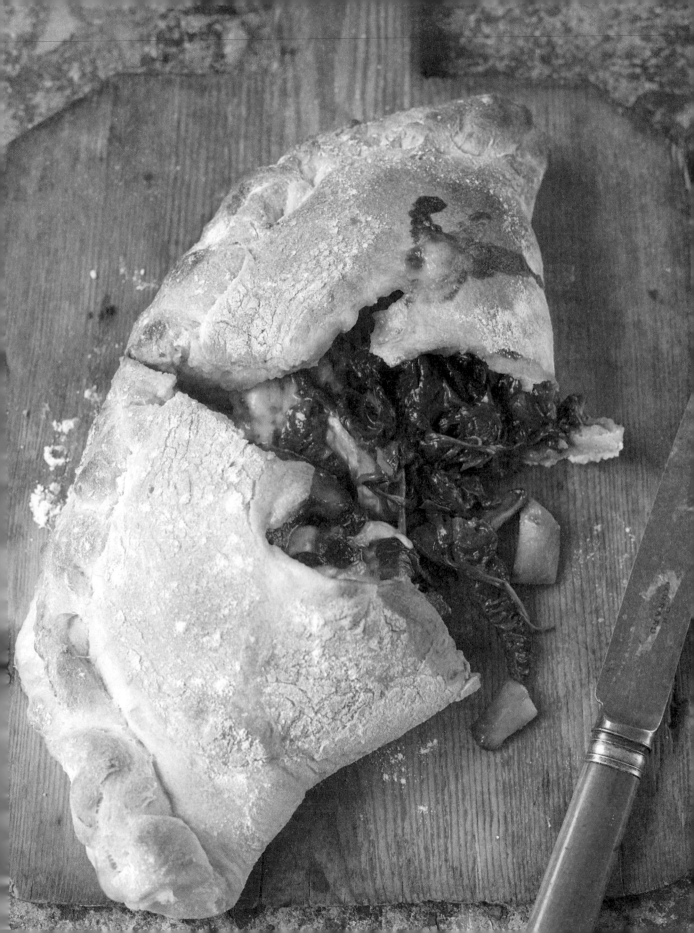

# Pizza dough

This is a fantastic, reliable, everyday pizza dough, which can also be used to make bread. It's best made with Italian Tipo '00' flour, which is finer ground than normal flour, and it will give your dough an incredible super-smooth texture. Look for it in Italian delis and good supermarkets. If using white bread flour instead, make sure it's a strong one that's high in gluten, as this will transform into a lovely, elastic dough, which is what you want. Mix in some semolina flour for a bit of colour and flavour if you like.

Sieve the flour/s and salt on to a clean work surface and make a well in the middle. In a jug, mix the yeast, sugar and olive oil into the water and leave for a few minutes, then pour into the well. Using a fork, bring the flour in gradually from the sides and swirl it into the liquid. Keep mixing, drawing larger amounts of flour in, and when it all starts to come together, work the rest of the flour in with your clean, flour-dusted hands. Knead until you have a smooth, springy dough.

Place the ball of dough in a large flour-dusted bowl and flour the top of it. Cover the bowl with a damp cloth and place in a warm room for about an hour until the dough has doubled in size.

Now remove the dough to a flour-dusted surface and knead it around a bit to push the air out with your hands – this is called knocking back the dough. You can either use it immediately, or keep it, wrapped in clingfilm, in the fridge (or freezer) until required. If using straight away, divide the dough up into as many little balls as you want to make pizzas – this amount of dough is enough to make about six to eight medium pizzas.

Timing-wise, it's a good idea to roll the pizzas out about 15 to 20 minutes before you want to cook them. Don't roll them out and leave them hanging around for a few hours, though – if you are working in advance like this it's better to leave your dough, covered with clingfilm, in the fridge. However, if you want to get them rolled out so there's one less thing to do when your guests are round, simply roll the dough out into rough circles, about 0.5cm thick, and place them on slightly larger pieces of olive-oil-rubbed and flour-dusted tinfoil. You can then stack the pizzas, cover them with clingfilm, and pop them into the fridge.

**makes 6 to 8 medium-sized thin pizza bases**

**1kg strong white bread flour or Tipo '00' flour**
*or*
**800g strong white bread flour or Tipo '00' flour, plus 200g finely ground semolina flour**
**1 level tablespoon fine sea salt**
**2 x 7g sachets of dried yeast**
**1 tablespoon golden caster sugar**
**4 tablespoons extra virgin olive oil**
**650ml lukewarm water**

# The quickest tomato sauce

I learnt this recipe from my mate and mentor Gennaro Contaldo. It's a brilliant, basic tomato sauce for using on pizza and it's also great with pasta or to serve alongside meat or fish – quick, fresh, fragrant and sweet.

Place a large non-stick frying pan on the heat and pour in 4 generous glugs of olive oil. Add the garlic, shake the pan around a bit and, once the garlic begins to colour lightly, add the basil and the tomatoes. Using the back of a wooden spoon, mush and squash the tomatoes as much as you can.

Season the sauce with salt and pepper. As soon as it comes to the boil, remove the pan from the heat. Strain the sauce through a coarse sieve into a bowl, using your wooden spoon to push any larger bits of tomato through. Discard the basil and garlic that will be left in the sieve, but make sure you scrape any of the tomatoey goodness off the back of the sieve into the bowl.

Pour the sauce back into the pan, bring to the boil, then turn the heat down and simmer for 5 minutes to concentrate the flavours. It will be ready when it's the perfect consistency for spreading on your pizza.

Store the sauce in a clean jar in the fridge – it'll keep for a week or so. Also great to freeze in batches or even in an ice cube tray, so you can defrost exactly the amount you need. But to be honest, it's so quick to make, you might as well make it on the day you need it.

**makes 500ml**

olive oil
**4 cloves of garlic, peeled
   and finely sliced**
**a bunch of fresh basil,
   leaves picked and torn**
**3 x 400g tins of good-
   quality, whole
   plum tomatoes**
**sea salt and freshly
   ground black pepper**

pizza

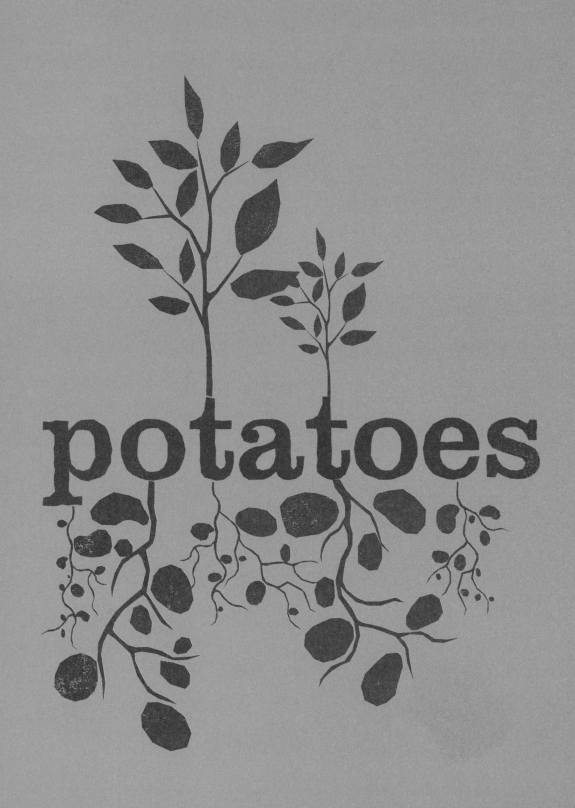

potatoes

Everyone loves potatoes! They're one vegetable you should definitely try growing, as they're so easy to look after. Home-grown potatoes also taste a million times better than any shop-bought variety you can get. And when you dig them up it's like finding treasure, because they look like little jewels! A complete joy. Their skins will be so soft that you'll be able to rub them off without having to scrub them clean before cooking. This is because they're so fresh that the skins don't have time to set firm like most potatoes you buy from the supermarket. Not only that, but they take about half the amount of time to cook when they're this fresh. Their texture is so buttery and delicious and when straight from the ground all you really need to do is boil them and serve them simply with a knob of butter. They're also great when boiled, squashed up and roasted, or added to stews or soups to give body and thickness.

Potatoes are popular all over the world. They were first cultivated around 6,000 years ago in South America. The Incas in Peru thought they made childbirth easier and used them to treat injuries. They must have been an important food source then, because historians have found more than 1,000 Inca words for them!

The first potatoes reached England in the late sixteenth century. The reason they're still so popular today is probably because you can grow a large number of them in a fairly small area and they provide good, high-energy food. Did you know that a single medium-sized spud contains nearly half our recommended daily intake of vitamin C?

However, you might be surprised to know that potatoes belong to the deadly nightshade family, along with aubergines and tomatoes. The fruits – small green growths that appear among the leaves – can cause diarrhoea, headaches and cramps and mustn't be eaten. Sprouted or green potatoes also cause these conditions, so don't eat those either as they are poisonous.

Potatoes are often referred to by their growing and cropping seasons, with each season offering a wide range of varieties, textures and flavours. Those that are dug up earliest are called 'new' or 'earlies'. Next come 'second earlies', and the ones harvested later in the year are known as 'maincrop'. Have a go at growing some, because once you've tasted a potato straight from the garden you'll be reluctant to go back to shop-bought ones. You may be lucky enough to have an allotment or a big garden, but if not, there are other ways to grow them. Potatoes are dead easy to grow in pots or growbags, so as long as you have a balcony, a little veranda, a flat roof or some space in your garden you can have your own home-grown crop.

# Potato salad with smoked salmon and horseradish crème fraîche

I've always loved smoked salmon, ever since I was a little kid. As I grew up living above my parents' pub, I could pretty much choose whatever I wanted for my packed lunch so I would ask Mum for extra smoked salmon sandwiches, saying that I was a growing boy. But instead of eating them myself I used to sell them to other kids at school. What a great son!

Anyway, this is a great little recipe – smoked salmon, potatoes and horseradish are best mates, so you can't go wrong! There are two key things to remember, though. The first is that you must try to get hold of some good-quality smoked salmon. Some supermarkets now offer a selection of wonderful smoked salmon with fantastic flavour and texture, without being too oily. The second is that it's best to dress your potatoes while they're still warm, so they suck up all the lovely juices. Let them cool down in the dressing before adding any fresh herbs or they'll wilt and lose their colour and flavour.

Pick out the larger potatoes and halve them, making them roughly the same size as the smaller ones. Put all the potatoes into a pan of boiling salted water. Boil for 15 to 20 minutes until the potatoes are just cooked, and drain in a colander.

Put the lemon zest and half the lemon juice into a bowl and add the vinegar. Normally, when making a dressing, I stick to one type of acid, but in this case using vinegar and lemon juice together gives the dish a lovely zinginess. Pour in three times as much extra virgin olive oil as vinegar, and add the capers. Season the dressing with salt and pepper. Mix everything well, then add the warm potatoes and toss around until they are all well coated.

Finely grate the horseradish into a bowl – be confident with the amount you use as you need the heat to go with the salmon and potatoes – and mix it into the crème fraîche with the remaining lemon juice and some salt and pepper. Sprinkle most of the dill or fennel over the cooled potatoes and toss again.

Lay your smoked salmon out on a big plate or platter. Don't be too neat – I want you to make it look rustic! Just pinch it up here and there so that it looks wavy and pile the dressed potatoes on top. Dollop over the horseradish crème fraîche, drizzle with some olive oil and sprinkle over the rest of the dill or fennel. Served with a glass of wine and some nice bread, this makes a delicious lunch.

serves 4

600g new potatoes, washed
sea salt and freshly
  ground black pepper
zest and juice of
  1 large lemon
a splash of red
  wine vinegar
extra virgin olive oil
2 tablespoons capers,
  soaked and drained
1 x 3cm piece of fresh
  horseradish, peeled,
  or grated horseradish
  from a jar, to taste
150ml crème fraîche
a small bunch of fresh
  dill or fennel tops,
  roughly chopped
400g sliced smoked salmon

potatoes

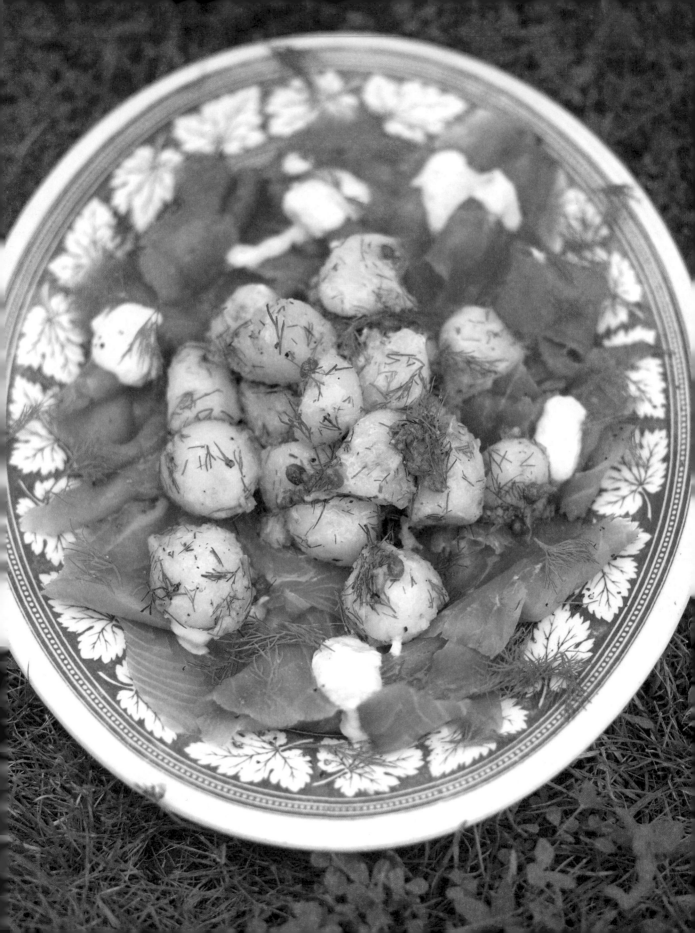

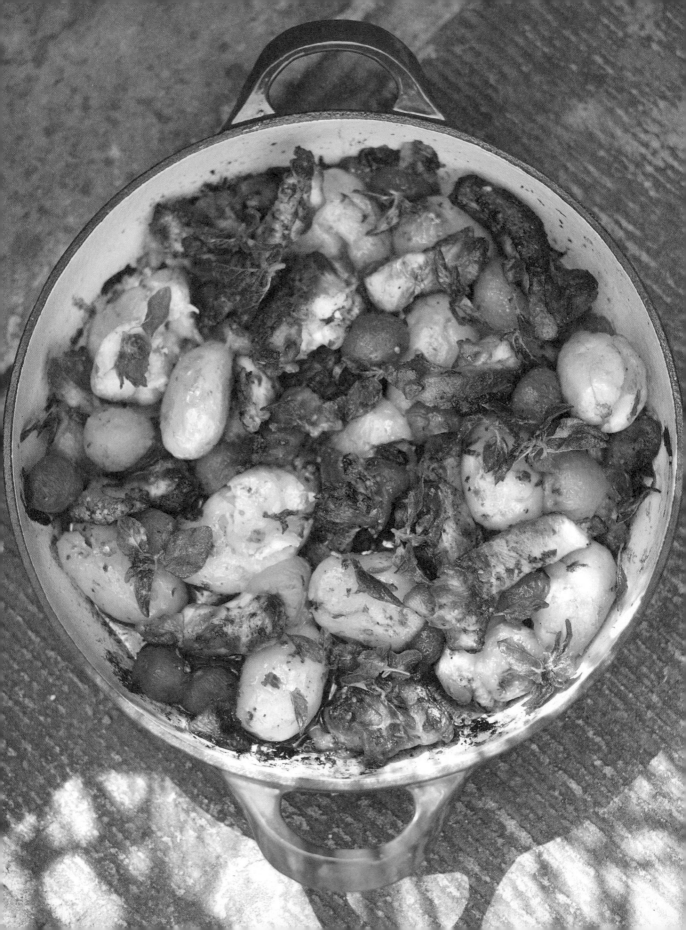

# Crispy and sticky chicken thighs with squashed new potatoes and tomatoes

This is a simple tray-baked chicken dish – the sort of food I absolutely love to eat. As everything cooks together in one tray, all the beautiful flavours get mixed up. This is what it's all about! With a green salad, it's an easy dinner.

Put the potatoes into a large saucepan of salted boiling water and boil until cooked.

While the potatoes are cooking, preheat your oven to 200°C/400°F/gas 6. Cut each chicken thigh into three strips and place in a bowl. Rub the meat all over with olive oil and sprinkle with salt and pepper, then toss. Heat a large frying pan, big enough to hold all the chicken pieces snugly in one layer, and put the chicken into the pan, skin side down. If you don't have a pan that's big enough, feel free to cook the chicken in two batches. Toss and fry over a high heat for 10 minutes or so, until almost cooked, then remove with a slotted spoon to an ovenproof pan or dish.

Prick the tomatoes with a sharp knife. Place them in a bowl, cover with boiling water and leave for a minute or so. Drain and, when cool enough to handle, pinch off their skins. You don't have to, but by doing this they will become lovely and sweet when cooked, and their intense flavour will infuse the potatoes. By now the potatoes will be cooked. Drain them in a colander, then lightly crush them by pushing down on them with your thumb.

Bash up most of the oregano leaves with a pinch of salt in a pestle and mortar, or a Flavour Shaker if you have one. Add 4 tablespoons of extra virgin olive oil, a good splash of red wine vinegar and some pepper and give everything another bash. Add to the chicken with the potatoes, the tomatoes and the rest of the oregano leaves. Toss everything together carefully. Spread out in a single layer in an appropriately sized roasting tray, and bake for 40 minutes in the preheated oven until golden.

Lovely served with a rocket salad dressed with some lemon juice and extra virgin olive oil, and a nice glass of white wine.

serves 4

800g new potatoes, scrubbed
sea salt and freshly ground black pepper
12 boned chicken thighs, skin on, preferably free-range or organic
olive oil
600g cherry tomatoes, different shapes and colours if you can find them
a bunch of fresh oregano, leaves picked
extra virgin olive oil
red wine vinegar

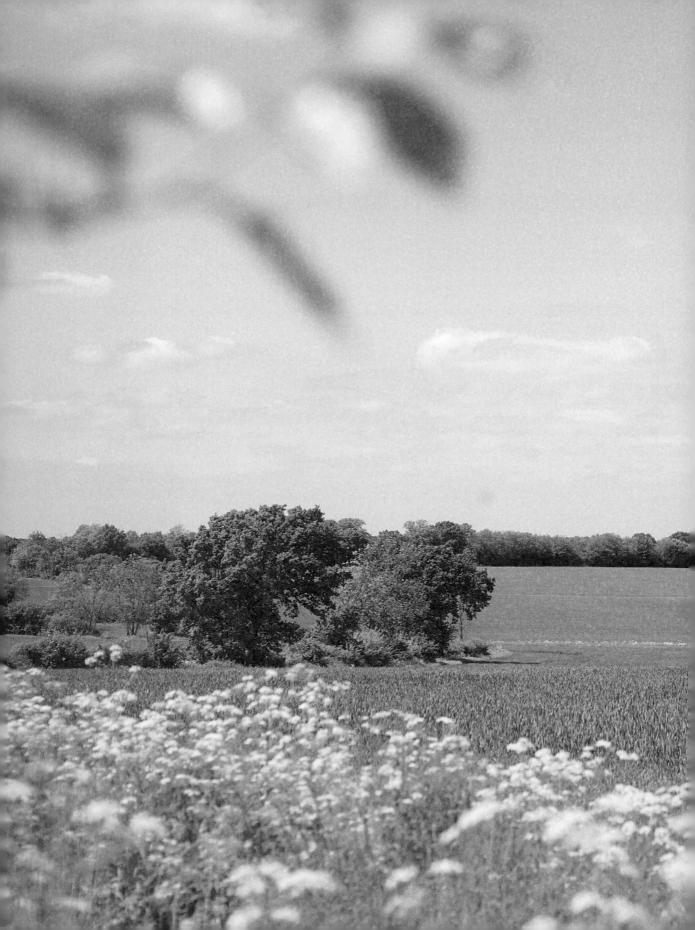

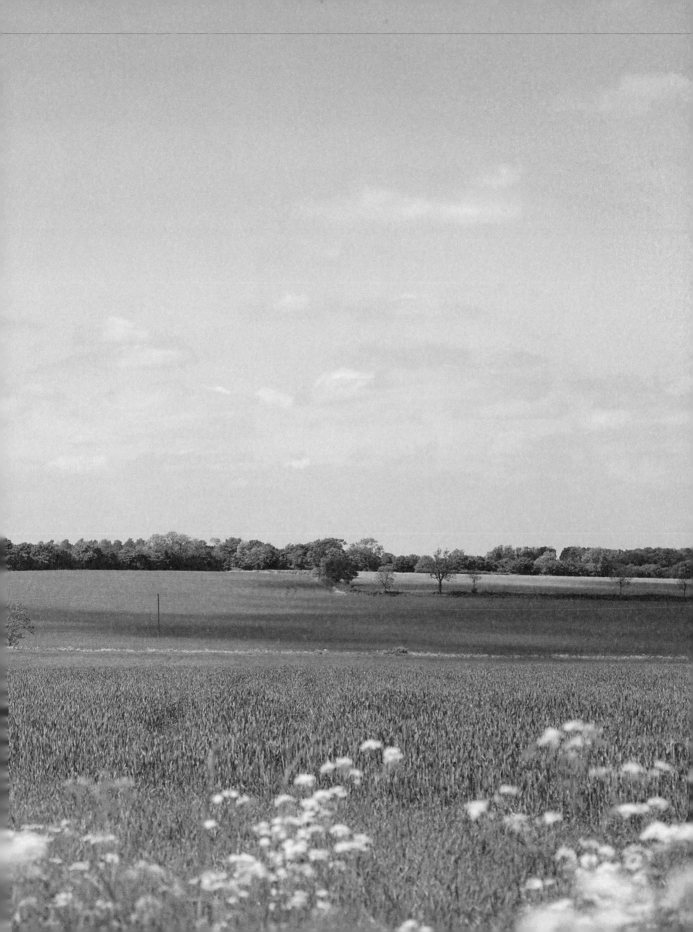

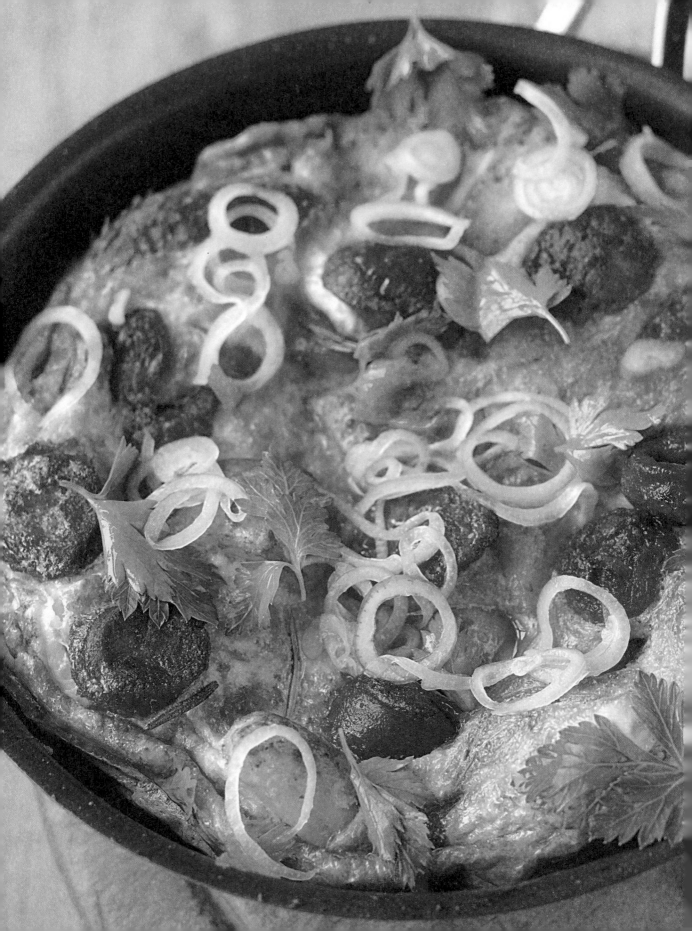

# Potato and chorizo omelette with a kinda parsley salad

This omelette is a cross between a Spanish tortilla and an Italian frittata. It's Spanish because of the chorizo and potato, but a little Italian too because I like to finish it off in the oven instead of on the hob, so it puffs up like a soufflé. It has all the things I love in it – potatoes, sausage and eggs.

Preheat your oven to full whack, or get your grill nice and hot. Put the potatoes into a saucepan of boiling salted water and simmer them until cooked, then drain in a colander and leave them to steam dry. Beat the eggs with a fork in a large mixing bowl, season well with salt and pepper, and put to one side.

Heat a 20cm non-stick, ovenproof frying pan. Add the chorizo slices and the potato chunks. The chorizo will start to sizzle, releasing all its tasty oils and spices. After a couple of minutes, when everything's lightly golden and crisp, remove from the pan with a slotted spoon and put to one side. Sprinkle the rosemary leaves into the hot fat. As soon as they hit the pan, they'll start to crisp up. Pour the beaten eggs on top immediately, adding the potatoes and chorizo and spreading everything out evenly. Place the whole pan in the preheated oven or under the grill until the omelette is golden brown on top and just cooked through in the middle.

While the omelette is cooking, put the shallots into a bowl with the lemon juice, some salt and pepper and a glug of extra virgin olive oil. Toss and pinch the shallots with your fingertips to soften them slightly, then mix in the parsley leaves. Serve a little on top of the omelette and tuck in!

serves 2

4 small waxy potatoes, scrubbed and cut into chunks
sea salt and freshly ground black pepper
6 large free-range or organic eggs
2 x 60g good-quality Spanish chorizo sausages, cut into 1cm thick slices
2 sprigs of fresh rosemary, leaves picked
2 shallots, peeled and very finely sliced
juice of 1 lemon
extra virgin olive oil
a bunch of fresh flat-leaf parsley, leaves picked

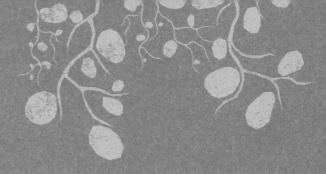

# How I grow potatoes

### Soil

If you're a beginner gardener, spuds are reasonably simple to grow. They like a rich, well-prepared soil, so you can help them along by adding loads of well-rotted manure or compost over the winter. Either dig it in or leave it on the surface for the worms and rain to work it in. They'll grow just fine in light parts of the garden as long as there's no heavy drought or mad waterlogging.

### Planting

I start off by planting organically grown seed potatoes, which you can buy from good garden centres or from my favourite seed suppliers on the internet (see page 395). These will give you a huge choice of variety and will have been carefully grown, ready for planting.

If you don't have a garden, you can grow potatoes in pots instead. You can do this from January as long as you keep them in a light, sheltered, frost-free place like a shed or greenhouse. Get yourself a pot about 30 to 45cm wide. Fill it with good rich organic potting compost and plant three to five seed potatoes about 10 to 15cm deep. You can plant them the same way in a growbag or bucket. Cover over with soil and keep moist by watering well. When the weather warms up, put the pots outside to continue growing. I like to plant some every few weeks until early summer so my crop's not all ready at the same time.

Most of the potatoes I grow are planted directly outside from March to May. Personally, I just watch nature and look out for when the grass starts to grow. It's like a natural thermometer telling you it's time to get going. New potatoes (earlies) can be planted in March and will be ready in June. Second earlies should be planted in April and come into season July to August. Maincrop can go into the ground in May and will be ready around September.

To plant, I just dig a hole about 15 to 20cm deep and plop a potato into it with the sprouting bits facing up. Potatoes do need space to grow, so I place them 45cm apart.

Make sure the soil is well watered, especially when the plants start to flower, as this is when the new seed potatoes will appreciate a bit of help to start swelling into a huge crop.

### Harvesting and storing

Earlies can be pulled up when the plant starts to flower. Maincrops are left for as long as possible, until the leaves on the surface die. All you need to do then is lift them out of the soil and let them dry in the sun for a few hours. They can be stored in thick paper bags out of the light. Stored potatoes should be checked every week and any mouldy ones thrown out.

### My growing tips

- You can grow even more potatoes by 'earthing up'. As soon as the plants are about 15cm high, pile more soil, compost or straw on them to cover them up, leaving about 6 to 7cm of stalk exposed. By blocking out the light you will trick the plant to encourage more offshoots from the main stem under the ground, meaning you'll get more clutches of potatoes growing off it. So instead of getting twenty or thirty potatoes off a plant, you can get 20 or 30 kilos!

- By carefully digging around a potato plant you can harvest some baby potatoes without pulling up the mother plant, which will continue growing and producing for longer. This works best with new potatoes and is called 'grabbling'. Pot-grown spuds can be harvested the same way if you're careful.

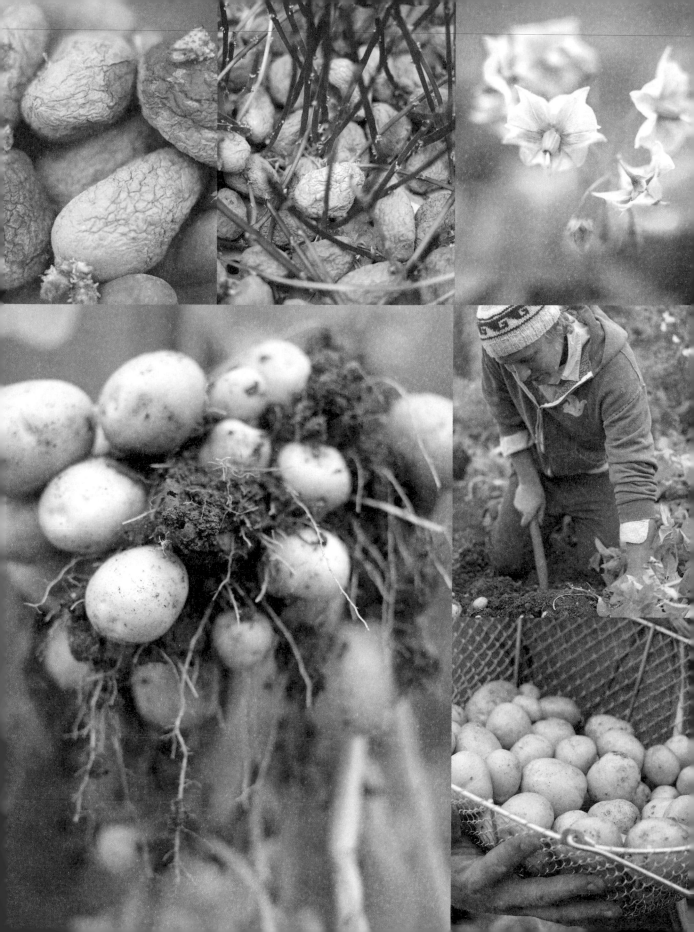

The beautiful strawberry is one of my favourite fruits in the world. Quintessentially British, strawberries represent for me a perfect summer's day and bring back so many childhood memories of squashing them up with vanilla ice cream or sticking them into a big lob of clotted cream on one of my mum's warm scones. When I was little, me and my mates loved strawberries, yet I've met loads of kids in the past few years who can't stand them. This is probably because strawberries are no longer eaten in season. Instead, they are available all year round, flown in from thousands of miles away across the world, and these imported strawberries just don't taste of anything.

Strawberries are always at their best from May to September in the UK and, in my opinion, they're particularly good in this country because of our climate. It means the fruit can develop and ripen slowly, which in turn intensifies the sweetness. Although we think of strawberries as being utterly British, I was amazed to find out that we've only been eating them since 1509. Back then, they were thought of as an aphrodisiac and given to newlyweds as a gift (yes, mother!). There's a bit of a debate about where the name comes from – could it be because strawberries were laid on straw to protect them during their journey from farm to market? Or from the word 'strewn', because the bushes climb and spread out all over the place?

The original strawberries in this country were a fraction of the size of those we get now – more like our wild strawberries. Well, size definitely does *not* count when it comes to strawberries, as the smaller ones can have three times as much flavour! It's not just the type of soil and the weather that determine whether a strawberry will have incredible flavour – largely it depends on the variety of strawberry being grown. It's a sad modern-day fact that mass-production of strawberries often means varieties without much flavour are championed over others that taste better, because they last longer on the shop shelf without going soft. If you want your strawberries to taste like heaven, the answer is to try to buy locally and in season and keep them out of the fridge.

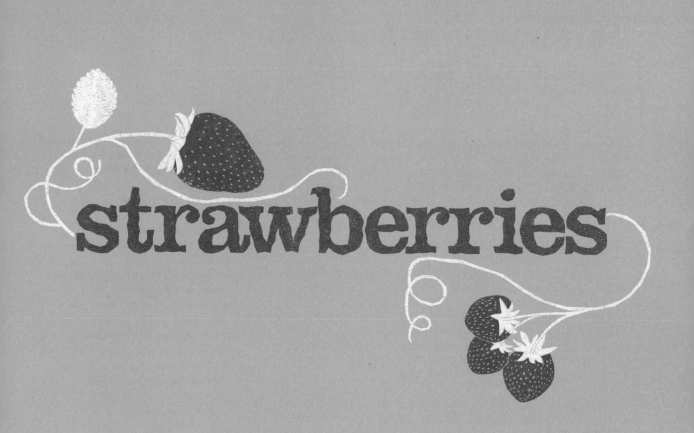

strawberries

# Strawberry salad with speck and halloumi

Most people think of strawberries as something they'd only eat for dessert, but they work so well in salads. Especially when paired with halloumi cheese, which I just love. It's a Cypriot cheese made from goat's or sheep's milk and you can get it from all good supermarkets. It's like a chewy feta but one you can cook with. When fried or grilled it goes all crispy on the outside and soft and slightly chewy on the inside. A brilliant thing to eat.

In a bowl, drizzle the sliced strawberries with a good splash of balsamic vinegar, the lemon juice and some extra virgin olive oil. Season with salt and pepper. This will draw out and flavour the lovely strawberry juices.

Preheat a large non-stick frying pan to medium hot and add a splash of olive oil. Press a basil leaf on to each slice of halloumi. Place the slices, leaf side down, in the frying pan and fry for a minute. Turn over carefully and fry for another minute until the halloumi is light golden and crisp.

Get yourself four plates and place a couple of pieces of the crispy halloumi on each. Put the mint, the rest of the basil leaves and the salad leaves into the bowl with the strawberries and toss together. Pile some of the strawberry mixture in the middle of each plate and drape the speck over the top. Finish with more salad leaves. To serve, drizzle with balsamic vinegar and extra virgin olive oil.

**serves 4**

**300g strawberries, hulled and cut into 0.5cm slices**
**good-quality balsamic vinegar**
**juice of ½ a lemon**
**extra virgin olive oil**
**sea salt and freshly ground black pepper**
**olive oil**
**a few sprigs of fresh basil, leaves picked**
**250g halloumi cheese, cut into 8 thin slices**
**a few sprigs of fresh mint, leaves picked**
**a handful of mixed salad leaves, washed and spun dry**
**8 slices of speck**

strawberries

198

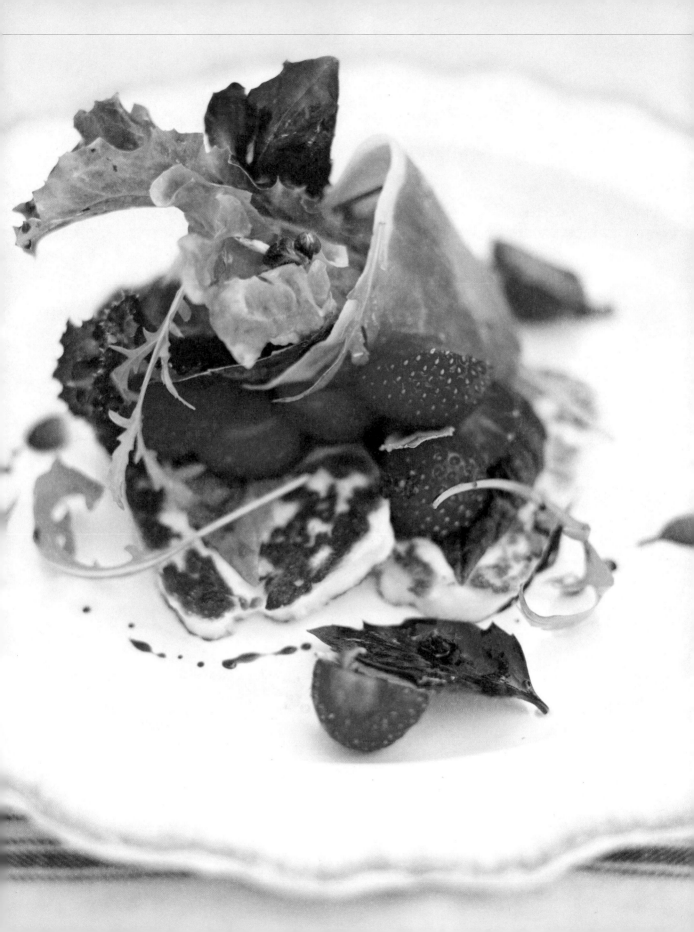

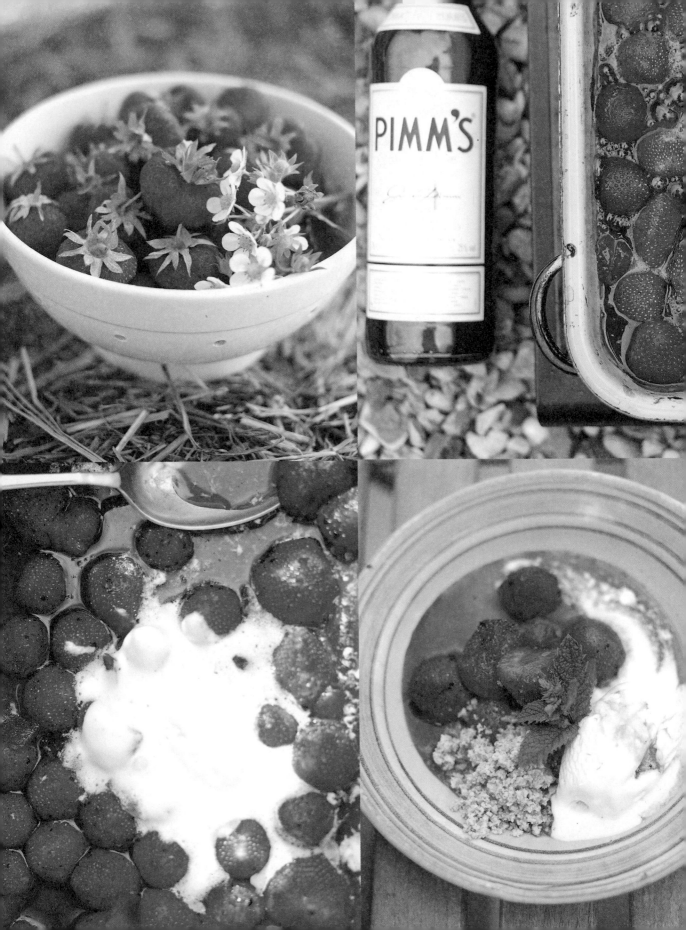

# Grilled strawberries with Pimm's and vanilla ice cream

This is an incredible dish based on the British Pimm's cocktail – a summertime classic. And it only takes about 10 minutes from start to finish! Flavourwise, vanilla and strawberries just love each other and the stem ginger gives the whole thing a brilliant extra tweak. When you eat it, there's a great mix of crunchy, cold, hot and sweet. You've got to give it a go.

Preheat your grill to high. Hull the strawberries with a knife, cutting off a bit of the flesh too so you get a flat base, and place them in a bowl. Mix in the stem ginger syrup, vanilla seeds, Pimm's and stem ginger chunks. Toss together, then place the strawberries on their flat bottoms in a snug-fitting shallow ovenproof dish, tips pointing up in the air. Pour over the juices and stem ginger pieces from the bowl. Place the vanilla pod on top and pop under the preheated grill for 3 to 5 minutes until bubbling and delicious-looking.

Wrap the shortbread in a tea towel or put it in a plastic bag and tie a knot in the end. Smash it with a rolling pin until you have quite fine crumbs. When the strawberries have softened and are hot all the way through, divide them between four bowls. Scrape up all the sticky bits on the bottom of the dish and carefully stir.

Pour the delicious juices over the strawberries and top with a dollop of soft vanilla ice cream. Sprinkle with the smashed shortbread and place a few mint leaves on top.

**serves 4**

500g strawberries, washed
a couple of pieces of stem ginger in syrup, chopped, plus 3 tablespoons of the ginger syrup from the jar
1 vanilla pod, split lengthways and seeds scraped out
a couple of splashes of Pimm's
8 butter shortbread biscuits
vanilla ice cream, to serve
a few sprigs of fresh mint

strawberries

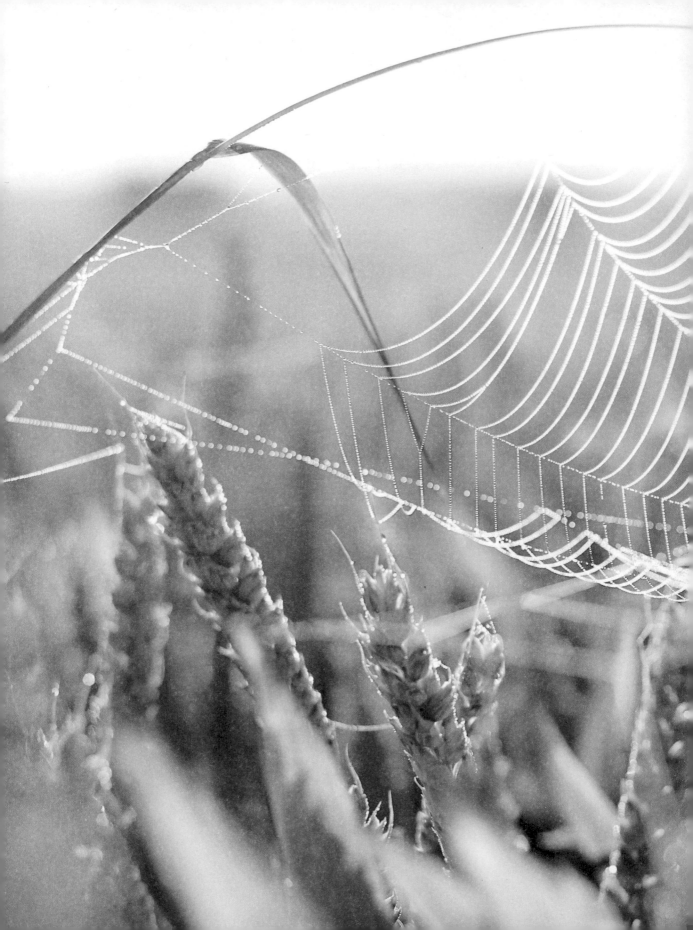

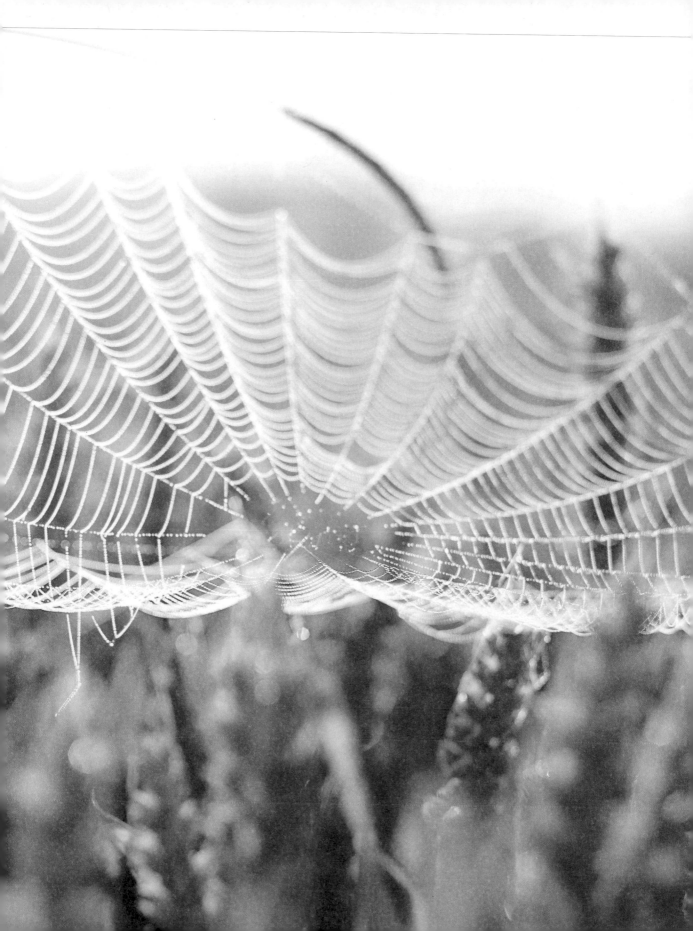

# Creamy rice pudding with the quickest strawberry jam

Rice pudding is loved by everyone, and it's one of my favourite desserts. Proper feel-good food, it's gorgeous served on its own or with whatever fruit you've got knocking around. For me, though, the best way of eating it, especially in the summer, is really cold with hot strawberry jam. As an alternative, you can grill or roast peaches and plums to serve with it. Beautiful!

I used to make jam with my mum when I was a kid. For a lovely fresh strawberry taste, I now use less sugar and I don't cook it for quite as long as my mum used to. Any leftover jam will keep in the fridge for a couple of weeks if you store it in a jar rinsed with boiling water, but you'll probably find it gets eaten way before that! It's great served as a sauce alongside a tart, drizzled over ice cream, or simply spread on a piece of toast or fresh bread.

Place the strawberries in a wide, stainless steel pan and sprinkle the sugar over the top. Scrunch the strawberries up with your hands, really pushing them between your fingers to pulp them up – the mixture will start to look like jam at this point. You want all the sugar to dissolve in the strawberry juice before you put the pan on the heat and bring it to the boil. Simmer for 20 to 30 minutes on a medium heat, and every 5 minutes or so come back to your jam to skim off the foam. Don't worry if it's still a bit liquid – it needs to be so you can swirl it into your rice pudding. Remove the pan from the heat and put to one side. There you have it – beautiful, quintessential strawberry jam!

Meanwhile, place the milk, rice and vanilla sugar in a deep saucepan. Bring to a medium simmer and put on the lid. Cook for half an hour, stirring occasionally, until the rice pudding is thick, creamy, oozy and moist. If it ends up being a bit too thick, you can thin it down by adding a little more milk.

To serve, divide the rice pudding between your bowls. Spoon over a big dollop of your beautiful strawberry jam, then slowly swirl it in so it marbles and ripples through the rice pudding. Sprinkle over the meringue pieces and scatter with a few wild strawberries, if you like.

**serves 6 to 8**

**50g ready-made meringues, crumbled**
**optional: a few wild strawberries, to serve**

*for the jam*
**1kg strawberries, hulled, washed and drained**
**150g caster sugar**

*for the rice pudding*
**1.2 litres organic whole milk**
**200g pudding rice**
**2 tablespoons vanilla sugar**

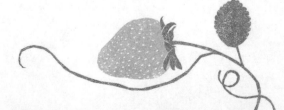

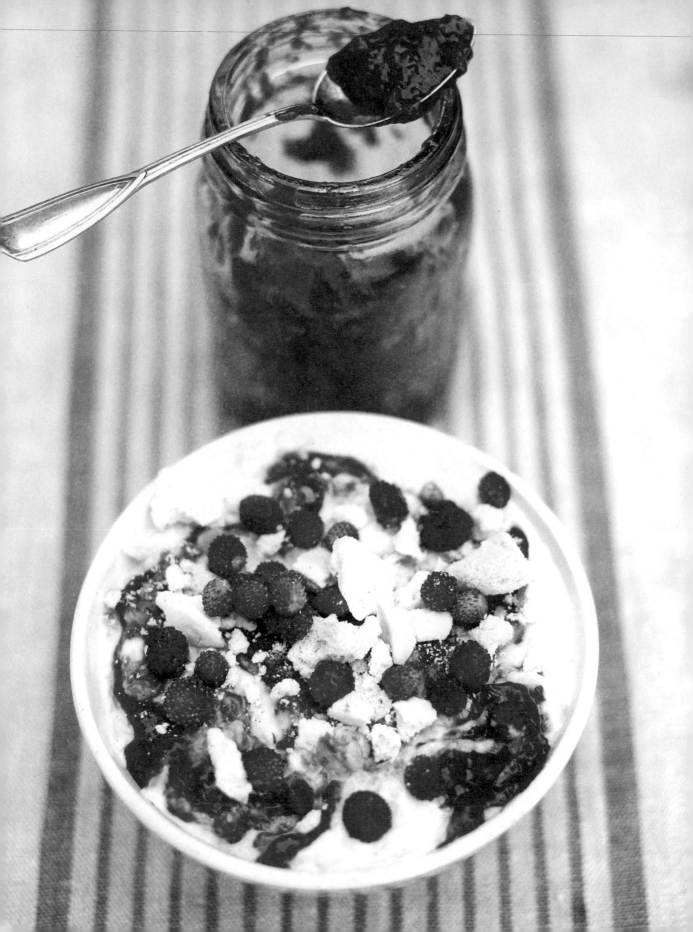

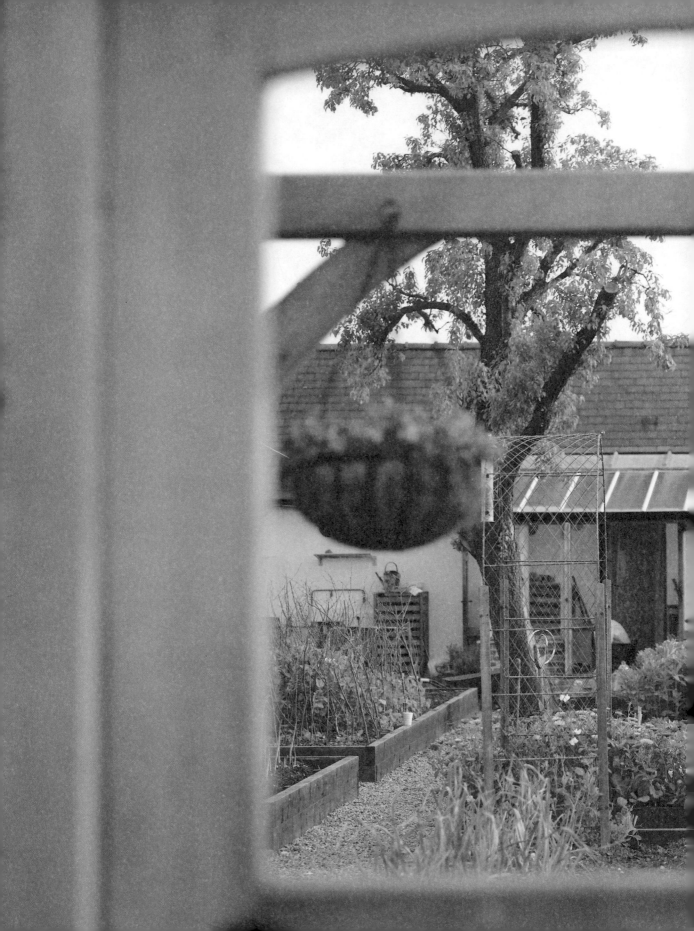

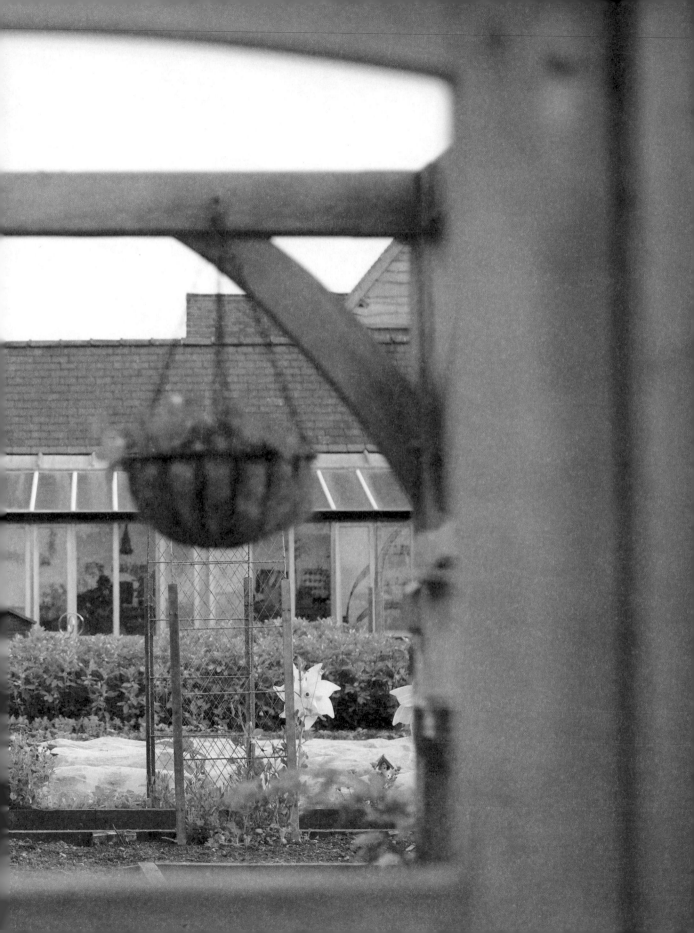

# Strawberry martini

Things like strawberry and lychee martinis are delicious but they can also be quite dangerous because you might not realize how much you're drinking, so beware. But enjoy!

Chill two martini glasses and your cocktail shaker in the freezer for half an hour until really really cold.

Put a few drops of dry vermouth into each glass and swirl it around. Put 3 strawberries into the bottom of each glass – if they're big ones, cut them into pieces first.

Throw the remaining strawberries and the mint into the cold cocktail shaker and squash them with the end of a rolling pin. Add the ice cubes and the gin or vodka, put the top on and shake it about. Strain into your two martini glasses.

**makes 2**

**a splash of dry vermouth**
**2 handfuls of sweet ripe**
**strawberries, preferably**
**wild ones, hulled**
**a sprig of fresh mint,**
**leaves picked**
**2 handfuls of ice cubes**
**150ml gin or vodka**

# Strawberry Champagne

This is the simplest recipe in the world and possibly one of the best Champagne cocktails I've ever tasted. A great way to start a summer dinner or party.

Place the mint leaf and the strawberries in a sieve. Push the strawberries through the sieve into a bowl, using the back of a spoon. (You're not really after the pulp, just the juice.) Chill until you are ready to serve your drinks.

Divide the strawberry purée between six Champagne glasses, carefully fill with bubbly and enjoy!

**serves 6**

**a leaf of fresh mint**
**3 large handfuls of
  strawberries, preferably
  wild ones, hulled,
  washed and drained**
**a bottle of bubbly, such as
  Prosecco or Champagne**

# How I grow strawberries

The best time to plant your strawberries is summer to early autumn. This way they'll have plenty of time to settle in and grow before the next fruiting period, the following summer. Strawberries like a bit of cold in winter, so don't be afraid to keep pots or hanging baskets outside throughout the winter. They will do better for it!

## Planting

Personally, I don't bother with seeds when it comes to growing strawberries. I just get some small good-quality strawberry plants from a nursery, garden centre or mail order company. Try to get a mixture of different strawberry hybrids. Not only will this give you different tastes, but as they have different fruiting times you'll end up with strawberries from May all the way through to the end of September if you play your cards right!

### In the ground

The only strawberries I plant in the ground in my garden are the original wild varieties, which, even though they're small and fiddly to pick, each have the flavour of ten ordinary strawberries. They look pretty, last for years and give wonderful ground cover to fill in all the gaps. I love lifting back the leaves in my strawberry patch to reveal a lovely little cluster of fruit underneath – the hens love it too when they're wandering around the garden!

To plant my wild strawberries in the soil, I usually build a little ridge so any excess water will drain off, meaning the plant won't rot away. Flatten the ridge off a little and keep a 30 to 45cm space between the plants, whether you're planting more strawberries next door or something else. Make a hole big enough to fit a plant in and lift the plant out of its plastic pot. As they've had no room to escape, the roots will have gathered together at the bottom, so pull some soil off to expose fresh root ends. Pop the plant into the hole, fill the gap with extra soil, pat to tighten and water well. Pull off any fruit that is already growing on your plant – you want it to pour all its energy into making a good root system for the long term, not into ripening those few bits of fruit.

### In hanging baskets and pots

After many experiments I now only ever plant medium to large hybrid strawberries in hanging baskets or in pots raised off the ground. Not only does this keep most pests and diseases at bay, including slugs and mildew, but you can tier the planting, which means you can get lots of plants into a small space. This also looks pretty unusual, with the berries trailing down overhead. But most important of all, by doing this you will get 40 per cent more yield (and you won't do your back in when you pick them!).

To plant strawberries off the ground, just pop your shop-bought plants out of their plastic pots and replant them into your hanging basket or container, filling it up with extra organic potting soil if necessary. Water them well, and stand or hang up in a warm sunny spot, preferably outside. Strawberries also grow very well in greenhouses, conservatories or on sunny windowsills.

## Some growing tips

- Strawberry plants in hanging baskets and pots need frequent watering when the weather is hot and dry.

- Don't be too generous with fertilizer – strawberries don't like to be overfed. You might get larger fruit but they won't taste of much.

- Once you've had the plants for a year or so, runners will start to grow in the autumn. If your strawberry plants are in the ground, you can peg the runners down with a wooden peg near the new little plant on the end. It will grow its own roots and you'll have a new plant for nothing!

- Strawberry plants have a life-cycle of about three years. The first year gives you a modest crop, the second year will be much better and after the third year the plant loses its oomph. Wild strawberries come back year after year.

- At the end of the picking season, cut all the leaves off the plant at about 7cm above the crown. This will keep your plants healthy during the cold season and, ultimately, will result in a better crop the following year.

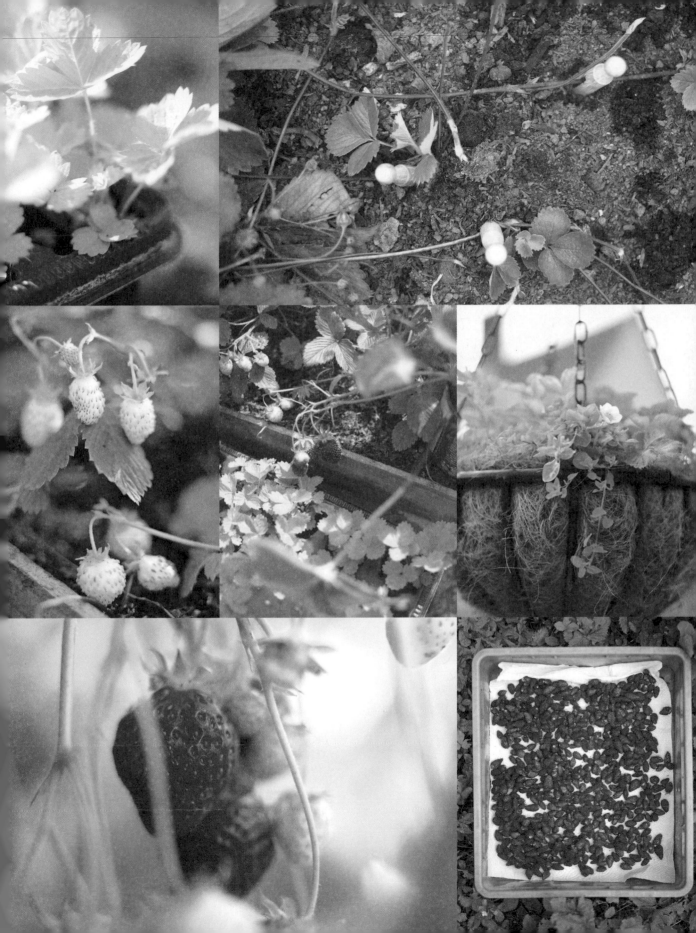

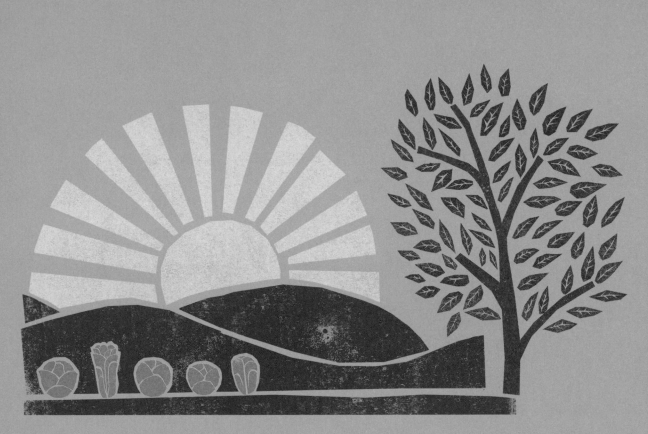

# summer
# salads

Salads are one of my favourite things to eat – there are so many different leaf varieties and combinations you can put together that there's no chance of ever becoming bored! I found out the other day that the first English-language book about salads was published in 1699 – how great is that? Written by the diarist John Evelyn, it was called *Acetaria: A Discourse on Sallets*, and describes new salad greens, like 'sellery', which were arriving from Italy and the Netherlands.

Back then, civilized people only ate meat and grains. Raw food was seen as the next best thing to suicide – it was thought to rot in your gut like it did on the compost heap and make you sick! Food handling and storage were unhygienic and people thought the best way to avoid getting sick from their food was to cook any 'disease' (along with the flavour, and the nutrients) right out of it. Raw greens and salads, with all their goodness, were therefore only eaten by peasants and animals.

Nowadays everyone seems obsessed with bagged salads. But did you know, most of those leaves have been washed in a chlorine solution? In some of our better supermarkets you can now buy salads washed in spring water, which is much better, but the best choice of all is to either buy five or six different organic heads of lettuce, or grow your own. All you need to do then is have a little five-minute wash-up – it's really important to wash your salad leaves.

Simply fill your sink with cold water and wash them well, then drain and spin in a salad spinner. You'll end up with lovely, healthy salad leaves that are ready to be dressed. Remember, though, that if you don't spin the leaves dry, your dressing will get watered down and the leaves will go off quicker, so it's really worth doing. I like to wash and spin dry a whole batch of leaves, then line the veg drawer of my fridge with a clean tea towel, put in the leaves and tuck the towel over them. They'll keep nicely for four days.

If you're a parent and you want to get your kids eating salad, plant it with them and watch it grow together. The other day I bought some mustard and cress seeds and the kids and I wrote their names in the soil with them. They absolutely love going into the garden to see how much their names have grown! Start them off on sweeter, softer leaves – we try to have a bowl of salad leaves on the table most dinner times as a matter of course. The girls have got used to it and think it's normal to eat salad, so it's worth a try.

Salad leaves are brilliant for beginners because they're so easy to look after. Just buy a few packets of seeds from your local garden centre or from a good website (see page 395), sprinkle them over a bit of soil, somewhere sunny, and give them some water. You'll probably be amazed how many times you get it right – I know I was!

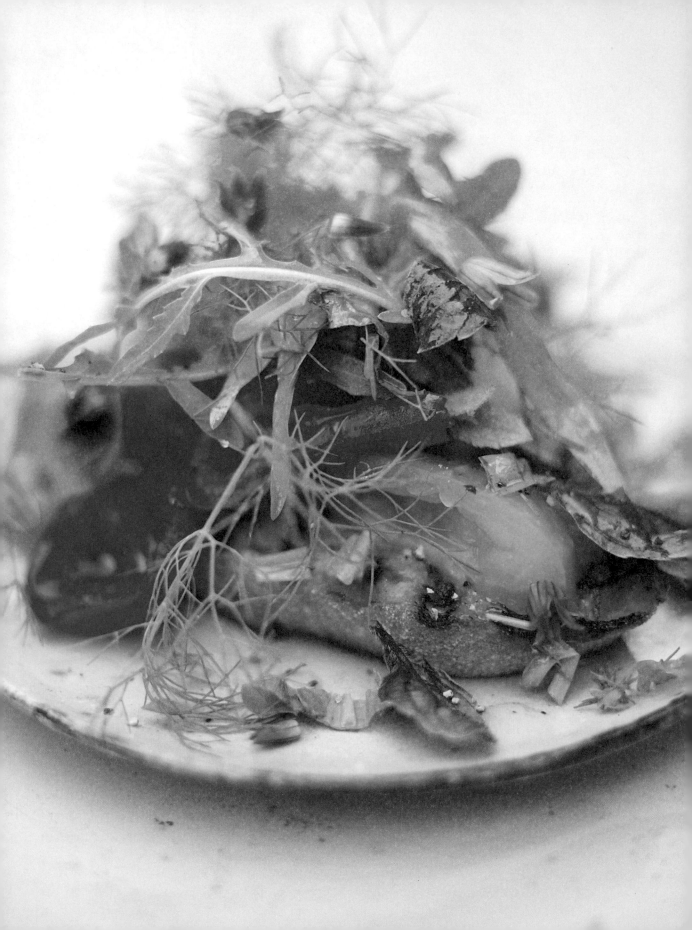

# Amazing herb salad on a tomato bruschetta

Fresh herbs are not only tasty, they can be exciting when used in a dish with some conviction and a bit of attitude! Whether you use delicate herbs mixed with leaves to make a lovely little salad, as I've done in this recipe, to accentuate some tomatoes, or whether you decide to serve them alongside a traditional roast or a grilled piece of fish, fresh herbs are amazing. If you haven't really used them in your cooking before, do try them from now on.

PS A little crumbled goat's cheese or grated Parmesan is nice sprinkled over just before serving.

If you have a griddle pan, put it on the heat and get it nice and hot. If you don't have one, you'll be using your toaster in a minute instead. Put your chopped tomatoes into a bowl with a glug of extra virgin olive oil and a swig of balsamic vinegar. Mix together and sprinkle with a little salt. I quite like to add a little chopped chilli too (but then again, I am obsessed with chilli!) and you can do the same if you like.

Toast the ciabatta slices in your hot griddle pan or a toaster for a minute or so on each side. Once the bread's nicely golden, rub each piece lightly with the cut side of the garlic.

Make a dressing by whisking together the lemon juice, three times as much extra virgin olive oil and salt and pepper to taste. Toss the rocket and herbs in the dressing.

Divide the ciabatta slices between four plates and top each one with a heap of chopped tomatoes. Press the tomatoes down into the bread and finish with a good pile of your herb and rocket salad.

**serves 4**

**3 or 4 ripe tomatoes, mixed colours if you like, roughly chopped**
**good-quality extra virgin olive oil**
**balsamic vinegar**
**sea salt and freshly ground black pepper**
**optional: 1 fresh red chilli, deseeded and chopped**
**4 slices of ciabatta bread, about 2.5cm thick**
**1 clove of garlic, unpeeled, cut in half**
**juice of ½ a lemon**
**a small handful of rocket, washed and spun dry**
**a few sprigs of fresh tarragon, leaves picked**
**a few sprigs of fresh herby fennel tops**
**a few sprigs of fresh mint, leaves picked**
**2 good handfuls of other interesting fresh herbs (use a mixture of sorrel, basil, parsley, dill or chive flowers), washed and spun dry**

# Green salad

I'm completely addicted to green salad. Even the most humble, basic one, with a few added herbs, can be a treat if dressed properly. You can tell a lot about a restaurant by the standard of its green salad – so many places get it wrong, but when they get it right, it's perfection. Although a great one doesn't need any extras, you can always toss in simple treasures such as cooked green beans, sweet raw peas, edible flowers, shaved fennel, or fresh mint, parsley, basil or tarragon leaves if you like. Great stuff.

So, to make your salad, get yourself a round lettuce and remove the leaves one by one. Wash them in plenty of cold water, spin them dry and pile them into a bowl. Make a basic dressing by mixing together three parts extra virgin olive oil, one part lemon juice and a pinch of sea salt and freshly ground black pepper. Drizzle the dressing over the leaves and use the tips of your fingers to gently mix the salad together. Be careful not to overdress it, though, or your leaves will go limp! That's it, your basic green salad.

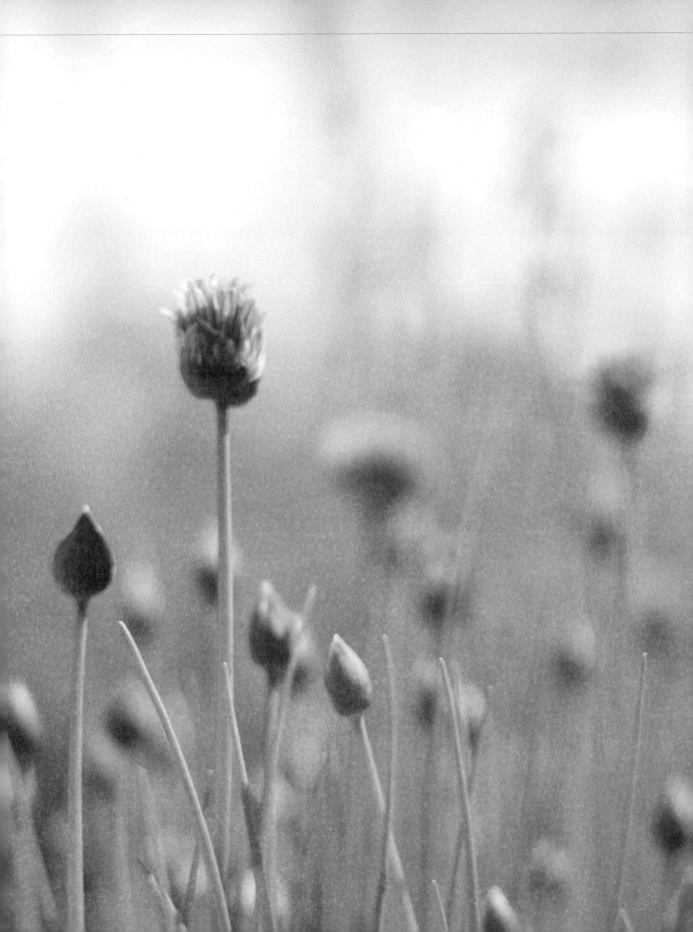

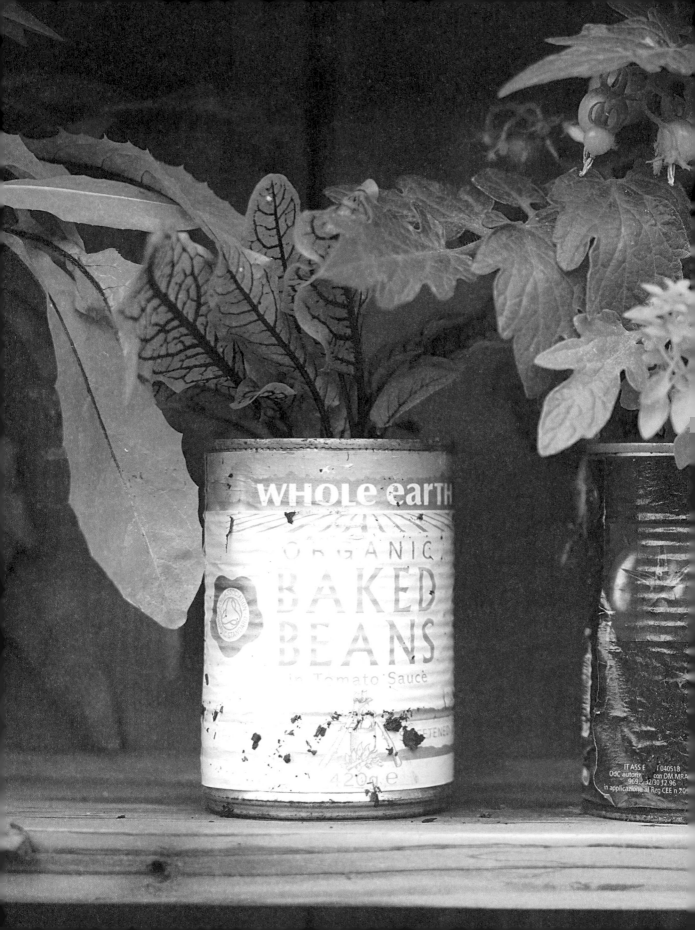

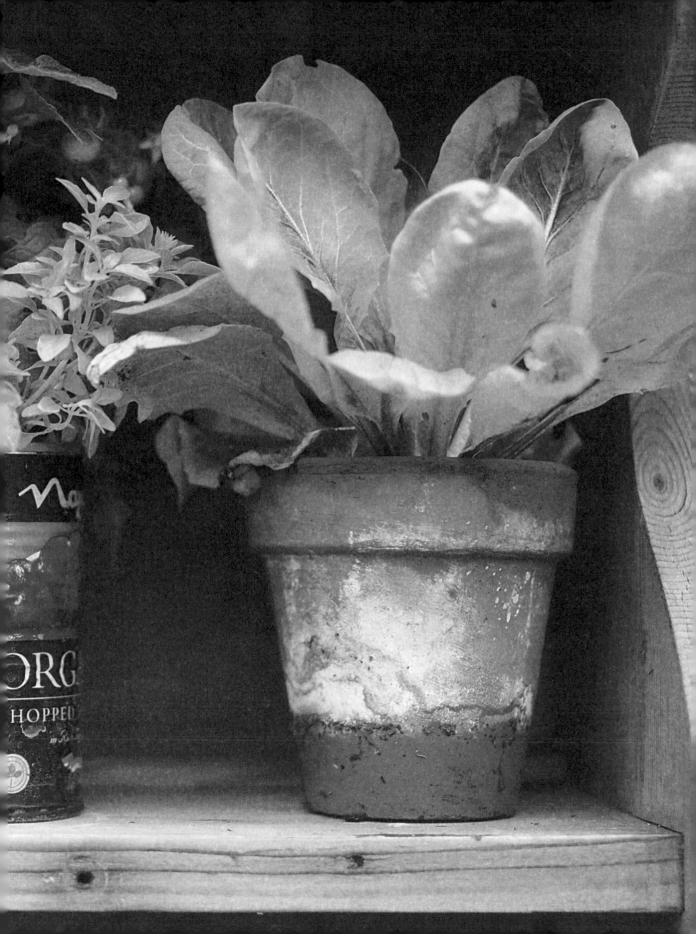

# Proper chicken Caesar salad

With my own versions of the classics, like Caesar salad, it's not about changing things entirely; it's about respecting the original while bigging up the flavours and textures where I can. My twists for this salad are to use chicken legs (not dry old breasts!), smoky pancetta and lovely rustic croutons to suck up all the juices. It's a lovely little salad with just a hint of attitude – and it's versatile, as you can serve it hot or cold.

PS Use your imagination – if you have any other unusual salad leaves, flowers or herb shoots lying around, chuck some in to make it look a little less predictable.

Preheat the oven to 200°C/400°F/gas 6. Place your chicken legs in a snug-fitting roasting tray with the pieces of torn-up bread. Sprinkle with the chopped rosemary, drizzle with olive oil and season with salt and pepper. Mix with your hands to make sure everything is well coated, then lift the chicken legs up to the top, so they sit above the bread. This way, the bread will soak up all the lovely juices from the chicken, giving you the best croutons! Pop the tray into your preheated oven.

After 45 minutes the chicken should be nicely cooked. Take the tray out of the oven, drape the pancetta or bacon over the chicken and croutons, and put back into the oven for another 15 to 20 minutes for everything to crisp up. Your chicken legs are ready when you can pinch the meat off the bone easily. When they're cooked, remove the tray from the oven and put it to one side for the chicken to cool down slightly.

Pound the garlic and anchovy fillets in a pestle and mortar or a Flavour Shaker until you have a pulp. Scrape into a bowl and whisk in the Parmesan, crème fraîche, lemon juice and three times as much extra virgin olive oil as lemon juice. Season your dressing to taste.

Pull the chicken meat off the leg bones – you can use two forks to do this, or your hands if you're tough like me – and tear it up roughly with the croutons and the bacon. Wash, spin dry and separate your lettuce leaves and red chicory, tear them up and toss with the chicken, croutons, bacon and creamy, cheesy dressing. Scatter with some Parmesan shavings.

**serves 4 to 6**

4 whole free-range or organic chicken legs, skin on

1 loaf of ciabatta bread (about 250g), torn into thumb-sized pieces

3 sprigs of fresh rosemary, leaves picked and roughly chopped

olive oil

sea salt and freshly ground black pepper

12 thin slices of pancetta or smoked streaky bacon

¼ of a clove of garlic, peeled

4 anchovy fillets in olive oil, drained

75g freshly grated Parmesan cheese, plus a few shavings to serve

1 heaped tablespoon crème fraîche

juice of 1 lemon

extra virgin olive oil

2 or 3 cos or romaine lettuces, outer leaves discarded

a couple of handfuls of red chicory

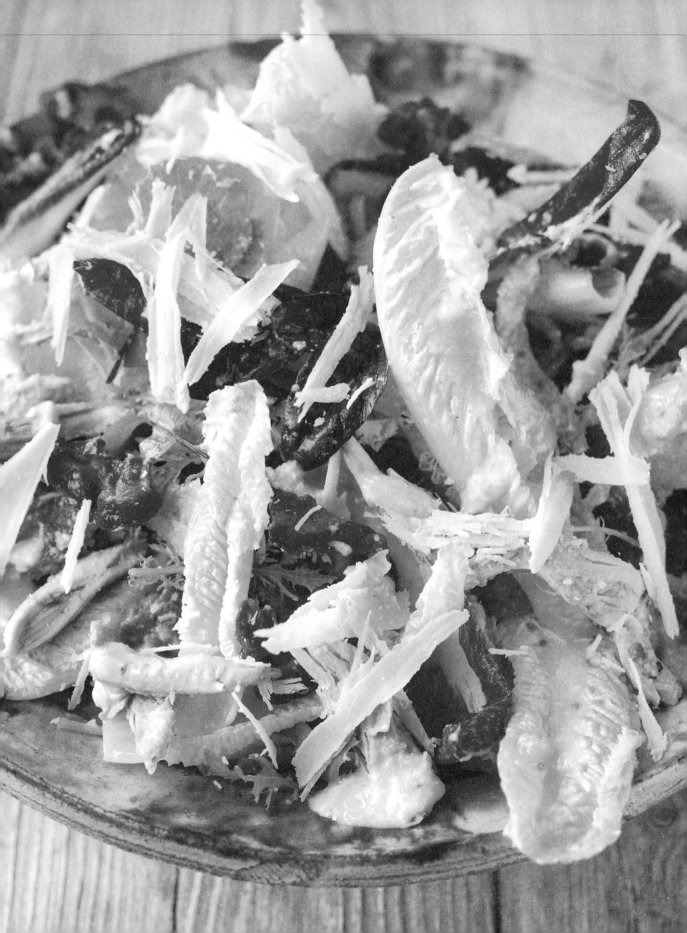

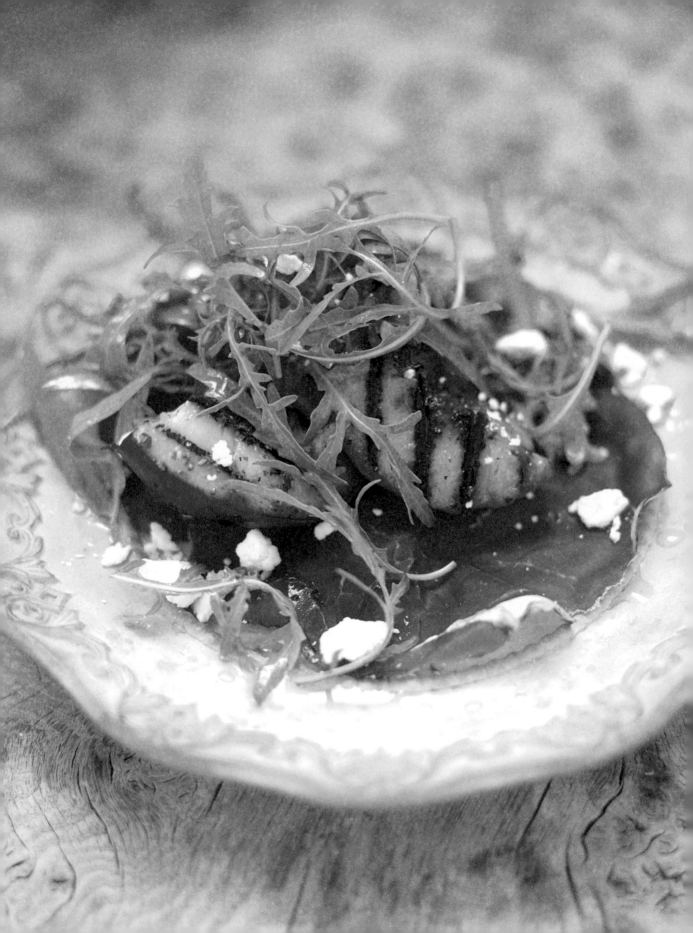

# Grilled peach salad with bresaola and a creamy dressing

In Italy fruit is often grilled – one of the best things I had when I was there was simply grilled stone fruit sprinkled with vanilla sugar and served with ice cream. So delicious! Peaches, pears, plums, apricots, even figs, are all good for grilling and don't just have to be eaten as a dessert. Here I'm serving grilled peaches with bresaola, which is very thinly sliced, cured, dried beef that you can get in Italian delis or good supermarkets. It's salty, savoury and goes with the peaches like a dream. This is my favourite little salad at the moment – dead nice!

Preheat a barbecue or griddle pan until hot. Cut the peaches in half, then twist them to remove the stones – don't worry if they break up when you do this. Toss them in a bowl with the chopped rosemary, a splash of olive oil and a little salt and pepper. If you're cooking on a barbecue, throw some herb branches on to the coals if you like – this will give the peaches a herby, smoky flavour. Grill the peaches for a couple of minutes on each side until nicely charred, but not burnt!

Pour the vinegar into a bowl or a Flavour Shaker and add three times as much extra virgin olive oil. Add the yoghurt or crème fraîche and a pinch of salt and pepper. Whisk or shake until mixed together well.

Drape the bresaola over four plates, pinching it up here and there so it's not lying flat. Place the peaches over the bresaola. Toss the tarragon leaves and rocket in the creamy dressing and pile the salad on top of the peaches. Drizzle with a little more extra virgin olive oil, scatter with the crumbled goat's cheese and tuck in!

serves 4

4 just-ripe peaches
a few fresh rosemary
   leaves, finely chopped
olive oil
sea salt and freshly
   ground black pepper
optional: some woody herb
   stalks or branches (such
   as rosemary or thyme)
1 tablespoon red
   wine vinegar
extra virgin olive oil
1 teaspoon natural yoghurt
   or crème fraîche
16 slices of bresaola
   or Parma ham
a few sprigs of fresh
   tarragon, leaves picked
2 handfuls of rocket,
   washed and spun dry
100g goat's cheese,
   crumbled

# How I grow summer salad leaves

## Soil

You can grow salad plants anywhere in the garden in a sunny or semi-shaded spot; there's no need to restrict them to your vegetable plot. The ones with frilly, ornately shaped or beautifully coloured leaves can be grown ornamentally as border edging or dotted in among other plants. If the soil is poor, enrich it with plenty of compost or well-rotted manure over winter, as this will add essential nutrients and increase its ability to retain moisture.

## Planting

First things first: all you need to do to grow salad leaves is buy some seeds, wait for mild weather, rough up some soil, add some compost, sprinkle on your seeds, cover them with soil and give them a good water. Believe me, it's that easy! When you see results you'll want to keep growing more and more stuff!

I start sowing outdoors from March onwards, using cloches or fleece for protection if the weather is still cold. By sowing small amounts of quick-growing varieties such as rocket and 'cut and come again' lettuce every fortnight you'll have a continuous supply of young tender leaves throughout the summer and autumn. Other crops can be sown indoors if they're slower-growing or frost-tender varieties, before being transplanted outside.

### Outside in the ground

Before sowing, rake the soil surface level, breaking up any big lumps, until the texture is like coarse breadcrumbs. The soil should be moist before sowing. If it's really soggy, wait a few days for it to dry out a bit. Make furrows about 30cm apart and 1 to 1.5cm deep, using a trowel or your finger, and sprinkle seed all along the row. Cover with soil and water gently using a fine rose on your watering can. When they come up, the seedlings may need thinning if you want some to grow big.

Leave a strong plant every 15 to 20cm. Don't waste those baby leaves – just throw them into a salad! Alternatively, scatter seed thinly over an area to give a solid block of small plants that can be used as 'cut and come again' leaves. Harvest them just above the lowest set of leaves when 3 to 6cm high, using scissors or shears – in a few weeks they will grow a new flush that you can cut again.

If you have bought, or have started your own, seedling plants in trays, keep them indoors or in the greenhouse until they look sturdy enough to plant out and you can see their roots through the bottom of the tray. Make a hole in the soil, ease the seedling out of the tray and place it in the hole. Gently firm it in. Space plants about 15 to 20cm apart and water in well. You can cover the rows with netting if you have a problem with birds or cats digging up the garden.

### Outside in pots

Salad leaves can also be grown in pots on a patio, a balcony or even a sunny windowsill – just fill them with good organic potting compost, sow the seeds thinly and cover with a little more compost. Tomato growbags are also a wonderfully easy way of growing things – I've used them loads of times and had success. Alternatively, transplant small seedlings into pots and harvest them when big enough. Don't forget to water them!

## My growing tips

- Plenty of water is essential. The soil should always be kept just moist as dry soil is likely to cause bolting, which means the plant starts to produce seeds too early, ruining the crop.

- It's always best to water plants at the end of the day. However, avoid watering peppery leaves like rocket and basil too much if you want to maintain their strong taste.

- Salad crops will bolt if left in the ground for too long after they're ready to harvest. If you sow seeds every fortnight, your whole crop will not run to seed at the same time.

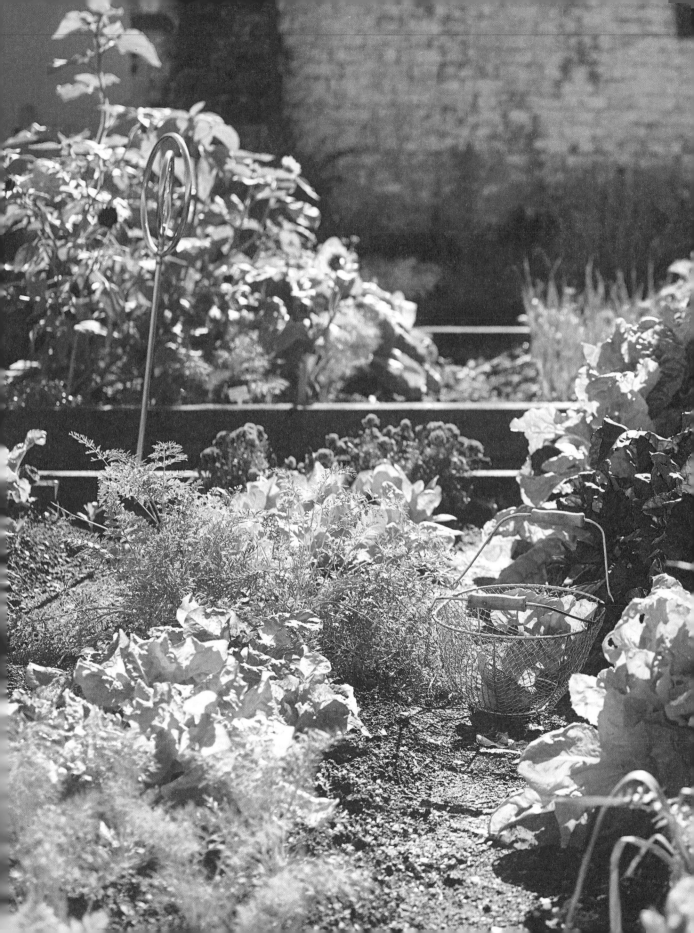

There are a few ingredients for me that if they didn't exist I'd give up cooking tomorrow and become a carpenter. Tomatoes are one of these, because you can vary your cooking so much with them. Their flavour can be so different – from a lovely fresh, limey, under-ripe tomato salsa, to an incredible tomato salad with lovely bread and mozzarella. Even historic brands like Heinz have built their reputation on tomatoes, and their tomato soup tastes great! I grew up on that stuff. I had a mug of it a few months ago and still love it as much as I did when I was a kid. So, whether under-ripe, perfectly ripe, raw, stewed in a sauce, or, most incredibly, slow-roasted on the vine with a sprinkling of sea salt and oregano, the range of flavours in the world of tomatoes is just incredible.

Tomatoes have to be one of the most exciting things to grow. I'm calling them 'things' because even though they are treated like a vegetable, a tomato is actually a fruit. And when you have a go yourself, the varieties, shapes, colours, tastes and smells are so completely different from what you can buy in the shops. The choice is incredible. And it's fascinating to watch them grow. Even in the supermarkets these days, or the farmers' markets, the choice is just getting better and better every year. If you tend to shop on autopilot for your normal red tomatoes, take a second and third look – I think you'll be amazed at all the different types available now.

Tomatoes first arrived in Europe from South America in the sixteenth century. Originally yellow and as small as cherries, they were called 'golden apples' in France and Italy. This translated as 'pomi d'oro' in Italian, which changed into the modern 'pomodoro'. It's hard to believe now, but tomatoes used to be considered deadly poisonous and were used only as decorative plants. It took a famine to force the peasants into trying them (imagine being so hungry that you would consider eating something poisonous…). Only then (after not keeling over!) did they realize how good tomatoes were and Europe went mad for them, using them in so many different ways. Now, of course, we know all about the benefits of tomatoes and they're far from poisonous. They're loaded with vitamins A, C and E, along with potassium and calcium for healthy bones and teeth. But most importantly of all, they contain lycopene, a potent antioxidant that helps to lower cholesterol and protect against heart attacks, strokes and cancer. So if we all eat a load of tomatoes, especially cooked tomato sauces and tomato ketchup because our bodies can use the lycopene in cooked tomatoes better (although you should watch the sugar content), it's a really positive thing.

In this little chapter the recipes are, quite frankly, what I felt like cooking when my tomatoes happened to be ripe and ready. Have a go at them all – even the slightly camp tomato consommé, because that really is the essence of tomato!

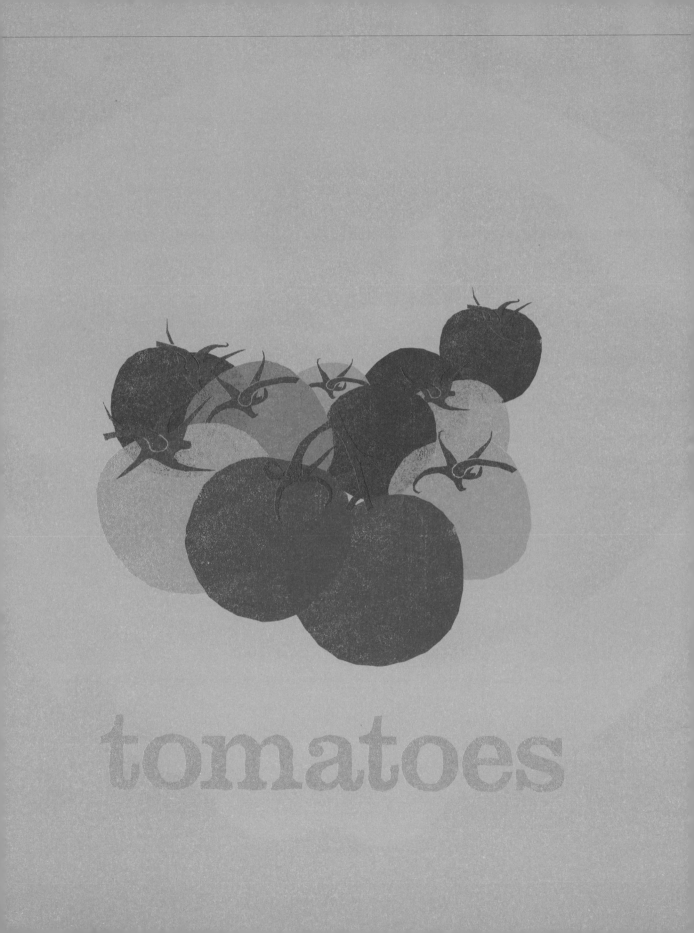

tomatoes

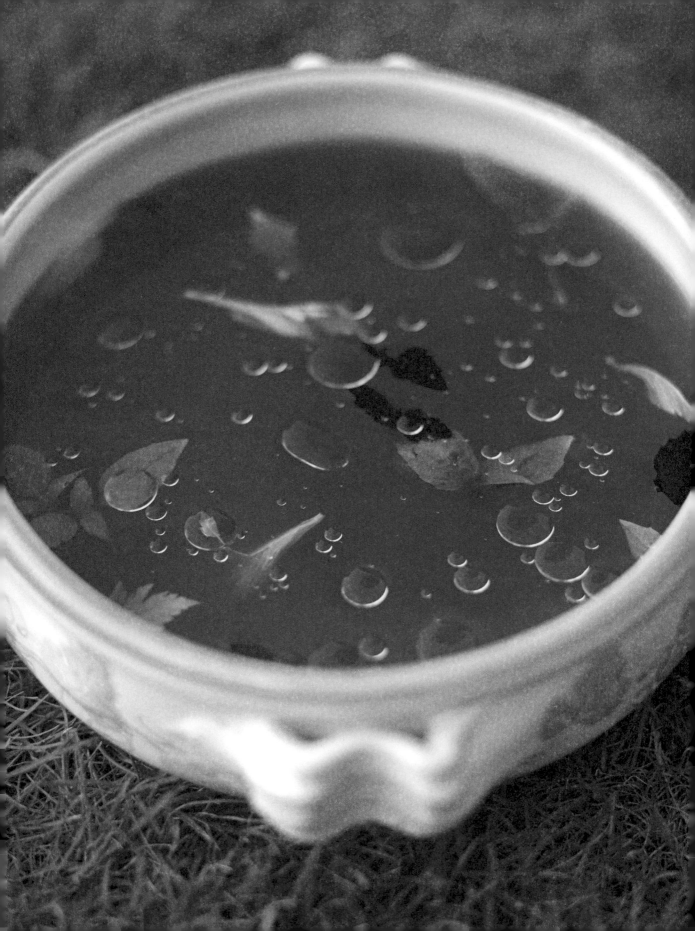

# Tomato consommé

I never thought I'd include this kind of recipe in one of my books, as it's more of a posh restaurant kind of dish. However, it's so simple to make and incredibly fresh and delicious, I didn't want to let personal style get in the way of a cracking recipe. I've based this soup on the same flavours as a Bloody Mary, as a real celebration of tomatoes. Serve this as a starter on a hot summer's day and it'll be like having a slap round the face – it really gets your tastebuds going!

PS You can only make this soup if you have a couple of layers of clean fine muslin (or a clean tea-towel) and a butcher's hook – you can get them from a good butcher's or cook shop.

First of all, pick out the tiny inner basil leaves and put them in a bowl in the fridge. Then put all the tomatoes, basil leaves and stalks, horseradish, garlic, vinegar, vodka, beetroot and a good pinch of salt and pepper into a food processor or blender (you may have to do this in batches) and whiz until you have a kind of slush. It'll smell great! Give it a stir, have a taste and season with salt. As horseradish varies in strength, you may need to add a little more – I would say it's better to slightly over-horseradish it – and whiz again.

Line a big mixing bowl with a double layer of muslin and pour the tomato pulp into it. Gather up the corners of the muslin and carefully, but securely, knot them together so you can lift the bundle up by the knot. Hang from a butcher's hook over a clean bowl to collect the juice that drips through the muslin and place in the fridge or a cool pantry. The liquid will be the most incredible crystal-clear rose-coloured essence.

Taste a spoonful and adjust the seasoning with sea salt only – don't use pepper now or you'll get little black bits in your lovely clear juice. Stir, season, taste until you feel you've got perfection – be confident, as now is not a time for blandness! One of the background tastes should be a subtle acidity from your red wine vinegar – add a little more if you like, but not too much. You could also swig in a little extra vodka at this point.

It will take about 5 to 7 hours for the juice to drip through. (If you think this sounds like a long time, you can gently push the muslin to force the juice out over the course of a minute, then let it drip for an hour or so from there. The longer you can let it drip naturally though, the clearer the consommé will be.) You'll know when it's done because you'll have 4 to 6 large ladles of juice in your bowl and the muslin pouch will be reasonably empty – discard what's left in it. Chill the soup in the fridge, along with your serving bowls.

When you're ready to serve, divide the soup between the bowls and sprinkle with the reserved basil leaves and a few small drips of quality extra virgin olive oil. Absolutely incredible!

serves 6

a large bunch of fresh
   basil, leaves picked,
   stalks reserved
2kg really nice, ripe
   tomatoes
1 x 5cm piece of fresh
   horseradish, peeled
   and roughly chopped,
   or 2-3 teaspoons grated
   horseradish from a
   jar (but not creamed
   horseradish!)
½ a clove of garlic, peeled
1-2 tablespoons good-
   quality red wine vinegar
a couple of shots of vodka
1 slice of beetroot (for
   colour)
sea salt and freshly
   ground black pepper

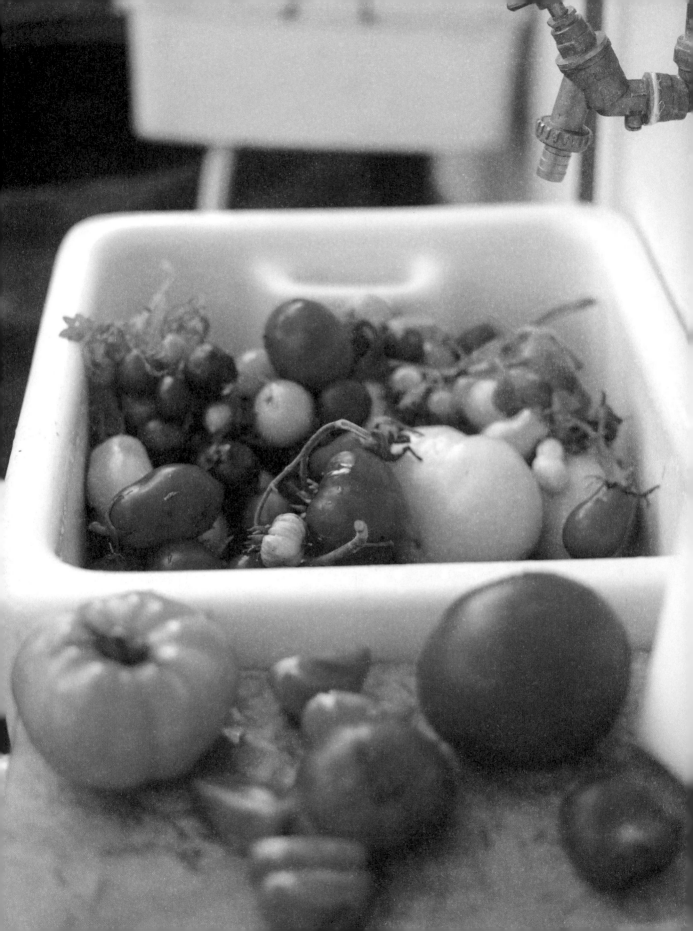

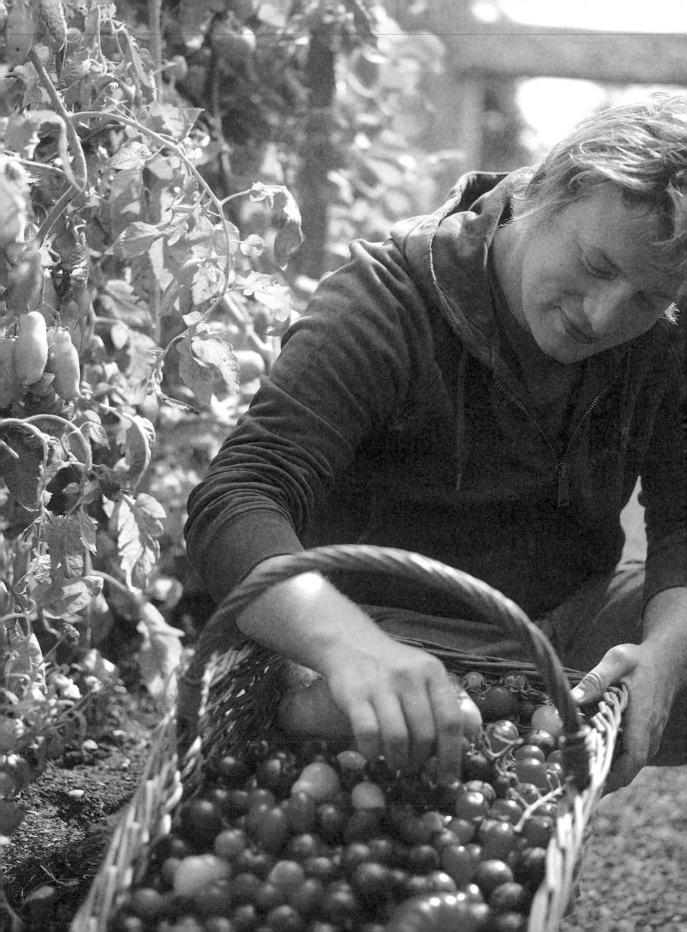

# The mothership tomato salad

This is an incredible tomato salad but there are two things to remember if you want to wow your guests with something so simple. The first is that you should try to get a mixture of different, tasty, local (if possible) tomatoes in all different shapes, sizes and colours. Second, the flavour is brought out by salting the tomatoes, so don't skip this bit. Some people get worried about putting this much salt on their food, but the bulk of it will drip off, leaving you with really beautiful, intensely flavoured tomatoes.

If you can get hold of some dried flowering oregano then do, as it has the most heavenly flavour. Feel free to use the dried stuff that you get in a little container, but it can taste a bit like sawdust when compared to the fruity, fragrant flavour you get from the flowering variety. Oregano is also great to grow in the garden.

Depending on the size of your tomatoes, slice some in half, some into quarters and others into uneven chunks. Straight away this will give you the beginnings of a tomato salad that's really brave and exciting to look at and eat. Put the tomatoes into a colander and season with a good pinch of sea salt. Give them a toss, season again and give a couple more tosses. The salt won't be drawn into the tomatoes; instead it will draw any excess moisture out, concentrating all the lovely flavours. Leave the tomatoes in the colander on top of a bowl to stand for around 15 minutes, then discard any juice that has come out of them.

Transfer the tomatoes to a large bowl and sprinkle over the oregano. Make a dressing using one part vinegar to three parts oil, the garlic and the chilli. Drizzle the tomatoes with enough dressing to coat everything nicely.

This is a fantastic tomato salad, which is totally delicious to eat on its own. It's also great served with some balls of mozzarella or some nice, grilled ciabatta bread.

**serves 4**

**1kg mixed ripe tomatoes, different shapes and colours**
**sea salt and freshly ground black pepper**
**a good pinch of dried oregano**
**red wine or balsamic vinegar**
**extra virgin olive oil**
**1 clove of garlic, peeled and grated**
**1 fresh red chilli, deseeded and chopped**

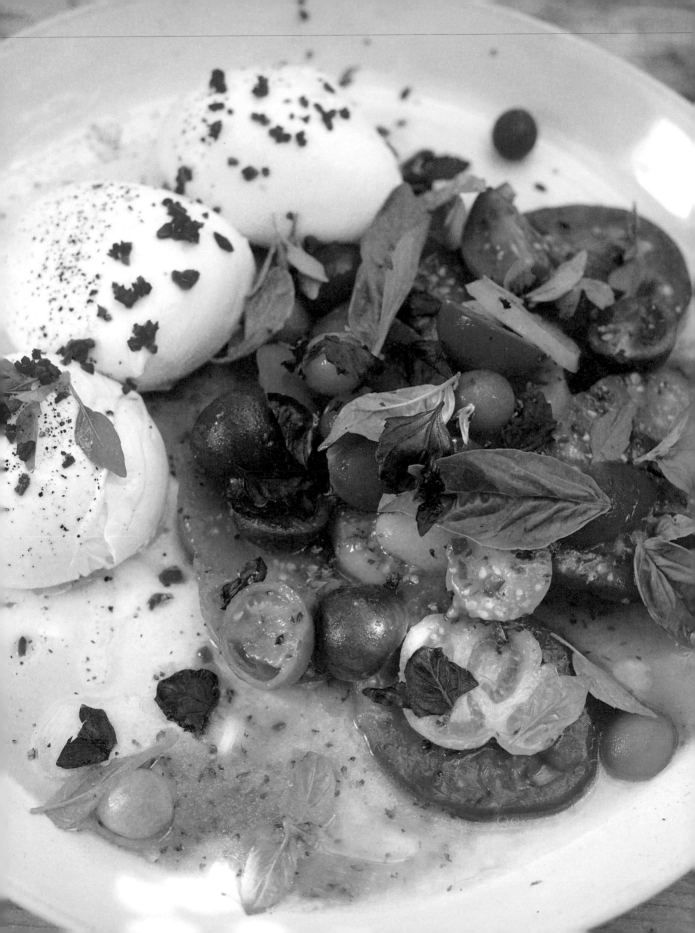

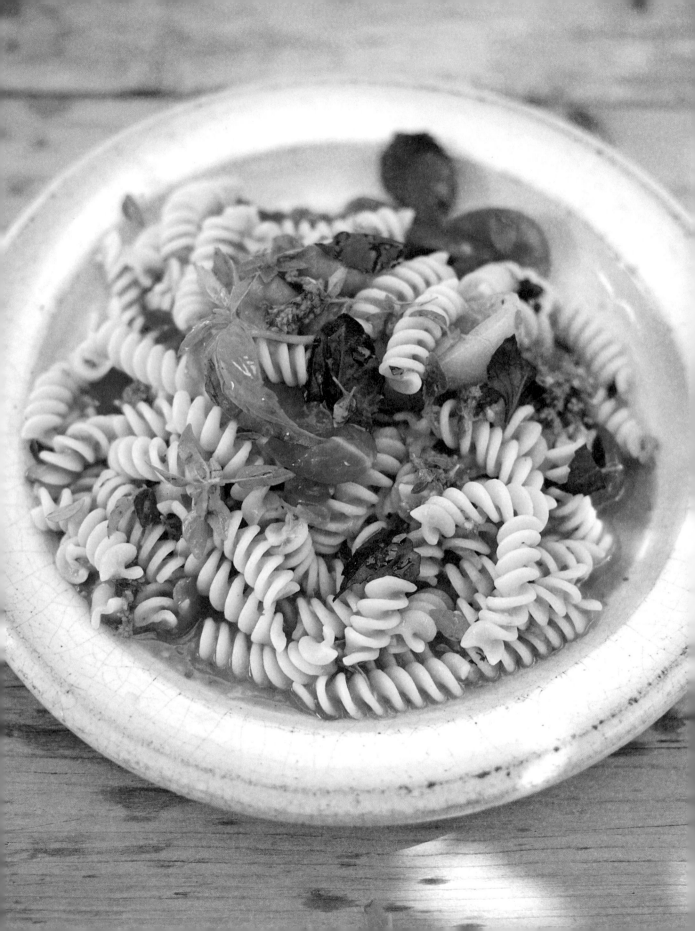

# Summer tomato pasta

I really enjoy making this pasta dish as it's so quick – the sauce doesn't need to be cooked, it just gets warmed through. It's dead simple and an absolute celebration of the summer months. Personally I like to use fusilli, but spaghetti, linguine, bucatini, farfalle or penne also work well, so feel free to use any of these types of pasta.

Pour some boiling water from the kettle into a pan over the heat and add the pasta and some salt. Place a large metal or earthenware bowl on top of the pan. Put the butter, balsamic vinegar and chopped herbs in the bowl and warm until the butter has melted. Now squeeze in the tomatoes, season with salt and pepper, then remove the bowl from the pan and put to one side. Give the pasta a stir.

With clean hands, really scrunch the tomatoes and all the flavours in the bowl together. Have a little taste and decide whether they need some more seasoning or vinegar.

When the pasta is cooked according to the packet instructions, drain it in a colander, reserving some of the cooking water. Tip the pasta into the bowl with your tomatoes and stir the sauce into the pasta. Drizzle with a good glug of extra virgin olive oil, loosen with some of the reserved cooking water if need be, and sprinkle over the reserved baby herb leaves. Serve with a block of Parmesan for grating over. Lovely with some olives thrown in.

**serves 4**

**500g dried fusilli**
**sea salt and freshly**
  **ground black pepper**
**75g butter, cubed**
**2 tablespoons balsamic**
  **vinegar**
**a large bunch of mixed**
  **soft fresh herbs (like**
  **green and purple basil,**
  **marjoram, flat-leaf**
  **parsley, thyme tips and**
  **oregano), leaves picked, a**
  **few baby leaves reserved,**
  **the rest roughly chopped**
**600g mixed cherry**
  **tomatoes, roughly**
  **chopped**
**extra virgin olive oil**
**a block of Parmesan**
  **cheese, for grating**

# Tomato coriander salsa with grilled tuna

If you understand what makes an incredible tomato salad, like the mothership one on page 232, you'll also understand how to make a great tomato salsa. The only slight difference is that with a tomato salad you're looking for balance but salsa can have a bit more attitude! In essence, you need great tomatoes, salt to make them sing, a twang of vinegar, a good hit of lemon or lime, a herb or mixture of herbs for fragrance, and chilli for background or in-your-face heat. Any of these factors can be tweaked or varied when you make this salsa. It will turn a simple roasted piece of chicken or a grilled pork chop or a piece of barbecued swordfish or tuna into an absolute flavour-fest. Bloody exciting stuff and damn quick to make.

PS When buying your fish, look out for whatever's fresh. Tuna and swordfish can be overfished in many parts of the world and we need to let their stocks grow – just be aware of this and go for fish that is plentiful and fished for in a responsible and sustainable way.

First of all, get your barbecue or griddle pan preheated and ready to go. Making the salsa is pretty easy – it just involves a lot of chopping! Get yourself a big board and finely slice the spring onions and half of the chillies on it. Then, on top of the spring onions, finely chop the coriander leaves with the upper parts of the stalks, and the mint leaves. On top of them, slice up your tomatoes and chop to the kind of consistency that you like – I like my salsas quite fine. By chopping everything on the same board it allows for better integration of the flavours.

Carefully scrape everything off the board into a nice serving bowl with all the juices. Season and balance the flavours confidently with sea salt, the lemon juice and the lime juice, bearing in mind that these vary in juiciness, size and sourness all over the world, so taste as you go and use common sense. To my mind, a salsa has to be pretty punchy and fragrant, so add, stir and taste, add, stir and taste, until you've got something good going on! If you want to add extra chilli to give it a bit more of a kick, chop some more on the board and add it to the bowl now.

Put the salsa to one side while you get your fish ready. Rub it on both sides with olive oil and season with salt and pepper, then grill or griddle to your liking on both sides. Serve the fish on a plate with a big dollop of the salsa on top, or to the side, and enjoy.

serves 6

6 spring onions, trimmed and finely chopped
1–2 fresh red chillies, deseeded and finely chopped to taste
a bunch of fresh coriander, leaves picked
a bunch of fresh mint, leaves picked
1kg beautifully ripe but firmish tomatoes
sea salt and freshly ground black pepper
juice of ½ a lemon
juice of 1 lime
6 fresh fish fillets (particularly Mediterranean fish like tuna, swordfish, marlin and any from the snapper family)
olive oil

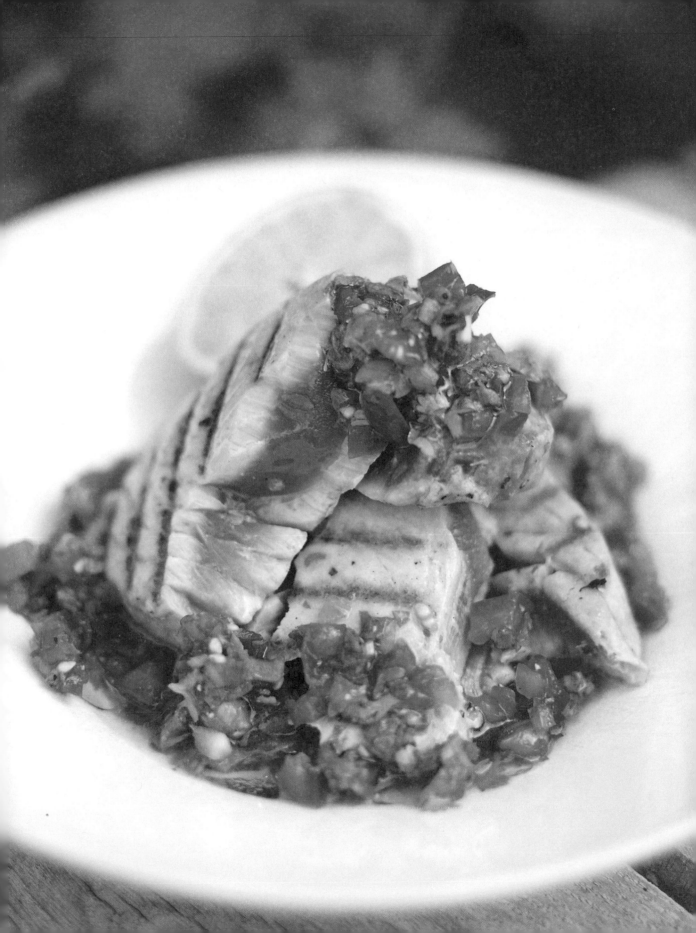

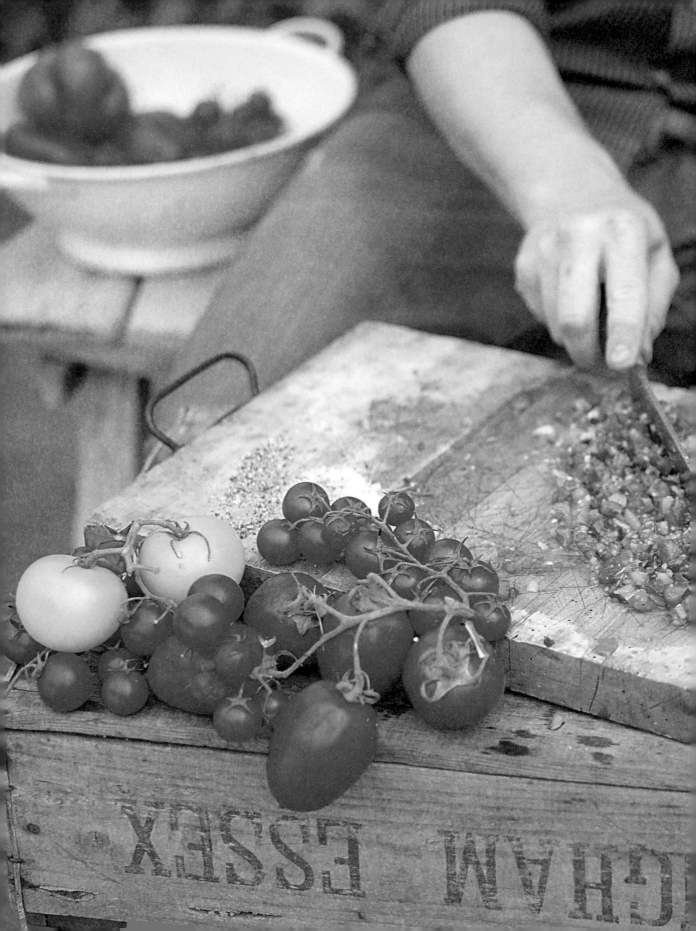

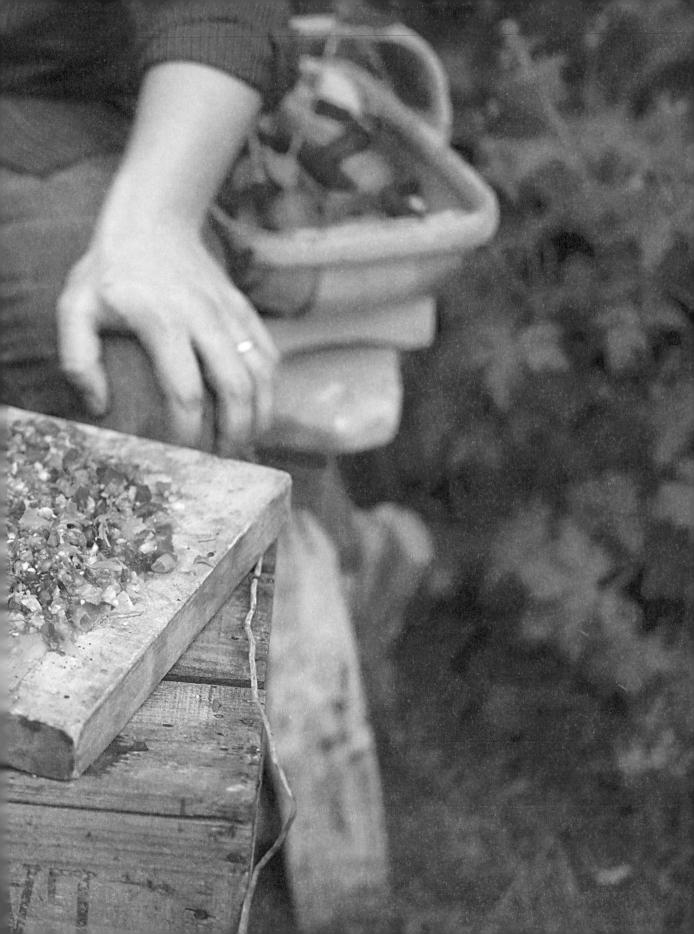

# Sweet cherry tomato and sausage bake

There are so many things I love about this dish: it's all cooked in one tray; we're using more robust herbs like thyme, rosemary and bay with the tomatoes, which work really well; the half-roasted, half-stewed fresh tomatoes turn into a lovely rich and chunky sauce which is miles better than anything you can get if using tinned tomatoes; and we're roasting the sausages, which I think is far better than frying or grilling them. Try to buy the best fresh coarsely ground sausages you can.

PS Any leftovers can be chopped up and made into a wonderful chunky pasta dish, using penne or rigatoni, the next day.

Preheat the oven to 190°C/375°F/gas 5. Get yourself an appropriately sized roasting tray, large enough to take the tomatoes in one snug-fitting layer. Put in all your tomatoes, the herb sprigs, oregano, garlic and sausages. Drizzle well with extra virgin olive oil and balsamic vinegar and season with salt and pepper. Toss together, then make sure the sausages are on top and pop the tray into the oven for half an hour. After this time, give it a shake and turn the sausages over. Put back into the oven for 15 to 30 minutes, depending on how golden and sticky you like your sausages.

Once it's cooked, you'll have an intense, tomatoey sauce. If it's a little too thin, lift out the sausages and place the tray on the hob to cook it down to the consistency you like – I tend to make mine quite thick – then put the sausages back in. Check the seasoning and serve either with a good-quality loaf of bread warmed through in a low oven for 10 minutes (great for mopping up the sauce!) or with mashed potato, rice or polenta, a green salad and a nice glass of wine.

serves 6

2kg lovely ripe cherry tomatoes, mixed colours if you can find them
2 sprigs each of fresh thyme, rosemary and bay
1 tablespoon dried oregano
3 cloves of garlic, peeled and chopped
12 good-quality Cumberland or coarse Italian pork sausages
extra virgin olive oil
balsamic vinegar
sea salt and freshly ground black pepper

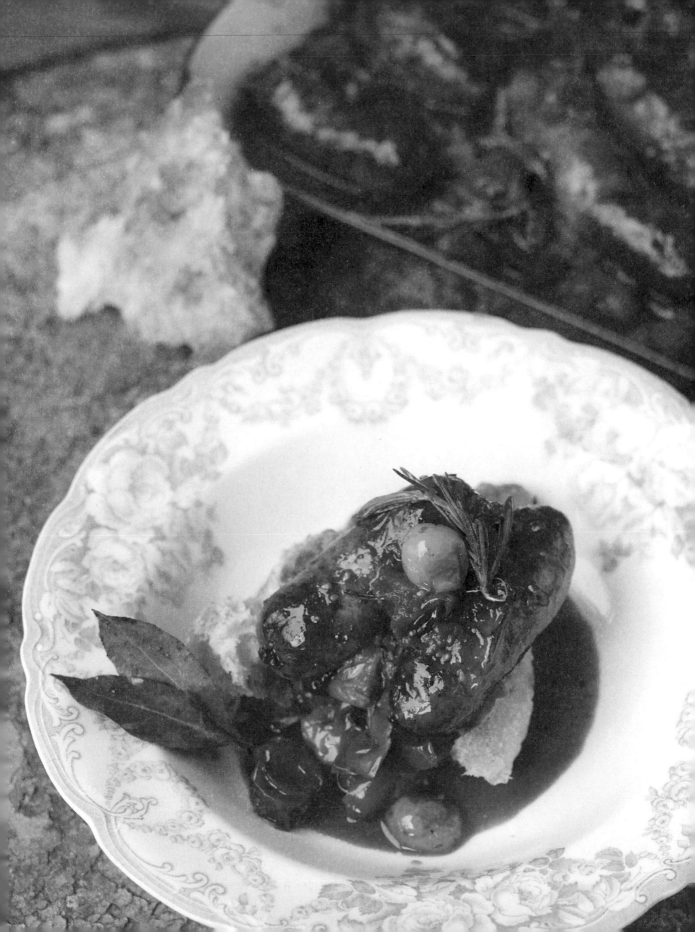

# How I grow tomatoes

## Soil

Tomatoes love growbags – they have the right soil mix, with some nutrients already mixed in. They're dead easy to use and you can sow seeds directly into them when it's warm. Two or three tomato plants will easily fit into one bag, and a couple of bags will give you more than enough tomatoes for the family.

## Planting

In February or early March I like to sow my tomato seeds in small pots (about 5 to 7cm diameter) filled with a good organic seed compost. I'll keep these indoors in a fairly warm place (anything from 15 to 20°C) to get them going. A sunny windowsill or a greenhouse are good places. I sow one or two seeds per pot about 1cm deep, and then give them a good watering. After a few weeks, when the seedlings have grown into plants about 6 to 9cm tall I've found that it's really handy to transfer them individually into bigger pots just for a month or so, until they've grown into sturdy little plants strong enough to go into growbags in a greenhouse, or outside in late spring, early summer. Remember that tomatoes need warm summers to succeed outside. They cannot stand cold weather. If you don't want to do the whole sowing thing, you can always buy little tomato plants at a garden centre and go from there. This is a great way of trying out different varieties.

When it's time to put the plants outside in May, after the last frosts, you need to choose a warm, sunny spot in the garden. You simply place your growbags where you want them, or you can use any number of other containers or big pots, as long as they're filled with good rich soil. Carefully transplant two tomato plants into one growbag or large pot. You will start to get tomatoes after about ten to twelve weeks. The plants will continue to produce tomatoes for several months and the number you get will depend on the temperature, the amount of sunlight and the strength of the plant.

## Harvesting and storing

To get the best flavour from your tomatoes, let them ripen fully before you pick them, however tempting it may be to pick them sooner! With artificial ripening, which some supermarkets do, the tomatoes are picked when they're still a bit green and sprayed with a gas called ethylene to speed up the ripening process. Bananas actually give off this same gas, so if you've got some green tomatoes that have fallen off your plants, or you have some that are still green right at the end of the season, put them next to a bunch of bananas and they'll ripen.

Tomatoes should never be stored in the fridge. Did you know, they actually go off quicker if you do this? They'll keep ripening as long as they are kept above 12.5°C, so if you put hard, unripe tomatoes in the fridge they will come out hard and unripe. If you store them in a cool place, out of the sun, they'll remain at their best. However, if you have any that are already over-ripe they will last a little longer in the fridge.

## My growing tips

* I sometimes half-fill a big pot with manure, then top it up with potting compost and stick in a tomato plant or two ... when the roots hit the manure the plants go crazy!

* Tomatoes like to go into the ground, but remember not to plant them in the same place year after year – it helps prevent disease.

* This year I tried planting a load of basil, marigolds and garlic between my tomato plants to ward off whitefly and other pests. They act as insect repellents because of the strong smells they give off. Basil and garlic are also thought to enhance the flavour of tomatoes, if you plant them close by. Chives, carrots, roses, borage, asparagus and many others are also sometimes used in a similar way. This is known as 'companion planting'.

* As long as they have good soil, a sunny spot, regular watering, a bit of feeding and some means of supporting the plant off the ground (like a bamboo cane structure or a trellis), you will get a great crop of tomatoes with very little effort.

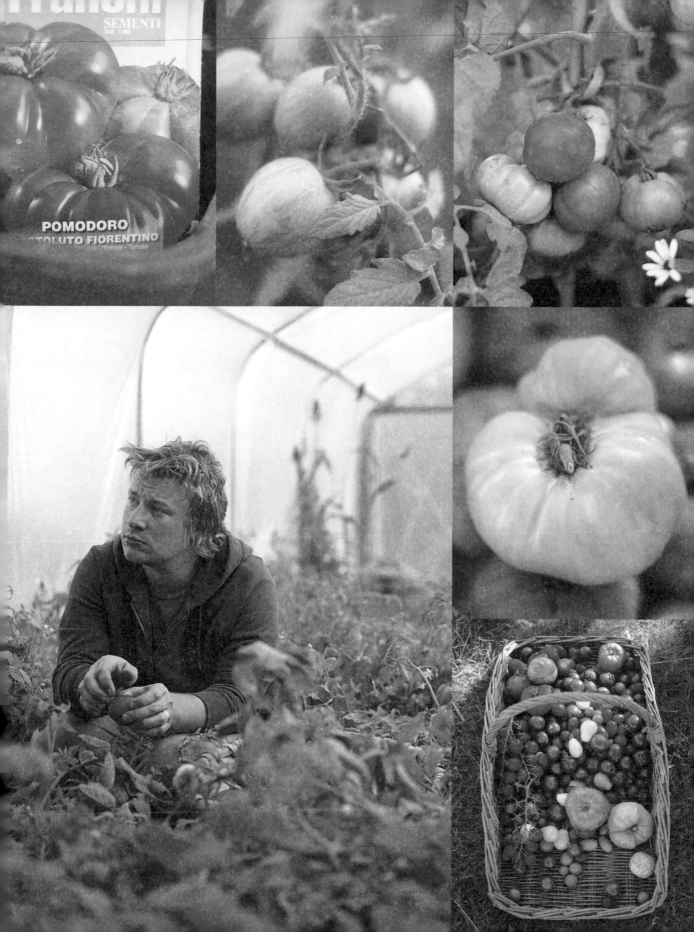

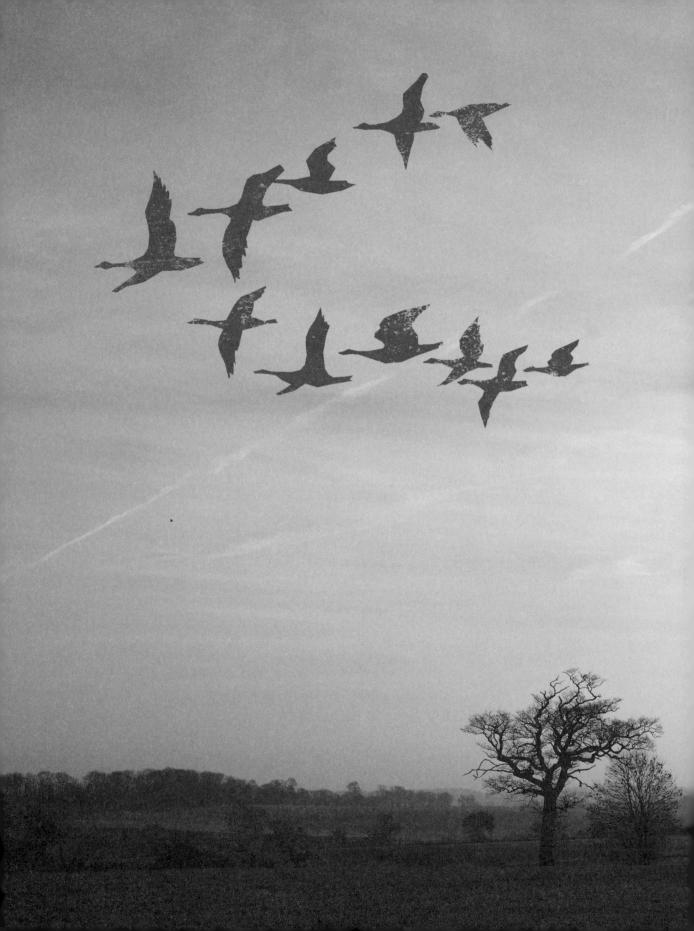

# autumn

chillies and peppers / feathered game /
furred game / mushrooms /
orchard fruit / pickles

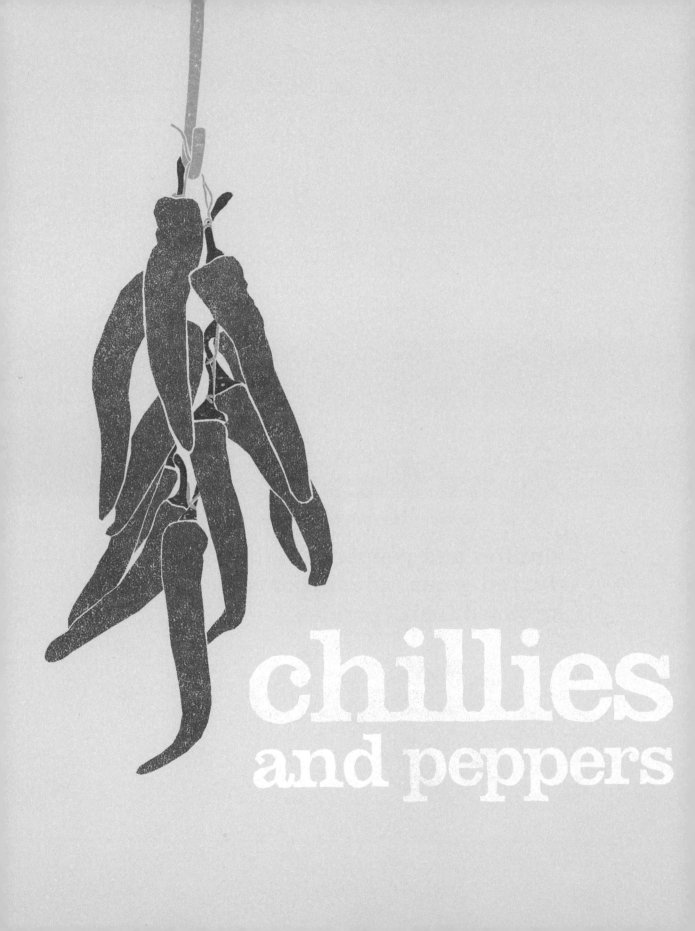

# chillies
## and peppers

I love chillies so much that I have withdrawal symptoms and feel a bit miserable and lethargic if I go without them for a while! When I think about chilli, even on a cold winter's day, the back of my tongue starts to tingle. In fact, my mouth is watering while I'm writing this ... Now you might be thinking this is all very strange, but actually it's not. Eating chillies gets the endorphins going in your body, giving you a rush of blood, making you sweat, while also causing a sense of vigour and well-being. Eating chillies also speeds up your metabolism by 25 per cent, helping you to burn off calories quicker and not store them as fat in your body. But, most importantly, chillies taste great.

I used to think that chillies were chillies, but I now know that's like saying a glass of wine is a glass of wine. There are hundreds of varieties to choose from, differing in heat and possessing a whole range of flavours, from an intense peachiness to crisp apple. They can be petally, perfumy, fragrant and fruity. They can have a clean, short-lived heat, or a really robust, chunky, concentrated, long-living heat. Basically, with chillies you can tweak, change and improve all kinds of dishes. And when you smash up fresh chillies with fragrant things like kaffir lime leaves and fresh ginger, you can create the most incredible cocktail of smells and perfumes known to cooking. This type of Asian-style flavour mix is brilliant, whether for smearing over a piece of roasted fish or for using in a curry.

You might be someone who doesn't like 'hot' food, but just because you're using chilli in your cooking doesn't mean you have to use loads – you can be subtle. The big rule about eating a chilli is to lick it first, then try a tiny bite to find out its heat. If you ever do get caught out eating chillies, don't drink beer or alcohol as these will exaggerate the pain. Have a glass of milk or some yoghurt instead.

It might sound bizarre, but the tiniest hint of chilli heat in any chocolate dish is incredible. Shellfish and vegetables are jaw-droppingly delicious when tossed in a little chopped chilli, mint and lemon oil. Anything crunchy or crispy and salty, be it poppadoms or crisps or flatbreads, with a hellishly hot chilli salsa or sauce is just brilliant.

### Tips for handling chillies

- It's not the seeds or the flesh that contain the heat of a chilli – it's the fine white membrane that holds the seeds. As soon as you cut through it, the heat is released. So, when you deseed a chilli, you need to scrape out this membrane as well as the seeds.

- If you're handling really hot chillies, it's always a good idea to wear kitchen gloves. And don't rub your eyes afterwards! Always wash your hands straight away.

PS Oh, and peppers are quite nice too! They're part of the same family as chillies; they come in different colours, shapes and sizes, but they don't have the heat of chillies.

# Hot smoked salmon with an amazing chilli salsa

I'm really excited about this one. There are two processes when it comes to smoking food: 'cold smoking', where things like raw fish, meats and cheeses are put into a smoky environment with no heat source, and 'hot smoking', which has the added heat source. It gives great results. All you need is an old biscuit tin with a lid, a wire rack that fits inside it or a bit of chicken wire and some uncoated sawdust (the type you get for putting in pets' cages). When you put the tin on your heat source, it will act like a kind of oven – don't get nervous if it seems a bit radical to you, because it's so easy. And imagine how impressed your mates will be when you tell them you've hot smoked the food yourself!

PS A word of warning: this will make your house a bit smoky, so either open the windows to get some fresh air through, put the fan on or have a go at doing it outside on your barbie.

Get your biscuit tin and place a handful or two of wood shavings into the tin, followed by your rosemary and sage sprigs. Place your wire rack in the tin, so it sits about halfway down, or bend some chicken wire to fit. Carefully pierce the lid of the tin five or six times with a screwdriver.

Most salmon fillets come around the same size and thickness, so their cooking times are similar. Sprinkle the salmon fillets with salt and rub with a drizzle of olive oil. Then lay them skin side down on top of the wire (this acts like a grill rack) and put the lid on the tin. Place it on the hob, over a medium heat, and cook for 8 to 10 minutes. After a couple of minutes it will start to smoke a bit.

While the fish is cooking, mix all the salsa ingredients together – you can go as light or as heavy on the chillies as you like. When the fish is ready, turn the heat off and leave it to sit for 3 minutes before opening the tin. This will allow any residual smoke and heat to penetrate the fish. Lift the salmon fillets out and place on to individual serving plates. Spoon over some chilli salsa and sprinkle with your whole coriander leaves. Drizzle over some extra virgin olive oil and serve with the lime halves and the rest of the salsa in a little bowl. Lovely with some new potatoes and a green salad for lunch.

serves 2

a sprig of fresh rosemary
a few sprigs of fresh sage
2 x 200g wild or organic
  salmon fillets, skin on
sea salt
olive oil
1 lime, halved
a few whole coriander
  leaves

*for the chilli salsa*
1–2 fresh red chillies,
  deseeded and finely
  chopped
2–3 medium-sized ripe
  tomatoes, deseeded
  and diced
½ a cucumber, peeled
  and finely diced
juice of 1 lime
2 spring onions, trimmed
  and finely sliced
a small handful of fresh
  coriander, leaves
  picked and chopped
1 avocado, stoned,
  peeled and chopped
extra virgin olive oil

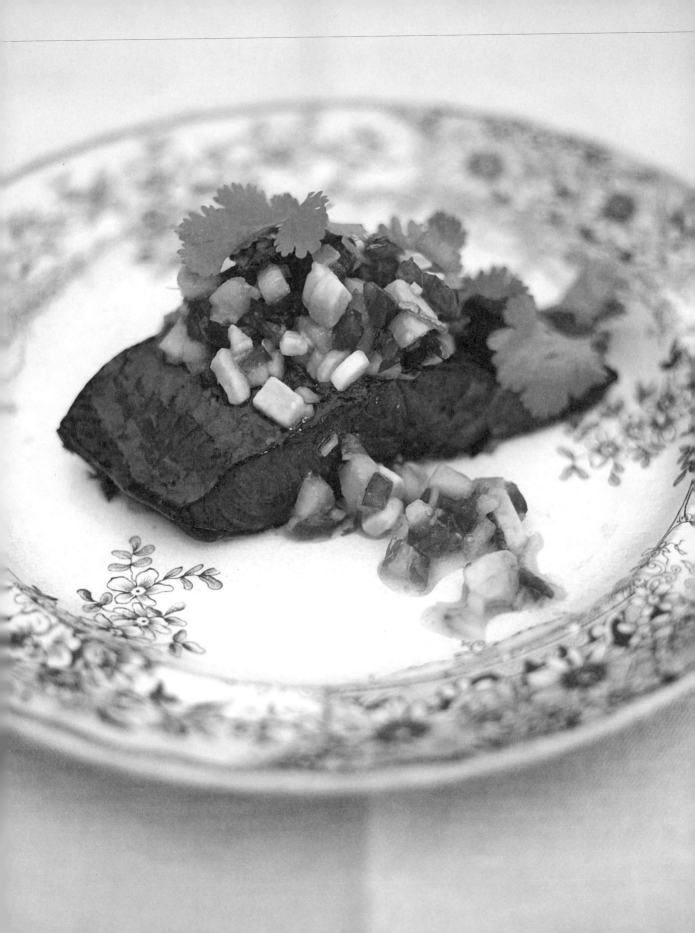

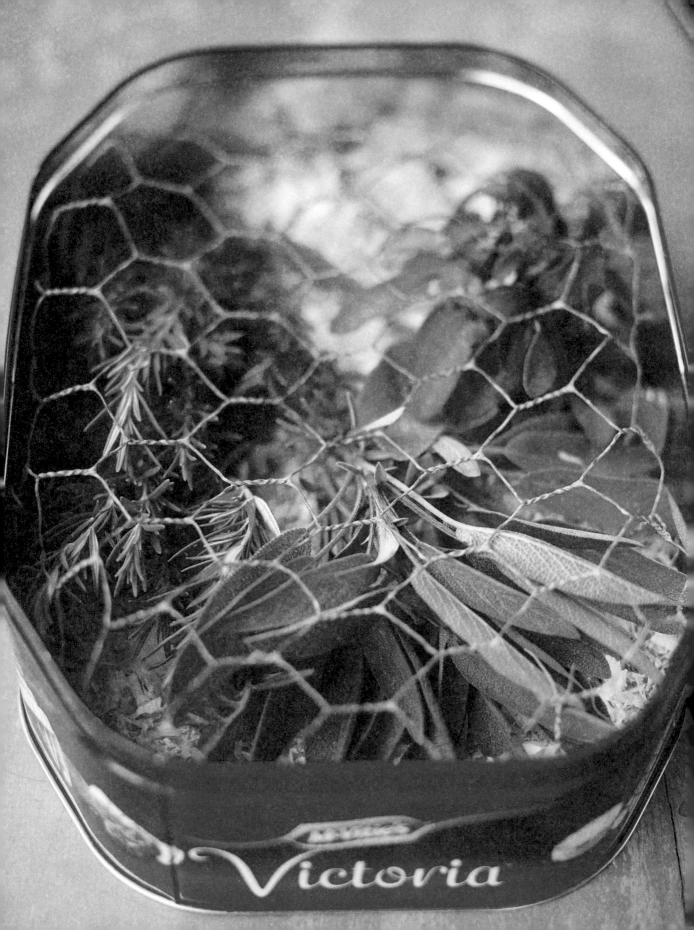

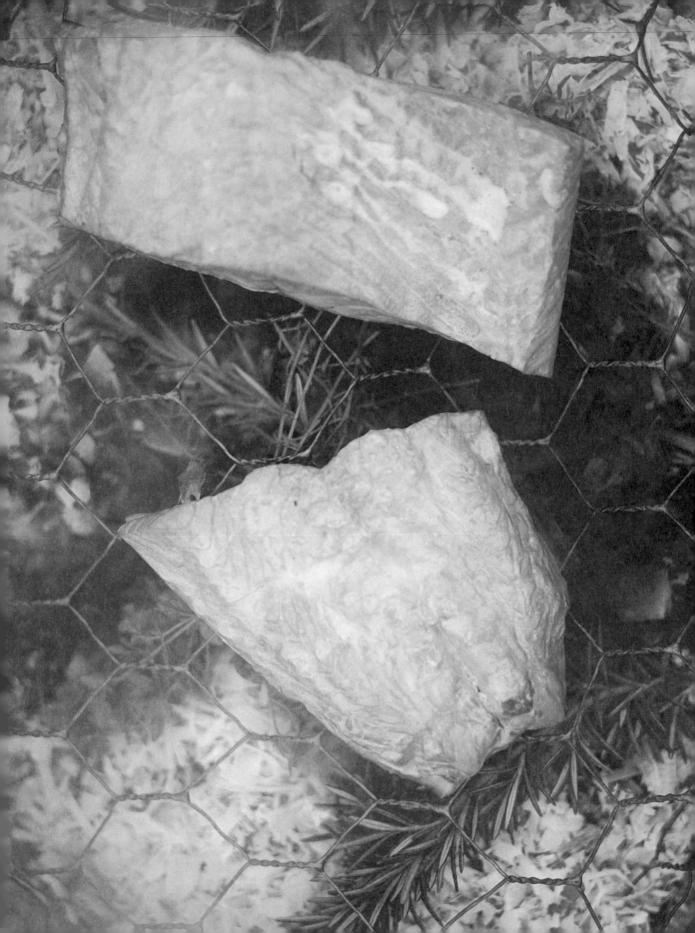

# Roasted peppers with chillies and tomatoes

There's something about peppers, chillies and tomatoes that works so well – together they do a great job. Try to get hold of different colours for all three and the finished dish will look amazing. This recipe gives you a basic way of roasting which is very easy to do. With regard to the amount of chilli you use, if you want to use less than I suggest, feel free.

Preheat the oven to 200°C/400°F/gas 6. Season the peppers, inside and out, with salt. Spread them out on a baking tray, side by side, with the cut side up.

In a bowl, mix together the garlic, cherry tomatoes, sliced chillies, capers, olives and basil leaves. Season with a pinch of salt and pepper. Add the vinegar and 4 tablespoons of extra virgin olive oil. Use your hands to mix and toss everything together.

Stuff each pepper half with a couple of spoonfuls of the filling, pushing it right down inside and making sure there's a little bit of everything in each pepper. Pour the juices left in the bowl over the peppers. You can either roast the peppers like this for a lovely vegetarian dish, or, as I like to do, you can drape 2 slices of pancetta over each pepper.

Cover the tray with tinfoil and bake in the preheated oven for 20 minutes. The peppers will steam inside the foil, softening nicely. Then remove the foil and place the peppers back in the oven for a further 20 to 30 minutes, until they are crisp and golden brown around the edges. If using pancetta, it should be lovely and crisp.

Toast your slices of sourdough bread. Divide the toasted bread between your serving plates and top with the roasted peppers. If you stab through the peppers into the bread with a sharp knife, the lovely juices will soak through. Serve with a torn ball of mozzarella, some rocket and, if you like, a tiny sprinkling of chopped chilli to give it an edge. Finish with sea salt and a drizzle of extra virgin olive oil.

PS These peppers are also lovely served with roasted fish or puréed and made into an amazing soup with chicken stock. Any leftovers are good tossed with pasta.

**serves 4**

**2 red peppers, halved lengthways, deseeded, stalk left on**
**2 yellow peppers, halved lengthways, deseeded, stalk left on**
**sea salt and freshly ground black pepper**
**1 clove of garlic, peeled and finely sliced**
**24 cherry tomatoes on the vine, halved**
**3 fresh red chillies, 2 sliced, 1 deseeded and finely chopped**
**2 tablespoons capers, soaked and drained**
**a handful of black olives, stoned**
**a bunch of fresh basil, leaves picked**
**2 tablespoons red or white wine vinegar**
**extra virgin olive oil**
**optional: 8 slices of pancetta or smoked bacon**
**4 slices of sourdough bread**
**4 balls of mozzarella cheese, torn in half**
**2 handfuls of rocket, washed and spun dry**

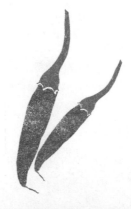

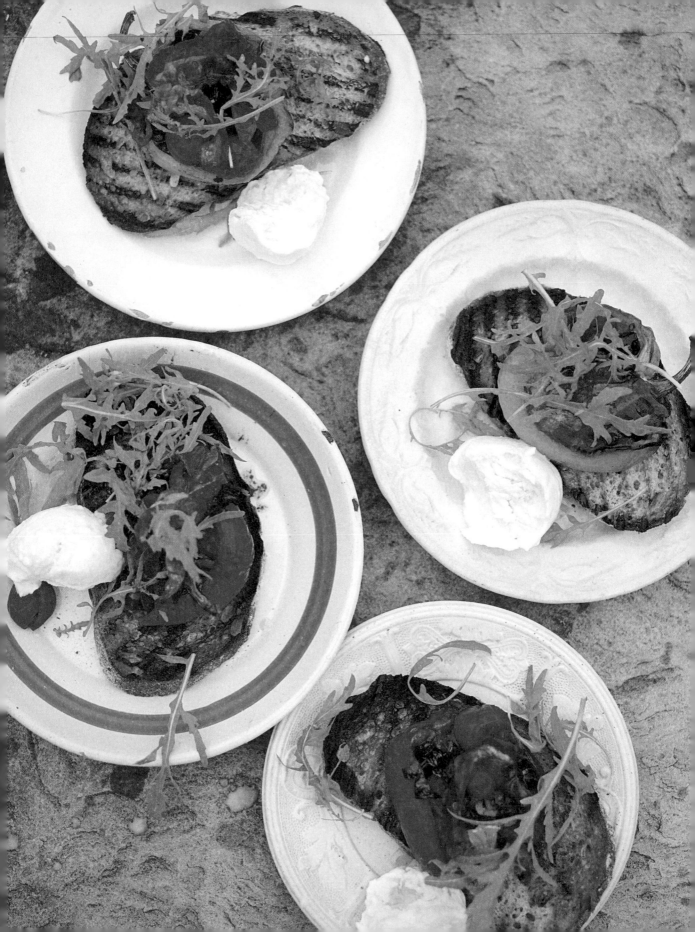

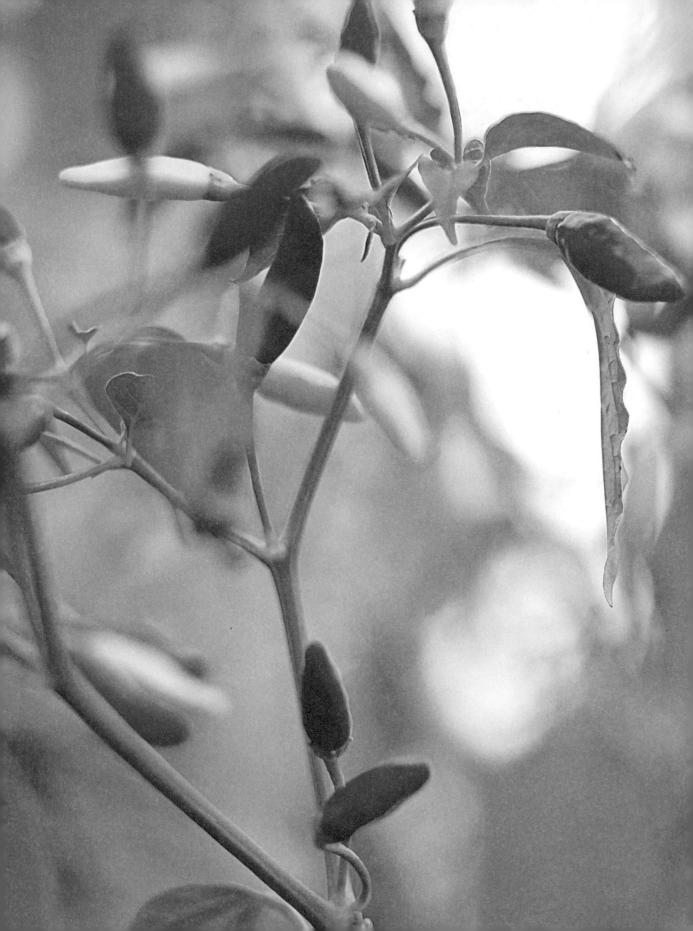

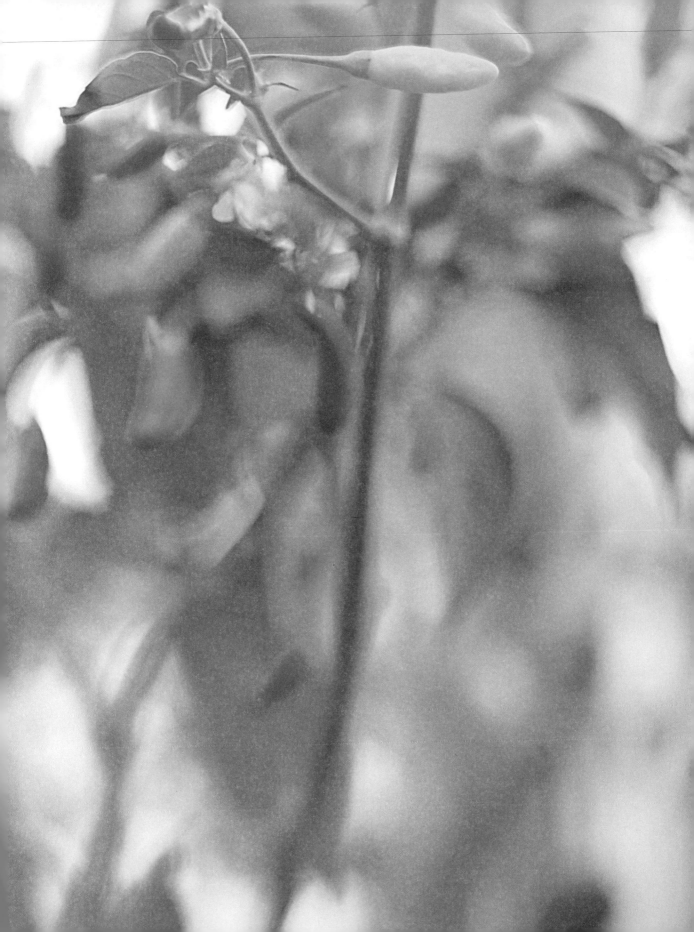

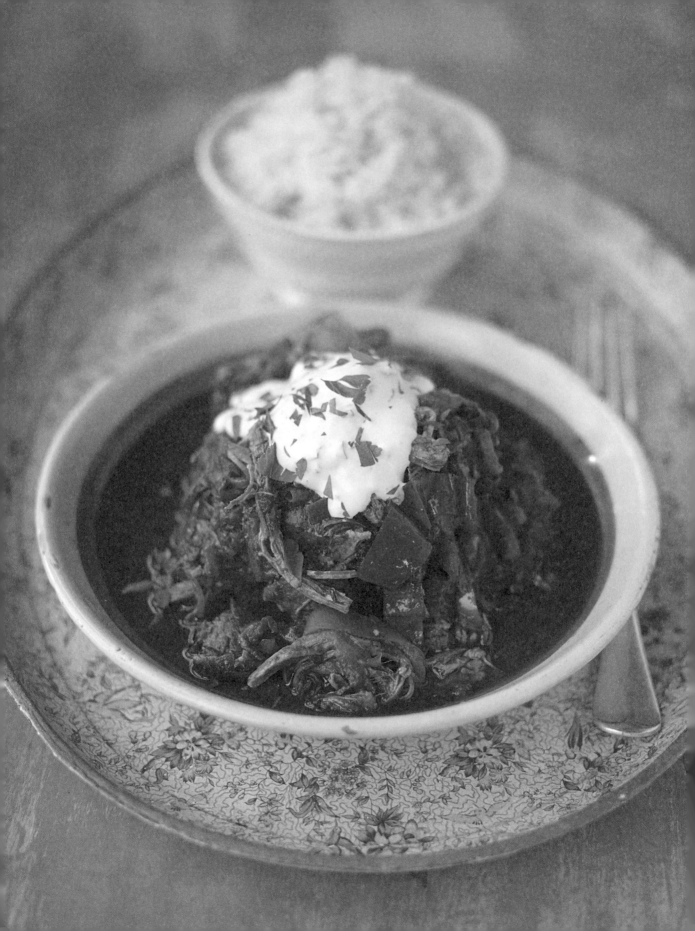

# Spicy pork and chilli-pepper goulash

The idea of cooking a tough piece of pork in a lovely pepper stew to make it extremely tender and melt-in-your-mouth is something I find quite exciting. This dish in particular is one of my favourites and, unless you've got a strange aversion to chillies and peppers, I know you'll end up making it again and again. It's a complete classic. It's also one of those dishes which tastes great when reheated the day after it's been made. You've got a whole range of chilli and pepper flavours going on; from smoked paprika to fresh chillies, and fresh peppers to sweet grilled and peeled ones. Delish!

Preheat the oven to 180°C/350°F/gas 4. Get yourself a deep, ovenproof stew pot with a lid and heat it on the hob. Score the fat on the pork in a criss-cross pattern all the way through to the meat, then season generously with salt and pepper. Pour a good glug of olive oil into the pot and add the pork, fat side down. Cook for about 15 minutes on a medium heat, to render out the fat, then remove the pork from the pot and put it to one side.

Add the onions, chilli, paprika, caraway seeds, marjoram or oregano and a good pinch of salt and pepper to the pot. Turn the heat down and gently cook the onions for 10 minutes, then add the sliced peppers, the grilled peppers and the tomatoes. Put the pork back into the pot, give everything a little shake, then pour in enough water to just cover the meat. Add the vinegar – this will give it a nice little twang. Bring to the boil, put the lid on top, then place in the preheated oven for 3 hours.

You'll know when the meat is cooked as it will be tender and sticky, and it will break up easily when pulled apart with two forks. If it's not quite there yet, put the pot back into the oven and just be patient for a little longer!

When the meat is nearly ready, cook the rice in salted, boiling water for 10 minutes until it's just undercooked, then drain in a colander, reserving some of the cooking water and pouring it back into the pan. Place the colander over the pan on a low heat and put a lid on. Leave to steam dry and cook through for 10 minutes – this will make the rice lovely and fluffy.

Stir the soured cream, lemon zest and most of the parsley together in a little bowl. When the meat is done, take the pot out of the oven and taste the goulash. You're after a balance of sweetness from the peppers and spiciness from the caraway seeds. Tear or break the meat up and serve the goulash in a big dish or bowl, with a bowl of your steaming rice and your flavoured soured cream. Sprinkle with the rest of the chopped parsley and tuck in!

serves 4 to 6

2kg pork shoulder off the bone, in one piece, skin off, fat left on
sea salt and freshly ground black pepper
olive oil
2 red onions, peeled and finely sliced
2 fresh red chillies, deseeded and finely chopped
2 generously heaped tablespoons mild smoked paprika, plus a little extra for serving
2 teaspoons ground caraway seeds
a small bunch of fresh marjoram or oregano, leaves picked
5 peppers (use a mixture of colours)
1 x 280g jar of grilled peppers, drained, peeled and chopped
1 x 400g tin of good-quality plum tomatoes
4 tablespoons red wine vinegar
400g basmati or long-grain rice, washed
1 x 142ml pot of soured cream
zest of 1 lemon
a small bunch of fresh flat-leaf parsley, chopped

# How I grow chillies and peppers

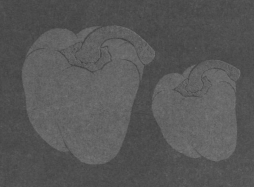

### Soil

In the UK, chillies and peppers usually don't grow too well in the garden – it's just not warm enough (although things seem to be getting hotter every year!). However, I've had great success growing mine in pots, using good organic potting compost, and keeping them inside – or in growbags in a hot, sunny spot, like a sheltered patio or against a south-facing wall. You must wait for the last frosts to be over before moving them outside. They should be brought back indoors when it turns cold again in the autumn.

### Planting

Chillies and peppers are grown in exactly the same way. You can use bought seeds or home-dried ones. The advantage of drying the seeds yourself is that you can find the varieties you like the taste (and, with chillies, the heat) of; the disadvantage is that your success rate will most likely be lower than with bought seeds.

There are literally hundreds of exciting and unusual seed varieties available to buy from specialist suppliers (see page 395), and starting them off early gives them the long growing season they need. You should sow them between January and March. If you're using seeds from a chilli or pepper that you've dried, just give it a shake. If it sounds like a maraca, you're in business! Simply break the chilli or pepper open and pour out the seeds. Get yourself a 5 to 10cm pot and fill it with your potting compost. Using your finger, make three little holes about 0.5cm deep in the compost and drop a couple of seeds into each hole. Cover over and water carefully.

If both seeds in each hole start to grow, you'll need to remove the weaker seedling to leave you with three strong ones in each pot. When they reach 8 to 12cm in height, transfer the whole lot into a larger pot (one that's 20cm wide should do them for the whole growing season). If they look a little under the weather at any time, give them an occasional feed with an organic liquid fertilizer. Tomato feed is great for chillies and peppers too.

### Harvesting and storing

Chillies and peppers will start forming soon after the first flowers fade. Most varieties are green at first and start changing colour as they ripen. They can actually be harvested at any stage once they've reached a reasonable size. Remember, though, that the heat of the chillies and the flavour of both will develop the riper they get.

Chillies are so versatile when it comes to storing and preserving. I usually dry them – all you need to do is get yourself a piece of thick cotton and a big needle, and thread it through the green stalks. Rack up as many as you've got and hang them up in your kitchen; it'll look really nice and rustic. They can also be turned into salsas, chutneys (see page 321) and rubs, or used to flavour oil. They're also really good when used to make flavoured salt.

### My growing tips

- Don't keep the plants too wet, and don't overfeed them, as this, believe it or not, gives you less tasty fruit!

- If you pick the fruit when green this often stimulates the plant into making new flowers, giving you more fruit.

- Just in case you're under threat from any rampaging elephants, large tropical chilli plants can be grown as hedges round your vegetable garden to keep them at bay!

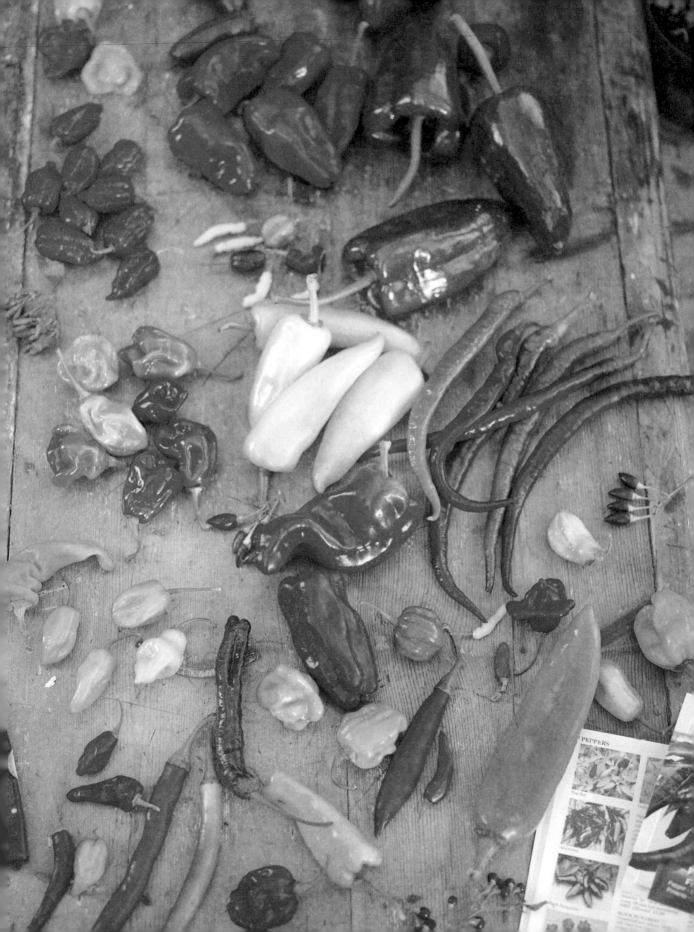

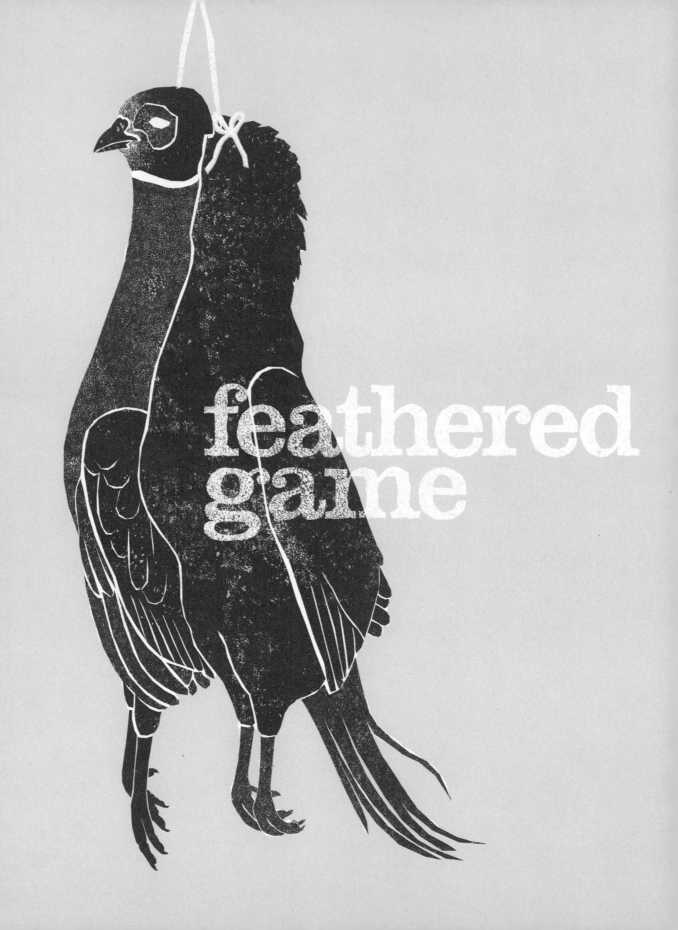

In the old days we used to eat loads of different types of birds – literally, anything that moved! But as time's gone by and life has changed, we've pretty much edited the list down to chicken, turkey and a bit of duck. Now these are all lovely, but there are so many other beautiful game birds out there that are delicious to eat as well: geese, partridge, pheasants, grouse, woodcock, pigeons and snipe. These are wild birds eating natural food, so, if you want to eat something fantastic and support an ethically sound food source, this is where it's at and I'd love you to have a try.

The natural flavours of game birds can be intensified or pulled back, depending on how long you hang them for, whether the guts are in or out, how old the animal is, how you choose to cook them and what flavours you put with them. Lighter game birds, like partridge and guinea fowl, can carry all sorts of flavours, but simply roasting them as you would a chicken is the best place to start. Personally, I love to boil up a load of garlic cloves, then I mush these up with chopped parsley and lemon zest and smear the mixture under the skin. I then roast the birds rubbed with butter – absolutely delicious.

Grouse and woodcock can be ordered in advance when in season and you can do so many things with them. Grouse should always be gutted but woodcock normally has its guts left in. The traditional way to cook and present woodcock is with its long neck bent round and the beak inserted through the side of the carcass. I love both these birds roasted pink and served with potatoes and vegetables, or with good mashed potato or polenta. I also love to eat a delicious coarse pâté made from the insides of a woodcock – sounds a bit hardcore but if you were to taste it I'm sure you'd love it served on a bit of toast! One of my favourite recipes, though, is a game pie, made with a melt-in-your-mouth stew using loads of root vegetables.

If you can get hold of some good wild wood pigeons (I'm not talking about the ones you see in Trafalgar Square in London!), they're delicious grilled on a barbecue with some smashed-up thyme, garlic and a little balsamic vinegar rubbed over them like a marinade. My mouth waters just thinking about it!

In this chapter I have given you a recipe using pigeon, one for partridge and a really rustic-style mixed game bird roast.

# Asian-style crispy pigeon with a sweet and sour dipping sauce

I absolutely love this dish. Bizarrely enough, there's something very delicate, simple and quick about the brash deep-frying method used for cooking these pigeons. Feel free to try the same method with quail or poussins. I really like to cook the pigeon until the meat is pink and slightly 'blushing'. I have eaten versions of this that have been cooked for a lot longer – so that even the bones become brittle and crisp so you can eat them – but the meat won't be as delicate. If you've never tried pigeon before, get down to the butcher's now and have a go at this recipe!

First you want to make a dry rub for the birds. In a pestle and mortar or a Flavour Shaker, bash up a good pinch of salt and a heaped teaspoon of Szechuan pepper with the five-spice. Wash the birds, inside and out, and pat them with kitchen paper until they are almost dry. Leaving them a little damp will help the rub to stick. Place your pigeons on a board and shake the rub over them, making sure you sprinkle it inside the birds as well as outside. Rub it in with your hands and try to get as much of it to stick as possible.

Pour the vegetable oil into a large saucepan or deep-fat fryer and heat it to 180°C. You can put the piece of potato into the oil as a temperature guide if you don't have a cooking thermometer – when it sizzles and floats, the oil is hot enough to start cooking.

While the oil is heating up you can make your delicious dipping sauce. Put the grated orange zest and juice into a small saucepan. Stir in the oyster sauce, sesame oil, honey and ginger, then add the lime juice and simmer for 5 minutes. Now taste it – there should be a balance of sweet, sour and salty. If you feel it needs a boost in any of these areas, this is your opportunity to do it by adding some extra lime juice, honey or salt. You'll end up with a really good sweet and sour sauce. Place the sauce in a dipping dish on a nice platter or board (it doesn't need to be kept warm).

When the oil is ready, remove the piece of potato and carefully add the pigeons to the pan. Cook for 4 to 5 minutes, after which time they should be golden on the outside and blushing pink, but not rare, on the inside. Remove the pigeons and allow any excess oil to drip off, then pat with some kitchen paper and place on a chopping board. Hold the pigeon down with the heel of your hand and carefully cut it in half lengthways, and then in quarters. Arrange the pigeon pieces on the platter or board with the dipping sauce and sprinkle with the chillies, spring onion and coriander. This is a fingerlicking, dipping kind of dinner so get yourself a finger bowl of hot water. Enjoy!

**serves 4**

sea salt and freshly
  ground Szechuan pepper
  (or black pepper if you
  can't get hold of any)
2 heaped teaspoons
  Chinese five-spice
4 wood pigeons
vegetable oil
optional: a piece of
  potato, peeled
2 fresh chillies, different
  colours if you have them,
  deseeded and sliced
4 spring onions, trimmed
  and sliced
a small bunch of fresh
  coriander, leaves picked

*for the dipping sauce*
2 oranges, zest of 1,
  juice of both
8 tablespoons oyster sauce
2 teaspoons sesame oil
1 teaspoon runny honey
a thumb-sized piece of fresh
  ginger, peeled and grated
juice of 1 lime

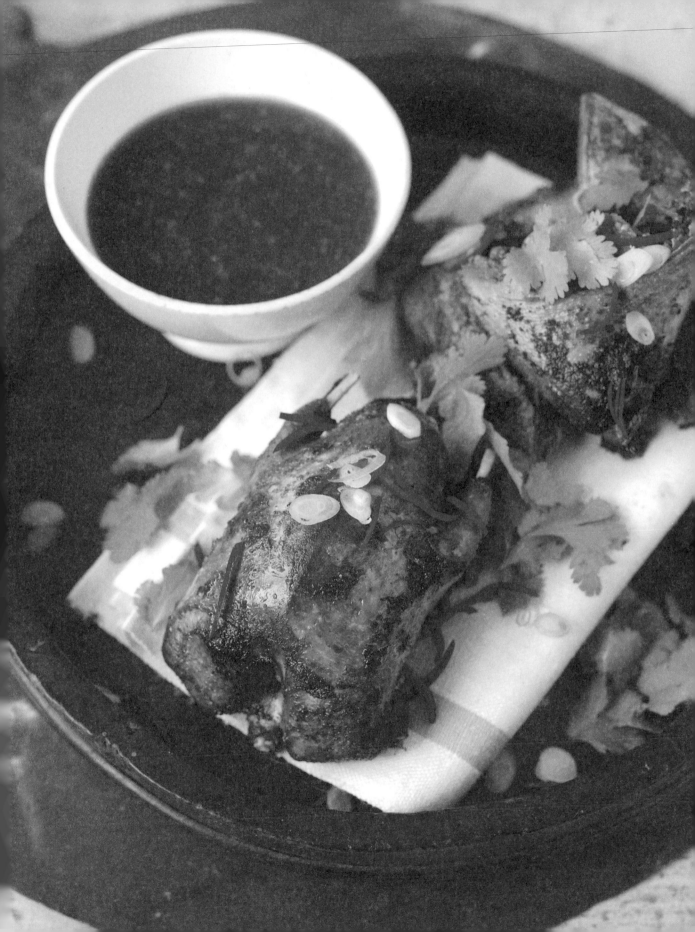

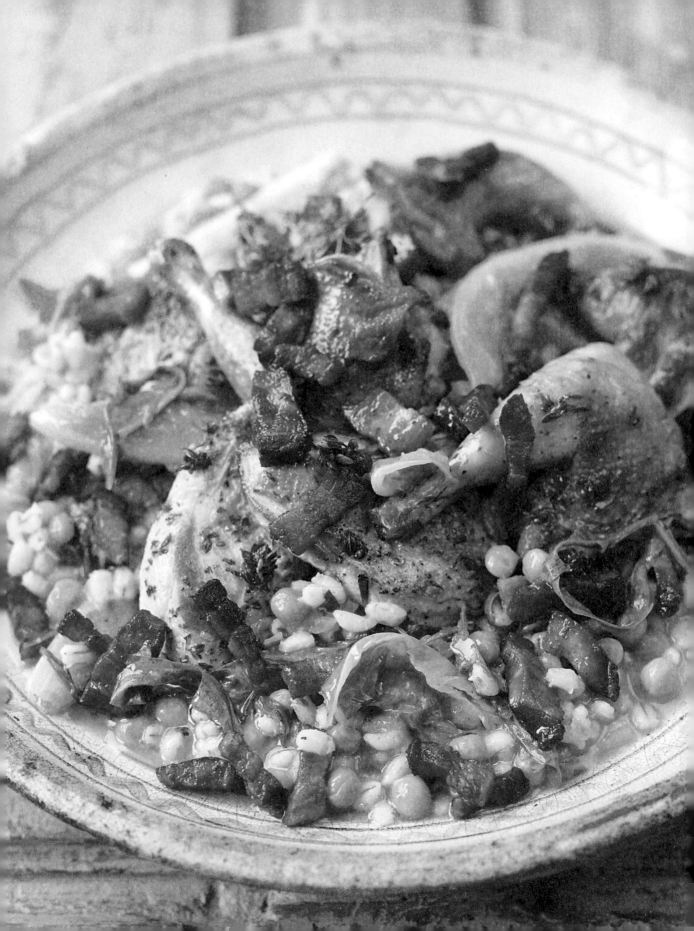

# Pan-fried partridge with a delicate pearl barley, pea and lettuce stew

What a simple, beautiful dish. Partridge is mild-flavoured, so it's a great introduction to game birds. Barley is an old English ingredient that isn't used so much these days, but it's fantastic in stews. Peas with lettuce is a French thing and they work so well together. And I love the pan-cooking method – not only is it quick but it's exciting too.

Cook the pearl barley in boiling, salted water for about 50 minutes, or until tender but still with a little bite, then drain and leave to steam dry. Next, heat a glug of olive oil in a frying pan and add the onion and a pinch of salt. Cook slowly on a low heat for about 10 minutes, without colouring too much. Add the barley and the peas. Cover with the stock and bring to the boil. Simmer for 10 minutes, stirring every now and then.

On a board, squash and mash the flour and butter together with a fork until you have a paste. This is called a 'beurre manié' and it's a great way of thickening stews or sauces without having to stir the flour in directly, which could give you lumps. Stir half of the dough into the peas and barley and continue to simmer until the liquid begins to thicken. If, after 5 minutes, it's not thick enough, add some more of your beurre manié. What you want to achieve is a silky smooth broth. Continue to simmer for another 10 minutes, adding a little extra stock if it gets too dry, while you cook your partridges.

Put some olive oil into another frying pan. Season the partridge legs with salt and pepper and add them to the pan. (The legs go in first because they're tougher than the breasts and need longer to cook.) Shake them about and, after a few minutes, when they're lightly golden, add the bacon bits and stir gently to stop them catching on the bottom. Meanwhile, lay the partridge breasts out, sprinkle over the chopped thyme and press on to both sides with a good pinch of seasoning. When the bacon is lightly golden, push it to one side of the pan with the partridge legs and lay the breasts in, skin side down. Cook for 4 minutes, then turn and cook on the other side for a minute to give you crispy skin and moist meat. You can cook them for longer if you like your meat well done.

When the breasts are done, taste the barley broth and adjust the seasoning, then stir in the lettuce and rocket – they only need a minute or so to cook. Serve the barley, peas and lettuce with the partridge breasts and legs on top and the bacon pieces sprinkled over. Spoon the broth juices over the top. Lovely homely cooking!

serves 2

100g pearl barley
olive oil
1 red onion, peeled and finely chopped
sea salt and freshly ground black pepper
200g frozen peas
500ml good chicken or vegetable stock
1 heaped tablespoon flour
25g butter
2 partridges, washed and patted dry, broken into legs and breasts
100g chunky smoked bacon or pancetta, rind off, cut into lardons
a few sprigs of fresh thyme, leaves picked and chopped
a handful of cos or romaine lettuce leaves, washed and spun dry
a handful of rocket, washed and spun dry

feathered game

265

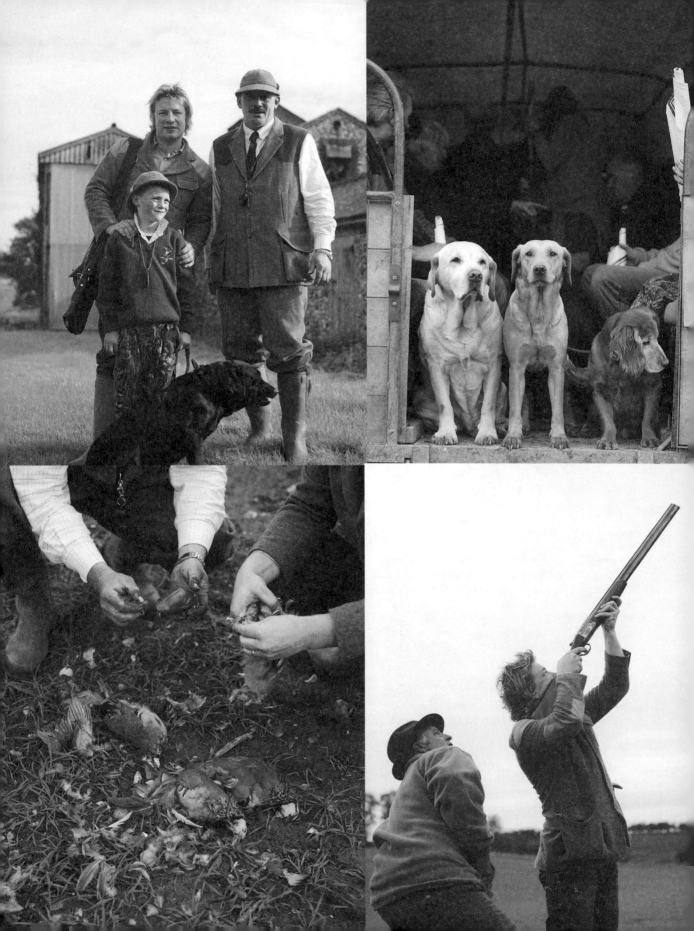

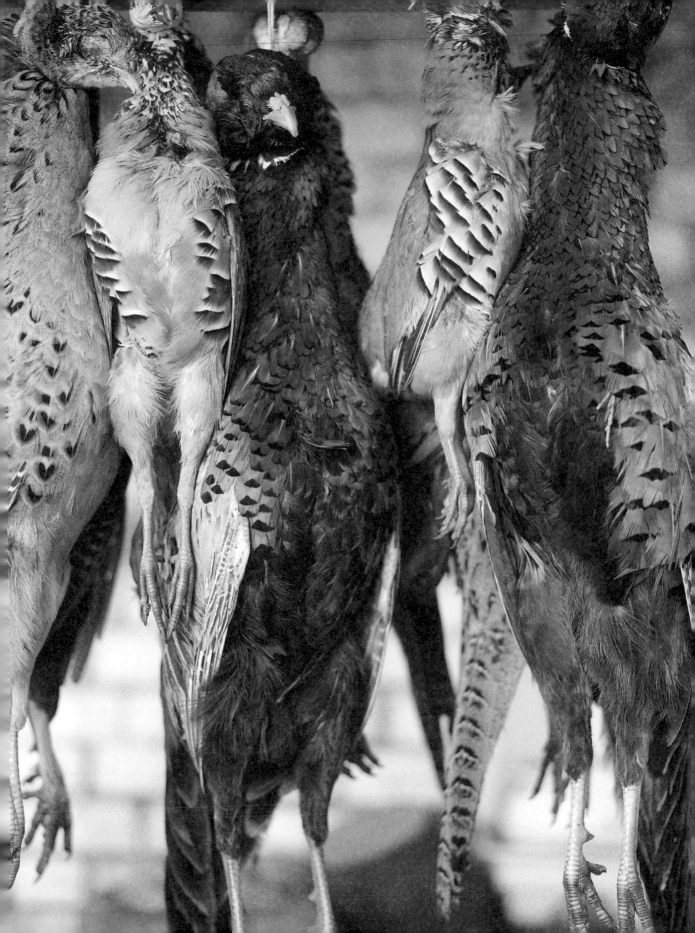

# Roast of incredible game birds with proper polenta

This Italian-style extravaganza is a luxury version of a Sunday roast. Use whatever game's available, or combine game birds with everyday chicken. If you give your butcher some notice, he can get you almost anything that's in season and prepare it for you!

Preheat your oven to full whack. Either ask your butcher to spatchcock the guinea fowl or chicken, and the pheasant for you, or have a go at doing it yourself. Turn the bird upside down and cut underneath the legs with a good pair of scissors. Remove the bony part of the carcass that has no meat on it (bearing in mind that you want to save the incredible meat around the legs) and open the bird out like a book. You can then stuff the cavities of the other birds with flavourings – a sprig of rosemary, a sprig of thyme and a little orange or lemon zest.

Place the onion, celery and carrots in a large roasting tray (or two small ones) and lay the sausages and birds on top. Throw in the bay leaves and the rest of the thyme and rosemary. Drizzle with olive oil and massage it into each bird. Season all the meat generously. Place in the preheated oven and immediately turn the temperature down to 180°C/350°F/gas 4. Cook for 1½ hours, turning the birds a few times, until the meat is juicy and cooked through to the bone.

After half an hour, bring 2 litres of salted water to the boil in a non-stick pan and whisk in the polenta. Turn the heat right down, place a lid on so it's ajar (otherwise the pan might spit hot polenta at you!) and simmer for 50 minutes, stirring it as often as you can. If it starts to become too thick, add some more hot water.

Remove the birds from the oven, lift them out of the tray and keep warm. Put the tray on the hob, pour in the wine and simmer gently to make a quick sauce. Then see to the polenta – it'll need some serious perking up now. Stir in about three-quarters of the butter and all the grated Parmesan. Once smooth, taste it and season if required. It should now be delicious! Spoon all the polenta on to a big board or platter, spread it out evenly and put to one side to firm up a little.

Give your sauce a stir and add the rest of the butter. Strain it through a sieve into a pan, pressing down hard. Cut the bigger birds into drumstick thighs and breast pieces and place with all the other birds on top of your polenta. Slice the sausages and add to the pile. Spoon the red wine sauce over the top and finish with a drizzle of extra virgin olive oil. Put the board in the middle of the table and let everyone dive in. A fantastic feast!

**serves 8**

1 pheasant, spatchcocked, washed and patted dry
1 guinea fowl or 1.2kg chicken, spatchcocked, washed and patted dry
1 partridge, washed and patted dry
2 wood pigeons, washed and patted dry
4 quails, washed and patted dry
a small bunch of fresh rosemary
a small bunch of fresh thyme
zest of 1 lemon or orange
1 red onion, peeled and roughly chopped
4 sticks of celery, trimmed and roughly chopped
4 carrots, peeled and roughly chopped
4 Italian sausages or 2 rings of Cumberland sausage
a few sprigs of fresh bay, leaves picked
olive oil
sea salt and freshly ground black pepper
500g polenta
a wineglass of red wine (Chianti is nice)
100g butter
2 handfuls of freshly grated Parmesan cheese
extra virgin olive oil

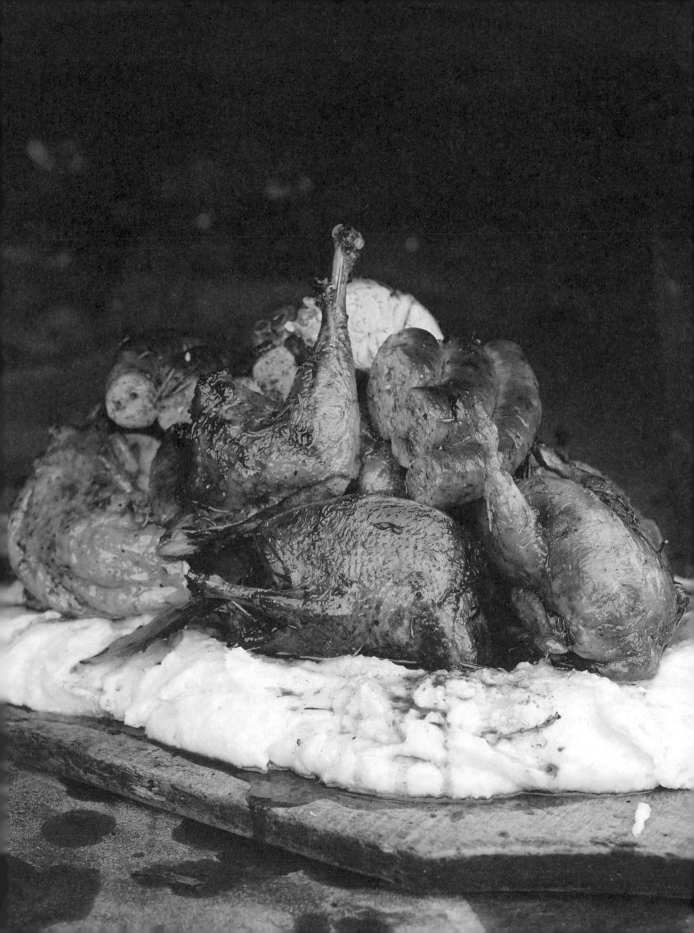

# What I've learned about shooting

My old man has always bought pheasants and pigeon, along with other game, to serve in his pub, from local shoots and hunts. So I've grown up being used to the whole thing. Now that I've been living in London for a while, I do feel that there's quite a lot of misunderstanding and misrepresentation about shoots and shooting. So as a publican's son from the countryside, here are my observations . . .

There's always going to be a bit of tension between those involved in the culling of animals and the vegetarians or animal-rights people. Of course, millions of people *do* eat meat – we're at the top of the food chain, so it would be unrealistic for us not to. However, I do have serious respect for vegetarians for not eating meat, and vegans for not even wearing any type of animal product – I think it's an amazing gesture to give up eating meat and I know I couldn't do it.

My second point is somewhat linked to the first. Formal shooting days, where hundreds of wild birds are coaxed into flying over shooters, are basically considered a sport, which really upsets protesters – they wonder how you can possibly enjoy a day out when the focus is on killing birds. Although I understand how they feel, there's something quite open and honest about the traditional British shoot. If you eat meat, and if the shoots are responsible and sell their birds to game dealers to be enjoyed and consumed in restaurants and homes, and if the long-standing basic manners or etiquette are embraced as part of the day, and if the amount of birds shot in a day is responsibly capped, the great British shoot is about as decent as any slaughter of food is ever going to be. The death of an animal is never ever a nice thing, but to me what happens at shoots is a hundred times more ethical than the conditions and treatment of battery-farmed poultry. I really think shooting is what it is: it's open for all to see.

I think many people consider shooting a posh person's sport and for some reason have a big aversion to this. In medieval times, game birds were a delicacy owned by the king, and the right to hunt game was given as a reward or bribe to nobles and clergy, so this is where the modern-day 'posh' association has probably come from. Whether people directly say it or not, I think there's still a historic lingering of the great British class issue here. Yet in my experience the reality is quite different. I've been on a number of shoots over the past few years and at each one there has been a total cross-section of people from all social backgrounds – plumbers, carpenters, builders. Even OAPs and young boys and girls join in, usually as 'beaters' to get some fresh air (they don't actually 'beat' the birds

– they just tap trees and disturb the birds so they fly up towards the shooters). The OAPs normally get a couple of birds for free, £20 tucked in their back pocket and a round down the pub afterwards.

A really good website for anyone who wants to understand more about shoots is run by the National Organization for Beaters and you can find it at www.nobs.org.uk (I promise it's not porn!). It will tell you all you need to know, with information about your nearest local shoots. Go and take a look.

# My tips for preparing game birds

## Buying and what to look for

- The age of a bird has a bearing on how good it will be to eat. Those below a year old will be very good, but any older than that and the meat starts to toughen up and dry out, especially with grouse.

- The bird should obviously look fresh, and if it has been plucked the skin should be dry, not moist. If it still has its feathers, look for bright eyes that are not sunken or dull. The feathers should have a lustre to them and not be dull and lifeless. If the bird smells strong, you may think it's off, but it is more likely to have been hung for a while. Some people prefer their game to be strong-tasting. You should be able to buy hung or reasonably fresh depending on what you prefer.

## Hanging

Pheasants and woodcock should be hung for five to seven days, snipe for up to five days, grouse and partridge for three to four days; a day is enough for wild duck, while quail doesn't need to be hung.

## Plucking and singeing

If you want to have a go at this, plucking a game bird is very easy. You need to hold the bird in one hand with the head away from you and the breast pointing upwards. Using your free hand, and starting at the neck, grasp a few feathers at a time and, giving a sharp tug towards the head, pull out the feathers. Never try to pull out too many feathers at once. If you keep the skin taut as you pluck, it'll be less likely to tear. Work your way back along the breasts, then the legs. Tail and wing feathers are much tougher and need to be removed one at a time. Once plucked, the bird needs to be singed to burn off any fine hairs not removed by plucking. Simply pass the bird over an open flame.

## Storing

Game can be frozen but you should prepare it as though you were going to cook it, discarding the insides (unless you're cooking woodcock), then freeze it.

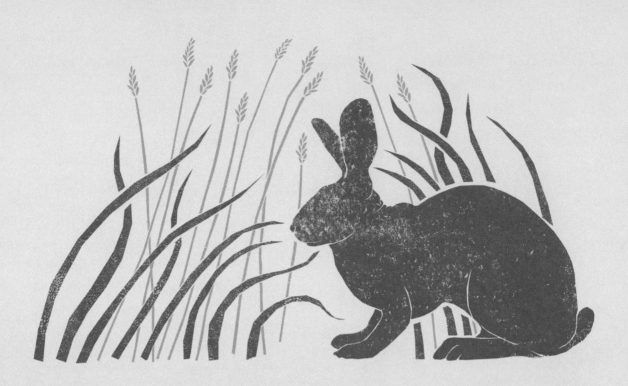

Furred game is really exciting to cook. Depending on the country you live in, 'game' essentially means wild animals that can be hunted or caught for food. In the UK, animals considered as furred game are deer (venison), rabbit and hare, although historically squirrels and badgers have also been eaten. I've always considered wild boar as game as well, although they haven't got game status in the UK. There aren't that many left in this country any more – just a few escapees that have bred!

The furred game of other countries might seem a bit odd to us, but totally normal to the locals. (Before I go any further, I want to make it clear that I'm talking about fully sustainable, unendangered species.) In Peru they eat guinea pigs, in Australia kangaroo and possums, in South Africa a type of buck called a kudu, along with buffalo, in Canada they eat moose and bear, and in parts of Asia they even eat various members of the monkey and dog families, but we won't go there in

this chapter! Extreme poverty, hunger and a natural survival instinct would have been the original incentives to eat these types of meat, but it wouldn't have taken long for the realization to set in that a lot of these animals were very tasty as well as being, nutritionally, a supreme natural food source. For all these reasons they would have become a major part of regular diets. That is, until modern times, especially in Britain, where game is now considered merely a small gastronomic part of the meat world compared to farmed animals. I'm not going to cook things like possums and kangaroos in this chapter, of course, as they are not animals that are local to me, but I *am* going to be cooking deer, rabbit and hare.

In simplest terms, meat is meat and it's there to be eaten. The proof of that comes from our own history. Most of our great-great-grandparents would have been tucking into animals like squirrels and badgers (which we would now consider odd) on quite a regular basis. And, yes, you can try eating rat, but I would never do that because of what they eat and where they live. Something like a squirrel, however, I totally get because they have an incredible diet of nuts and herbs and live in clean surroundings. Just a couple of months ago I ate a grilled spatchcocked squirrel at the famous St John restaurant in London and it was absolutely incredible! It tasted just like really good-quality chicken and had a confit rabbit leg texture – just brilliant.

Rabbit is a bloody gorgeous meat to eat and I love cooking it at home every now and then. It's fantastically lean, a bit like chicken, and a wonderful carrier of flavours, whether you're using it in a classic English dish or with stronger Asian-style flavourings. But my love for cooking and eating rabbit is not shared these days with the majority of you out there. The reality is that our choices of meat have decreased over the years, and the fact that there are thousands of recipes for rabbit which have never been passed down through the generations is a shame. Sixty-plus years ago it was more commonly eaten than chicken, which to me suggests that it's not because of the flavour but because we've lost the knowledge of how to cook it that it's not eaten so much these days. Hare is another delicious meat – it's more 'steaky', darker and richer than rabbit.

I do think views on eating furred game are changing, though, and it's very promising! I can slow-cook a shoulder of wild boar with red wine and veggies and shred it into the most incredible bolognese-style ragù. Or I can use a whole load of different game in a lasagne, or pot-roast a saddle of venison really hot and fast with some smoked bacon and beautiful veg from the garden. Or I can confit some rabbit legs in olive oil with bay and rosemary until the meat falls off the bone and toss it into a lovely warm salad with roasted cloves of garlic and balsamic vinegar. And if I put these on the menu in the restaurant, they'll sell out every time. So this is telling me something. And the customers are a total mix of people from all age groups, different classes and ethnic backgrounds. So the good news is that you lot love eating game, but you just might be a little nervous about cooking it. Well, I hope this chapter helps to get you trying a few dishes at home – they are some of my favourites.

# furred game

# Game ragù with pappardelle

The thing I love about this recipe is its flexibility. You can use different types of game and ask your butcher to prepare them for you. If you cut the meat big and chunky this makes a delicious stew, but if cut smaller, and cooked till it falls apart, it makes an amazing pasta sauce. I'm using pappardelle here, but any other robust pasta like rigatoni, tagliatelle or broken-up dried sheets of lasagne work well too.

In Italy, this sort of stewed meat would traditionally have been eaten on toast for breakfast by hunters or manual labourers who would have been up at the crack of dawn. It's probably a bit more appropriate for lunch though!

PS Red wine and game is a classic combination, but I'm using white wine here to lighten the flavours.

Preheat the oven to 180°C/350°F/gas 4. Pour a glug of olive oil into a casserole type pan and put it on the heat. Add the onion, carrots, swede, rosemary, thyme and bay leaves and cook gently for 10 minutes. Stir in the meat and the flour, pour in the wine and add a generous pinch of salt and pepper. Pour in the stock – there should be enough to just cover the meat. Bring to a gentle boil, put a lid on and place in the preheated oven for 1½ hours, until the meat falls apart easily.

When the stew looks good, bring a very large pan of salted water to the boil and stir in the pappardelle. Cook according to the packet instructions. While the pasta's cooking, you can get your ragù sauce rockin' and rollin'! Remove the bay leaves from the sauce and add the butter to it. Beat in half the Parmesan and half the orange zest – just a hint will make all the difference. Place the lid on top. Pick and chop your parsley leaves now – you want them to be nice and fresh, with as much colour and flavour as possible, so don't do this any earlier.

Drain the pasta in a colander, reserving some of the cooking water. Get everyone around the table, then toss the pasta with the sauce and the chopped parsley (you may have to do this in batches), adding some of the reserved cooking water if need be, to make the sauce silky and loose – very important for good texture. Taste and correct the seasoning. Serve with the remaining grated Parmesan and orange zest sprinkled over and a drizzle of good extra virgin olive oil. What an incredible pasta dish!

serves 6

olive oil
1 red onion, peeled and finely chopped
2 carrots, peeled and chopped
½ a swede, peeled and diced
a sprig of fresh rosemary, leaves picked and chopped
a small bunch of fresh thyme, leaves picked
2 bay leaves
1 rabbit or hare, boned and cut into 1cm dice
300g venison haunch, cut into 1cm dice
1 tablespoon flour
a large wineglass of white wine
sea salt and freshly ground black pepper
500ml good-quality chicken or vegetable stock
500g pappardelle
a knob of butter
75g freshly grated Parmesan cheese
zest of 1 orange
a bunch of fresh flat-leaf parsley
extra virgin olive oil

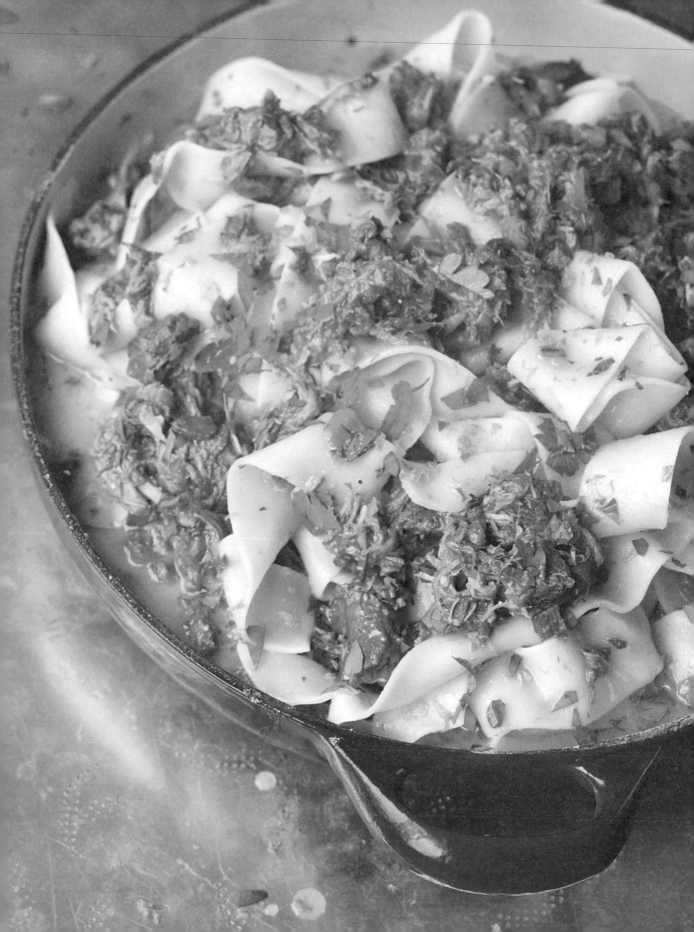

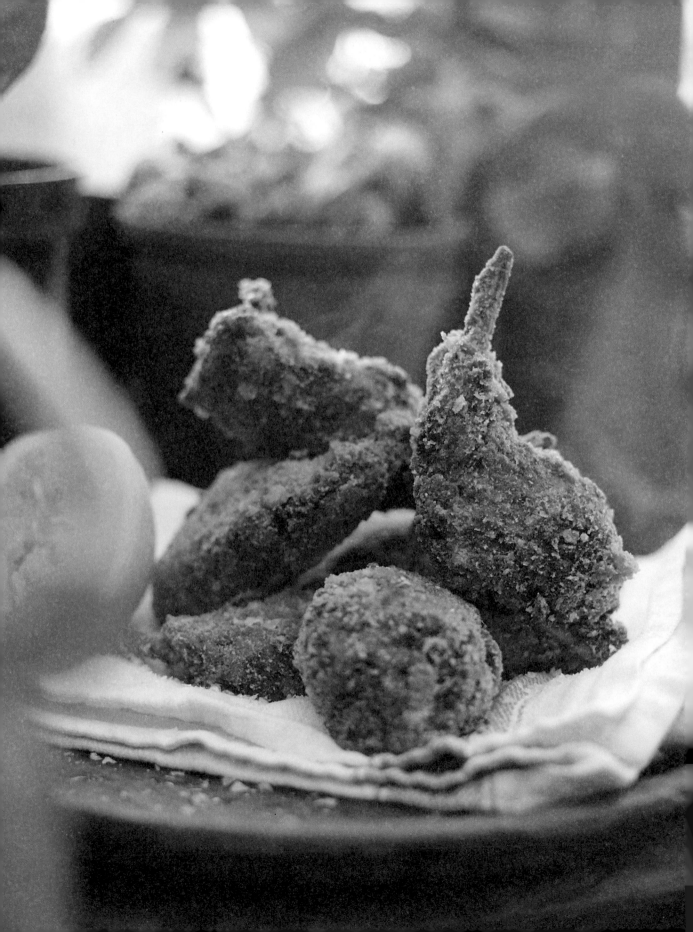

# E.F.R.

E.F.R.... Essex fried rabbit! If you've never tried rabbit before, this is a good place to start – this dish isn't particularly filling, so it's best as a starter or snack. Wild rabbit has a richer, gamier taste, but some people prefer the flavour of farmed. You can ask your butcher to prepare and joint the rabbit for you. And you can cook and breadcrumb the rabbit pieces in advance and put them in the fridge until you're ready to fry them.

Heat a saucepan big enough to hold all the rabbit pieces snugly in one layer. Pour in a glug of olive oil and add the rabbit, salt and pepper, the halved garlic bulb, 2 sprigs of rosemary and the wine and stock. Put a lid on the pan and simmer gently for 45 minutes to an hour, without colouring the rabbit too much. Check after half an hour, topping up with a little water if necessary. When done, the meat will just come off the bone if pulled gently. Allow to cool down.

While the rabbit is cooking, whiz the stale bread in a food processor with half the grated Parmesan until you have fine breadcrumbs. Have three wide shallow bowls or plates ready – fill the first one with sifted, seasoned flour, the second with the beaten eggs and the third with the breadcrumbs.

When cool enough to handle, put the cooked rabbit and garlic pieces into the flour and toss to coat. Shake off any excess flour and dip them into the egg. Let any excess drip off, then lay the pieces on top of the breadcrumbs. Before you cover them, sprinkle with the thyme leaves and remaining Parmesan. Now roll and pat the pieces in the breadcrumbs, put them on to a tray and keep in the fridge till you're ready to fry them.

Heat some vegetable oil to 180°C in a deep saucepan or deep fat fryer. You can place a piece of potato in the oil as a temperature guide – when it's golden and floats on the surface it's ready. Cover a plate with a double thickness of kitchen paper and put this to one side. Remove the potato from the oil, then fry the pieces of rabbit and garlic carefully (you can do this in batches) for 2 to 3 minutes, or until beautifully golden and crisp. For the last 20 seconds, drop in the remaining rosemary sprigs – they'll go deep green and crispy and lovely.

Lift everything out with a slotted spoon and drain on the kitchen paper. Dust with a little sea salt. Squeeze the garlic out of its skin into a bowl – it will be sweet, mild and delicious. Serve it with the rabbit, crispy rosemary and lemon halves.

serves 2

olive oil
1 wild rabbit, jointed into shoulders, legs and saddle split in half, washed and patted dry
sea salt and freshly ground black pepper
1 bulb of garlic, cut in half horizontally
4 sprigs of fresh rosemary
200ml white wine
200ml good-quality chicken or vegetable stock
a few slices of stale white bread, crusts removed
2 big handfuls of freshly grated Parmesan cheese
plain flour, for dusting
3 large organic or free-range eggs, beaten
a few sprigs of fresh thyme, leaves picked
optional: a small piece of potato, peeled
vegetable oil
1 lemon, halved

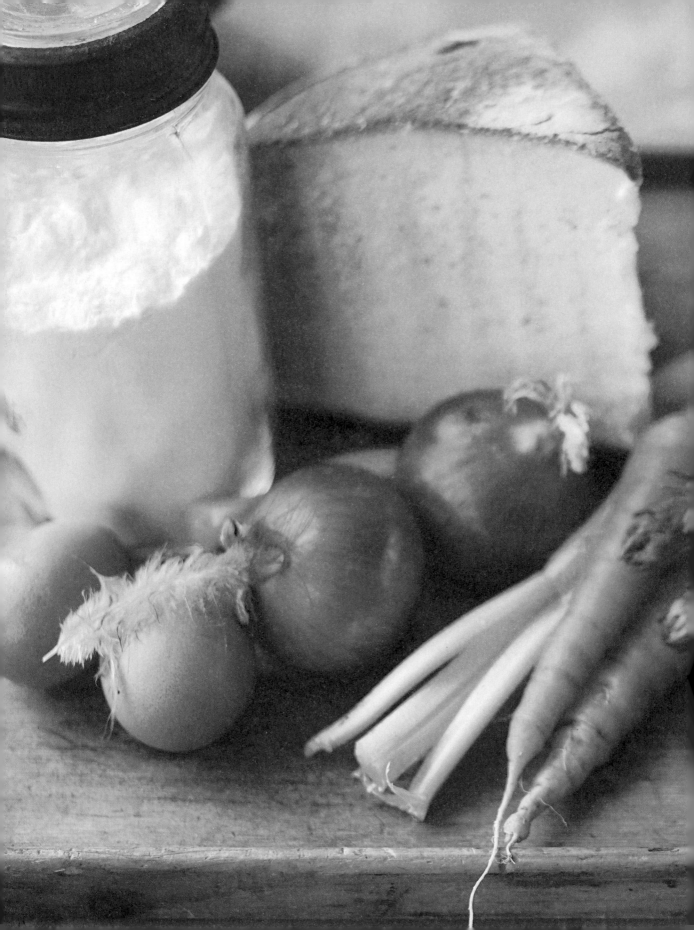

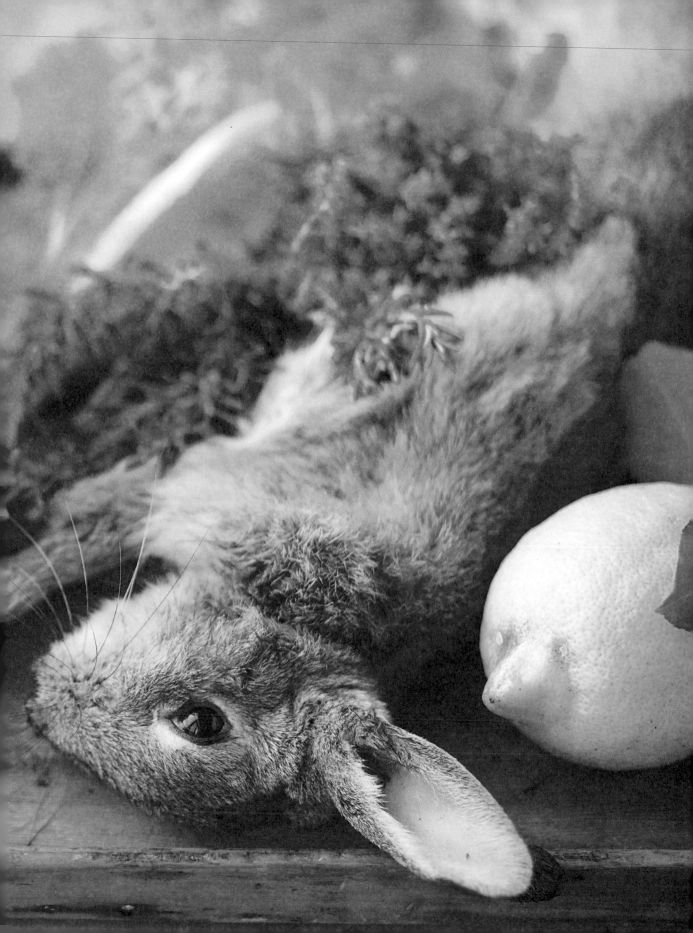

# Pan-roasted venison with creamy baked potato and celeriac

Venison is a fantastic lean dark meat. You can swap the celeriac for parsnips, Jerusalem artichokes or even fennel, but you must keep the ratio of potatoes in there so it tastes delish.

Preheat your oven to 180°C/350°F/gas 4 and butter a large, shallow baking dish. Slice the potatoes and celeriac into discs just under 0.5cm thick. Place the slices into a large pan, cover with cold water, season with salt and bring to the boil. Simmer for 5 minutes, then drain in a colander and allow the veg to steam dry for a minute or so. Put back into the pan with the cream, chopped garlic, sage, half the Parmesan and a good pinch of salt and pepper. Mix together, then tip into the buttered baking dish and spread out evenly. Pour any mixture left in the pan over the top. Cover tightly with tinfoil and cook in the preheated oven for 35 to 40 minutes until golden brown.

Chop your juniper berries and rosemary, add a pinch of salt and pepper, then sprinkle over a board. Rub the venison all over with olive oil before rolling it across the board and pressing it into the flavourings. Heat an ovenproof frying pan over a high heat and add a glug of olive oil. Sear the venison for a couple of minutes on all sides, then remove the pan from the heat. Add the smashed garlic bulb and any leftover flavourings from the chopping board. Shake everything together, pour in a splash of water to cool things down and place in the oven. Cook according to your liking – about 8 minutes will give you medium venison.

When the potatoes are cooked, take them out of the oven and remove the tinfoil. Return the dish to the oven, uncovered, and bake for another 10 to 15 minutes until bubbling and golden.

Take the venison out of the oven and let it rest on a plate, covered loosely with foil. Pour away any excess fat. Squash the garlic cloves with a fork and discard the skins. Mix the garlic with the herbs in the pan and place on the heat. Pour in the red wine, simmer until it has reduced by half and then add the butter. Stir with a wooden spoon, scraping up all the sticky meaty goodness from the bottom. As soon as the sauce comes together, take the pan off the heat, correct the seasoning and stir in another knob of butter. Carve the venison into 1cm thick slices. Pour any resting juices from the plate back into the pan, then pour your gravy through a sieve over the meat and serve with the potato and celeriac bake.

serves 4

50g butter, melted, plus a
  couple of extra knobs
1kg potatoes, peeled
1 small celeriac, peeled
  and halved
sea salt and freshly
  ground black pepper
500ml double cream
1 clove of garlic, peeled
  and finely chopped
½ a small bunch of fresh
  sage, leaves picked
  and roughly chopped
100g freshly grated
  Parmesan cheese
10 juniper berries, crushed
  with the side of a knife
3 sprigs of fresh rosemary,
  leaves picked
1kg venison loin in one
  fat piece, trimmed
olive oil
1 bulb of garlic, unpeeled
  and smashed, papery
  skin removed
a wineglass of good-quality
  red wine, like Pinot Noir

furred game

280

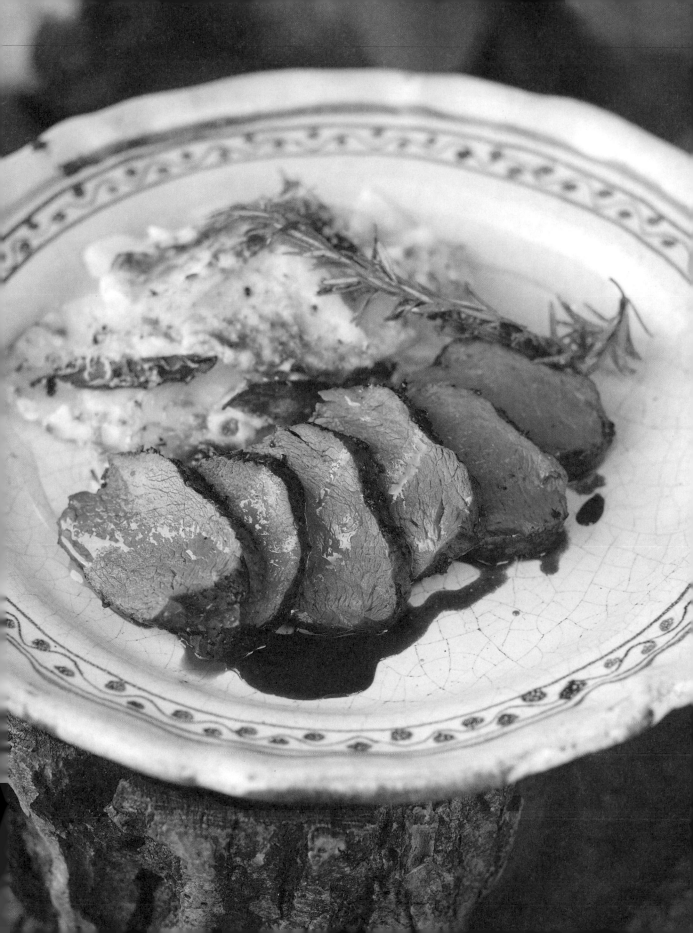

# Furred game

### Where does game come from?

In Britain, most of our furred game comes via game dealers from gamekeepers who look after large farming estates. I've met very few gamekeepers who just want to kill all their game and get rid of them (even if that was possible). However, they do need to control the numbers, otherwise they will destroy any new forests that are being planted by responsible landowners, as well as eat all the vegetables and cereals being grown for human consumption. If the numbers of game were not controlled, there would be a serious impact on farmers which would affect their products and their livelihood.

So the role of the gamekeeper is an incredibly important one. It might seem heartless to shoot animals and eat them, but it's actually instrumental in maintaining the countryside and making sure there is enough food for us. When the numbers of animals, particularly rabbits, grow, they run out of natural food and go looking for something else. They'll eat any new planting – I've seen trees completely stripped of bark round the base.

Also, firing bullets round the countryside is bloody dangerous and is a highly controlled and responsible job. I hold a shotgun licence and various rifle licences myself, and in all my years of growing up in the country and mixing with gamekeepers or locals who are out controlling pests I've never come across anyone with a gung-ho attitude towards shooting game. The whole process is perfectly aligned and is about controlling numbers and maintaining a balance of the countryside. And if there is a food source at the end of it, great.

So if you want to eat tasty meat, I think wild game, shot in season and bought from your local gamekeeper, butcher or game dealer, is about as ethical and nutritious a food source as you can get. On the whole the animals are completely wild, they feed on whatever is growing naturally and they've had unrestricted lives. It's Formula One meat!

### Buying game

You can buy oven-ready furred game from supermarkets but if you want to know a bit more about what you're buying, go to a specialist game dealer and don't be afraid to ask for advice. A game dealer will be able to tell you the age of the animal, when it was killed, and how long it has been hung for. They will often have a good supply of locally shot game of different ages that has been hung for different lengths of time. Any good local butcher worth his salt shouldn't have any trouble getting you some game on request. He will also skin and clean the animal for you and will joint it if you ask. Farm shops and farmers' markets often stock different kinds of furred game, and fine food fairs and the internet are other good sources.

### Hanging game

Game must be hung if it is to develop its flavour and become tender. The time required varies according to the age and type of the animal, but as a rule rabbits are gutted immediately then hung for two to three days, hares have their guts left in and need hanging for four to five days, and venison can be gutted immediately and will generally be at its best after seven to twenty days. They all need to be hung in a cold, well-ventilated area, away from other hanging animals. Leave hanging to the butcher or game keeper, unless you know what you're doing.

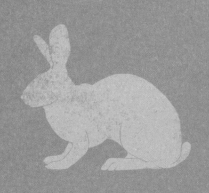

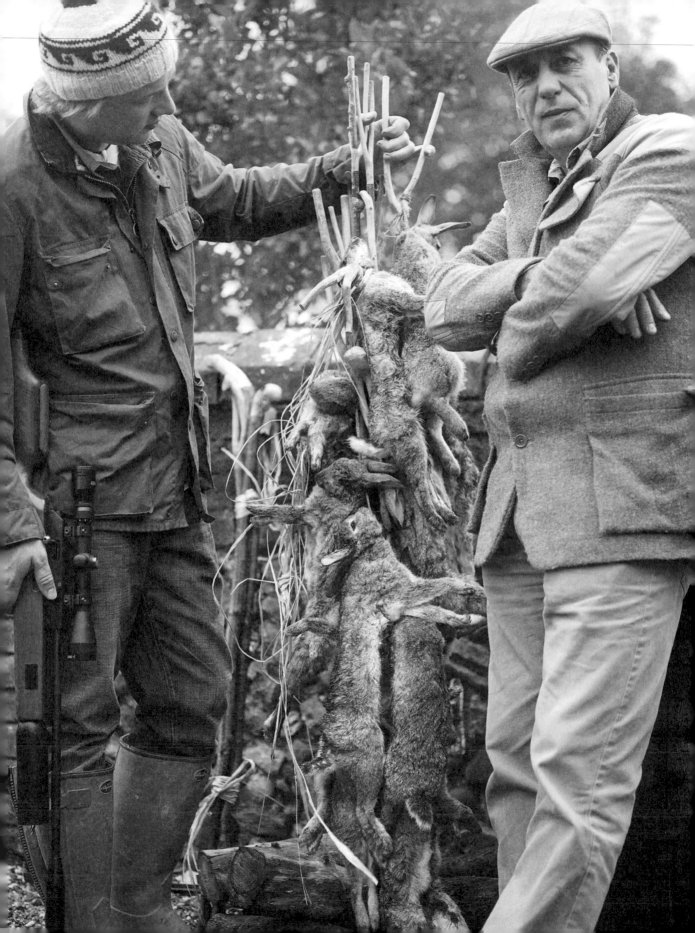

# mushrooms

I have a total soft spot for mushrooms, but it's hard for me to cook them at home because my wife can't stand them. So I have them when I'm cooking just for myself, whether in soups, simply pan-fried on toast or tossed into pastas and risottos. They're also brilliant with game, or as stuffings for wonderful roasts, shaved raw into salads or dry-grilled on the barbecue with just the tiniest pinch of salt and a squeeze of lemon juice. They're even great served alongside fish – now that's a winning surf and turf combination – a nice chunk of line-caught fish roasted in the oven with a pile of lovely buttered new potatoes and mushrooms cooked with herbs and a squeeze of lemon juice. There's nothing better. And the fact that I don't usually cook them at home because of the missus makes them even more of an indulgence for me.

Mushrooms come in all shapes and sizes. There are about 38,000 varieties in the world, with 3,000 of those growing in England. However, only about a hundred of them are edible, with twenty being seriously harmful – even fatal. With these odds, I wouldn't encourage any of you to go out foraging in the woods for mushrooms on your own. I do absolutely think everyone should have a go if they can, but make sure you have somebody with you who knows what they're doing. It's such a great way to spend a few hours.

I remember the first time I had a go at mushroom-hunting. It was with my mentor, Gennaro Contaldo, one of the UK's experts in wild mushrooms. As soon as we entered the forest, Gennaro got really excited, telling me to 'Look, look, look!' But I couldn't see a thing. He said, 'They're everywhere; get on the floor.' As soon as I crouched down I saw a whole sea of purple chanterelles, camouflaged on the woodland carpet. Being young, and far more shallow in those days, all I saw was about £300 in front of me, so I very carefully picked them all and packed them into my basket! It was so exciting. Very often when mushrooms grow somewhere they will be there the next year as well, so when Gennaro and I find a good place we will always go back the following year to monitor when the mushrooms are coming up.

If you're keen to go foraging for yourself, find a local expert or check on the internet to see if there's a local mushroom-picking society near you. Learn as much as you can, but remember that you don't have to know about every single mushroom. As long as you can recognize a few simple varieties that can't be mistaken for dangerous ones and you stay within your comfort zone, you'll be all right.

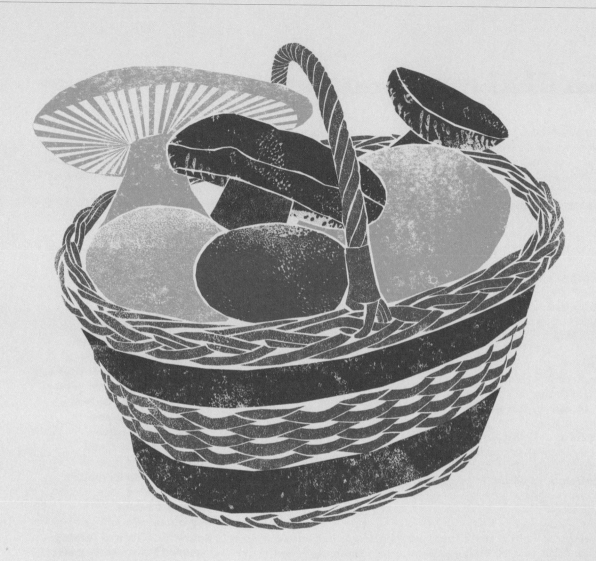

It may sound like a bit of a palaver and effort, and it is! The best things in life are never easy. But once you get into it, you'll never want to stop.

Most supermarkets now sell a great selection of farmed mushrooms: delicious varieties like chestnut, field, shiitake and oyster. Punnets of mixed wild mushrooms are also available to buy and include varieties like chanterelles, morels, pieds de mouton and trompettes de la mort. And then, of course, there are dried mushrooms like morels and porcini, which add an incredible, smoky flavour to dishes, so it's definitely worth keeping a pack of these in the cupboard.

Not only are mushrooms delicious but they also contain a similar vitamin mix to meat, making them a great substitute. They are high in fibre and protein and contain loads of minerals that are good for you, including selenium, which can help reduce the risk of cancer. They should definitely be part of your five-a-day!

# Grilled mushroom risotto

A mushroom risotto can be taken in many different ways, depending on what kind of mushrooms you have and whether they are introduced at the very beginning of cooking or just added at the end, as I'm going to do here. The inspiration for this recipe came when I was in Japan and saw mushrooms being cooked completely dry on a barbecue or griddle pan. This way of cooking brings out a really fresh and nutty flavour in them; perfect for being dressed lightly with olive oil, salt and lemon juice or stirred into a risotto at the last minute before serving.

Heat your stock in a saucepan and keep it on a low simmer. Place the porcini mushrooms in a bowl and pour in just enough hot stock to cover. Leave for a couple of minutes until they've softened. Fish them out of the stock and chop them, reserving the soaking liquid.

In a large pan, heat a glug of olive oil and add the onion and celery. Slowly fry without colouring them for at least 10 minutes, then turn the heat up and add the rice. Give it a stir. Stir in the vermouth or wine – it'll smell fantastic! Keep stirring until the liquid has cooked into the rice. Now pour the porcini soaking liquid through a sieve into the pan and add the chopped porcini, a good pinch of salt and your first ladle of hot stock. Turn the heat down to a simmer and keep adding ladlefuls of stock, stirring and massaging the starch out of the rice, allowing each ladleful to be absorbed before adding the next.

Carry on adding stock until the rice is soft but with a slight bite. This will take about 30 minutes. Meanwhile, get a dry griddle pan hot and grill the wild mushrooms until soft. If your pan isn't big enough, do this in batches. Put them into a bowl and add the chopped herbs, a pinch of salt and the lemon juice. Using your hands, get stuck in and toss everything together – this is going to be incredible!

Take the risotto off the heat and check the seasoning carefully. Stir in the butter and the Parmesan. You want it to be creamy and oozy in texture, so add a bit more stock if you think it needs it. Put a lid on and leave the risotto to relax for about 3 minutes.

Taste your risotto and add a little more seasoning or Parmesan if you like. Serve a good dollop of risotto topped with some grilled dressed mushrooms, a sprinkling of freshly grated Parmesan and a drizzle of extra virgin olive oil.

serves 4 to 6

1.5 litres hot chicken stock
a handful of dried porcini mushrooms
olive oil
1 small onion, peeled and finely chopped
2 sticks of celery, trimmed and finely chopped
400g risotto rice
150ml vermouth or white wine
sea salt and freshly ground black pepper
4 large handfuls of wild mushrooms (try shiitake, girolle, chestnut or oyster – definitely no button mushrooms, please!), cleaned and sliced
a few sprigs of fresh chervil, tarragon or parsley, leaves picked and chopped
juice of 1 lemon
25g butter
2 nice handfuls of freshly grated Parmesan cheese, plus extra for serving
extra virgin olive oil

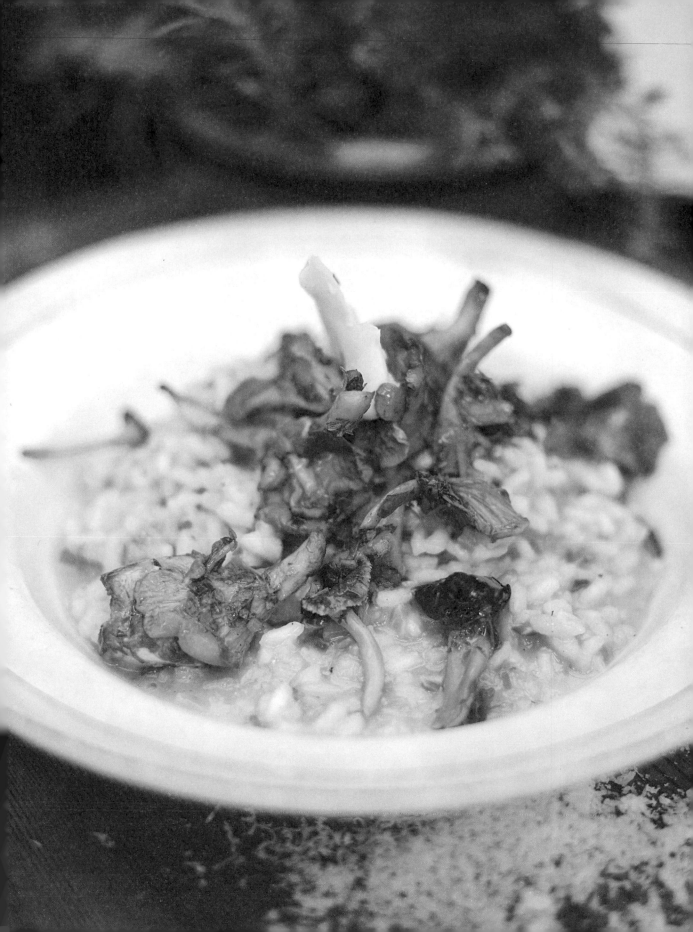

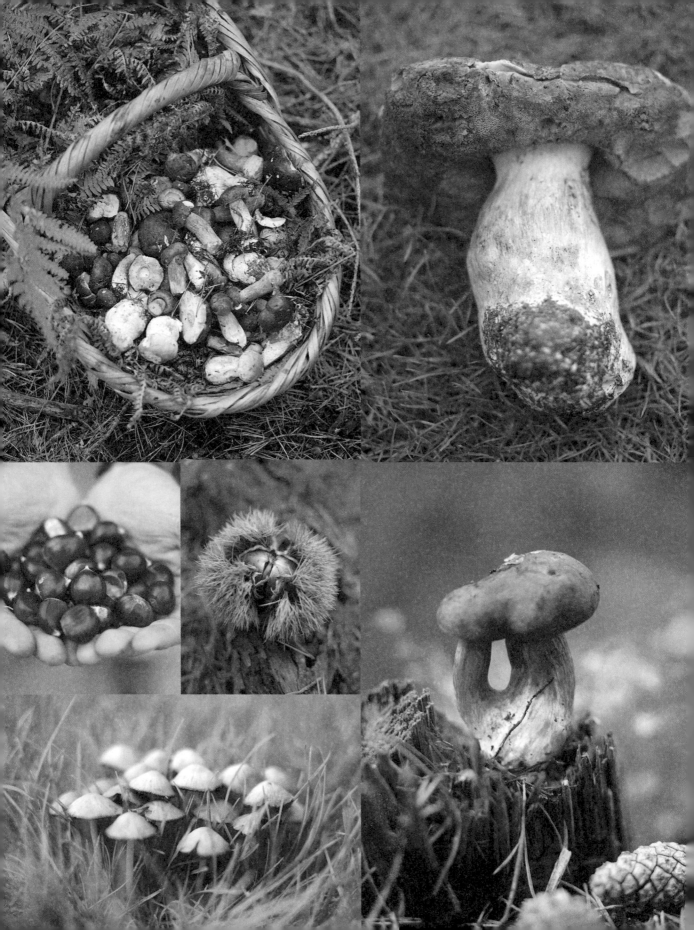

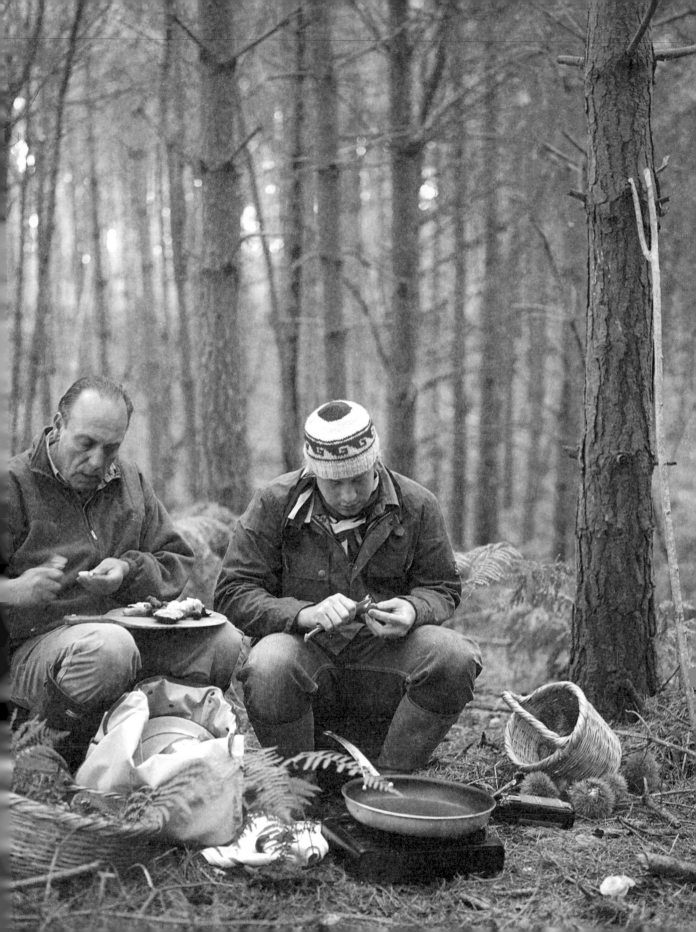

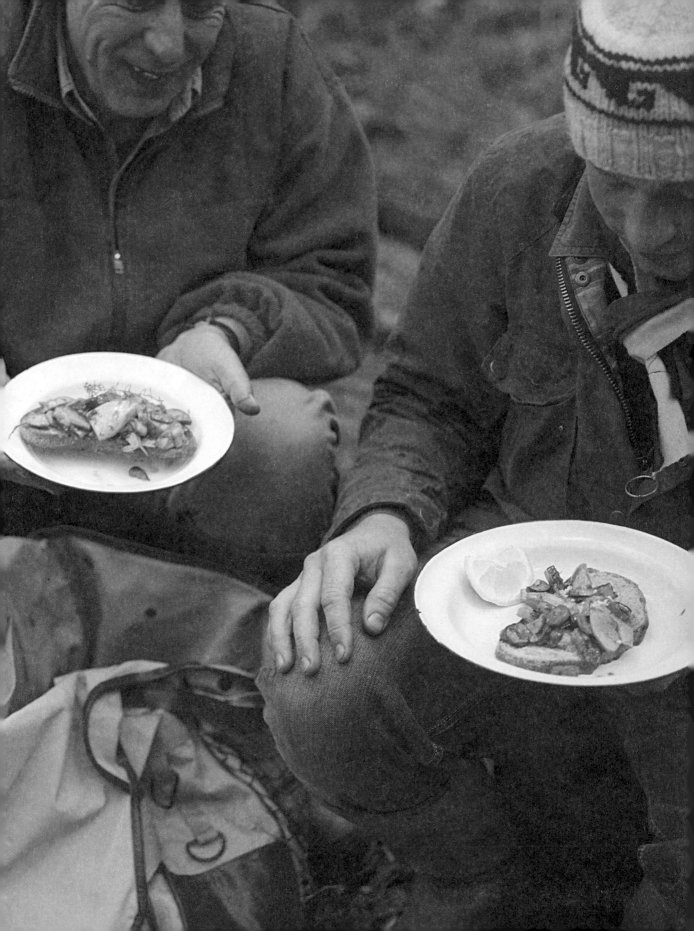

# Ultimate mushroom bruschetta

This bruschetta is brilliant for lunch, or as a snack or starter. In fact, during the game season (August to February), when it's easy to get hold of lovely birds like grouse, woodcock, pigeon, quail and partridge, this bruschetta would work really well with any of these birds simply roasted and served on top of it. The treat of the year!

Whether you're using farmed or wild mushrooms, or a combination of both, do your best to get hold of a nice interesting mixture. When it comes to frying them, make sure your pan is a large one so the moisture that comes out of them can evaporate easily. Otherwise they'll begin to boil in their own juices. Mushrooms cooked properly are so versatile – you can stir them into a risotto, sprinkle them on to a pizza or serve them with a grilled steak.

Put a large heavy frying pan, big enough to hold all the mushrooms in one layer, on the heat and add a couple of glugs of extra virgin olive oil. Depending on the size of your mushrooms, leave any small ones whole but tear, break or slice the larger ones up. Add them all to the pan and give it a shake to toss the mushrooms in the oil. Add the chopped garlic and fresh herbs and shake the pan again. Add a pinch of salt and pepper and the crumbled chilli and leave to fry gently for a few minutes. If the mixture becomes dry, pour in a little more oil.

Once the mushrooms have got some colour going on, after about 3 to 4 minutes, add the butter and a squeeze of lemon juice to give a nice twang – don't go overboard here, you don't need much – and toss again. To finish this off and make it into a lovely creamy sauce, spoon 2 to 3 tablespoons of water into the pan. Simmer for a little longer, until you have a lovely simple sauce that just loosely coats the mushrooms. Now toast your bread.

When toasted, rub the bread with the cut side of the remaining clove of garlic. Place each slice on a serving plate, pile the mushrooms and the creamy juices from the pan on top and tuck in. So good!

serves 2

extra virgin olive oil
300g mixed interesting
  mushrooms, wiped clean
2 cloves of garlic, 1 peeled
  and finely chopped, the
  other halved
a few sprigs of fresh
  thyme, leaves picked
a few sprigs of fresh
  parsley, leaves picked
optional: a sprig of summer
  savory, leaves picked
sea salt and freshly
  ground black pepper
1 dried red chilli, crumbled
a small knob of butter
1 lemon
2 slices of sourdough bread

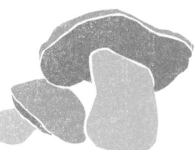

# Wild mushroom and venison stroganoff for two lucky people

This venison stroganoff is absolutely fantastic – of course, you can use the more traditional beef fillet instead of venison, and any mushrooms you like, but there's something about venison and wild mushrooms that works so well together. Have a go at this and you'll know what I mean!

The whole point of this dish is that by the time you start cooking the meat, it will all come together quickly. The meat will be quite pink – cook it for longer if you want but it will go slightly tougher.

Cook the rice according to the packet instructions until it's just undercooked and drain in a colander. Put the rice back in the pan, cover with tinfoil and leave to one side to steam – this will give you incredibly light and fluffy rice.

Heat a large frying pan on a medium heat and pour in a glug of extra virgin olive oil. Add the onions and garlic and cook for about 10 minutes until softened and golden. Remove from the heat and spoon the onions and garlic out of the pan on to a plate. Keep to one side.

Season the meat well with salt, pepper and the paprika. Rub and massage these flavourings into the meat. Place the frying pan back on a high heat and pour in some more olive oil. Add the mushrooms and fry for a few minutes until they start to brown. Then add the meat and fry for a minute or two before adding the parsley stalks (you can do this in two pans or in batches if your pan is not big enough) and the cooked onion and garlic. Toss and add the butter and brandy.

You don't have to set light to the hot brandy, but flaming does give an interesting flavour so I always like to do this. Once the flames die down, or after a couple of minutes of simmering, stir in the lemon zest and all but 1 tablespoon of the crème fraîche and season to taste. Continue simmering for a few minutes. Any longer than this and the meat will toughen up – it doesn't need long, as it's been cut up so small.

Serve your fluffy rice on one big plate and your stroganoff on another. Simply spoon the remaining crème fraîche over the stroganoff, then sprinkle over the sliced gherkins and the parsley leaves. Eat at once!

**serves 2**

200g white rice
extra virgin olive oil
1 medium red onion, peeled
  and finely chopped
1 clove of garlic, peeled
  and finely sliced
300g venison loin, fat
  and sinews removed,
  trimmed and sliced into
  finger-sized pieces
sea salt and freshly
  ground black pepper
1 tablespoon paprika
250g mixed exciting,
  robust mushrooms,
  wiped clean, torn into
  bite-sized pieces
a small bunch of fresh flat-
  leaf parsley, leaves picked
  and roughly chopped,
  stalks finely chopped
a knob of butter
a good splash of brandy
zest of ½ a lemon
150ml crème fraîche
  or soured cream
a few little gherkins, sliced

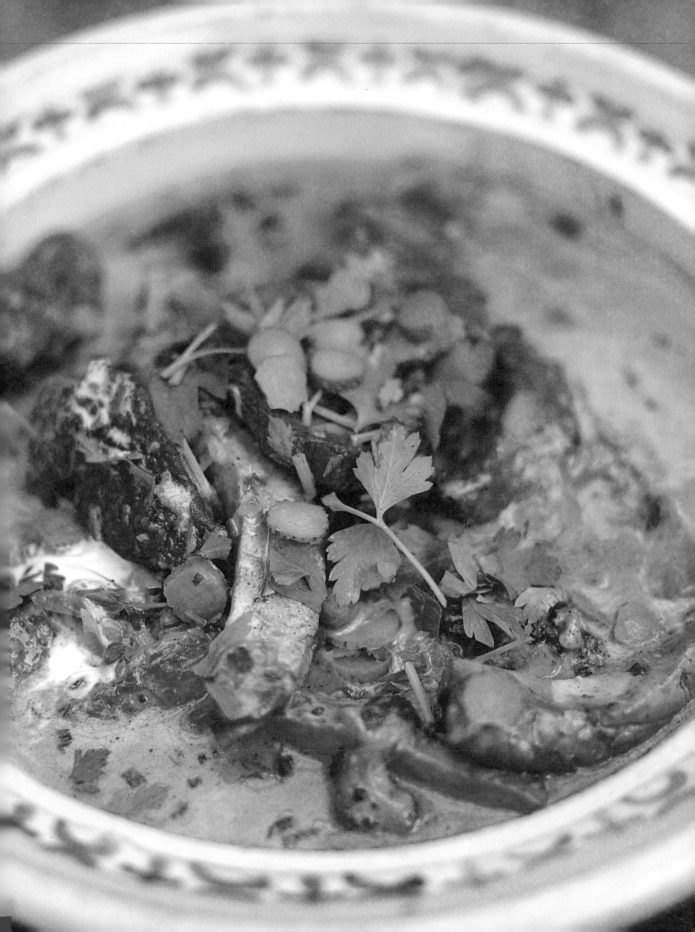

# How I grow mushrooms

It's quite easy to grow some kinds of mushrooms at home. However, unlike vegetables, mushrooms don't need to be planted. So here's a bit of a general chat about growing mushrooms, and I'll give you some tips as well.

## Growing

Although they prefer shady, moist environments, mushrooms don't necessarily need soil to grow in – some kinds, for example, are attracted to freshly cut wood, or wood chippings. One thing you can do is leave stacks of these around the garden. In time, different mushrooms will find these wood piles and start growing. You may be lucky and get some really good varieties but you must always check to make sure they are safe before eating them. If you want to control your mushroom growth a bit more, you can buy a special mushroom 'kit' which will contain all you need to get growing. These are available at good garden centres or on the internet. All you need to do is follow the instructions.

Another easy way to grow your own is to buy specially prepared 'mushroom logs'. These freshly cut logs have wooden dowels fixed into them which have been inoculated with types of mushroom. All you have to do is keep them moist in a shady part of the garden and crop the mushrooms whenever they grow. Some logs will crop several times a year for up to five years. Shiitake, oyster and lion's mane mushrooms can be grown this way.

It's also possible now to have a go at growing truffles in your own garden! Simply buy a young tree which has been inoculated with the black summer truffle fungus, plant it and wait for five or six years until it starts cropping. The trees are usually hazels which, if coppiced, can grow in quite small gardens and can last over fifty years.

## Cleaning and storing

The best way to clean mushrooms is to use a soft, dry brush. If you wash them they'll soak up the water and this will dilute their flavour. However, always wash morels just before cooking – as they're hollow they might have dirt and, possibly, bugs inside them!

Mushrooms should never be washed before being stored. Leave them in their punnet or paper bag and store inside a plastic bag to prevent them losing any moisture. Keep them in the bottom of your fridge, or in a cool place.

## My growing tips
- Mushrooms don't need light to grow. Give them moisture and a cool climate and they'll grow overnight.

- Mushrooms and other fungi could pop up anywhere in your garden, even without you trying to grow any, so please get them safely identified – if you're lucky they may be edible!

- If you're interested in having a go at growing your own, take a look at page 395 for three great websites, all of which offer a mail-order service for the mushroom kits and logs.

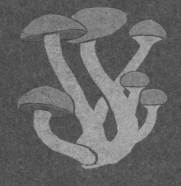

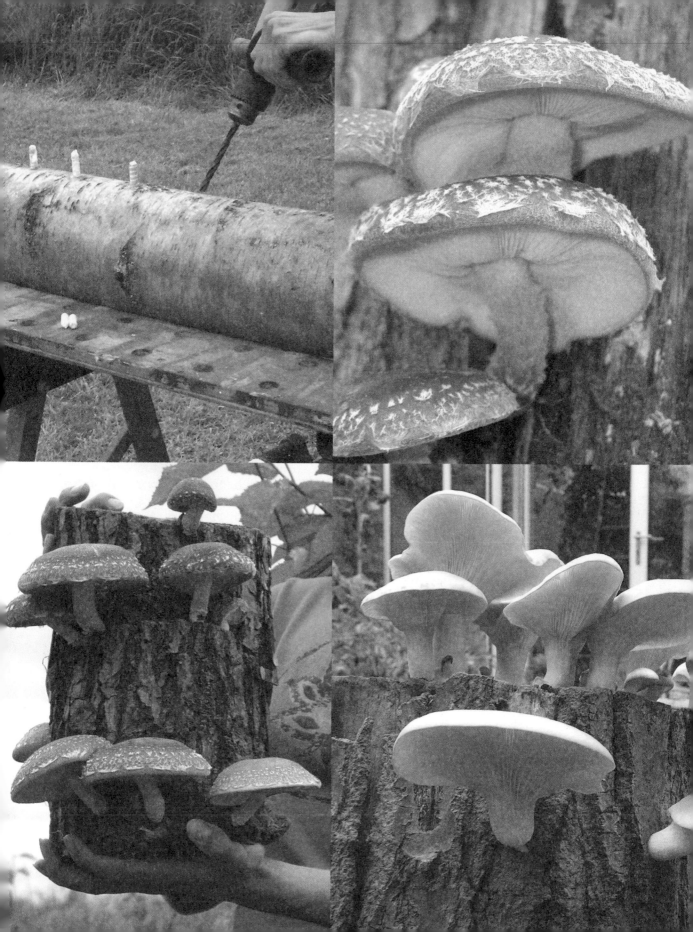

# orchard fruit

The word 'orchard' might conjure up images of a large field of fruit-bearing trees, but actually it can be a very small group of just four or five. For me, planting fruit trees is a nice little investment for a house, because as time goes by they'll grow bigger and become more beautiful. And of course the real bonus is that it's the easiest way to cultivate your own food. It may take them a little while to build up their production and quality of taste, but these trees need very little looking after – just the odd bit of pruning now and then.

What I find really exciting is that there are so many different varieties of orchard fruit. Like the world of vegetables, if you scratch the surface to find some of the more unusual apples or plums that are around, you'll be rewarded with fruit that is far tastier than any of the commercially grown supermarket equivalents. For instance, there are over 7,500 varieties of apple worldwide, yet we are only ever offered a small selection (think Cox's, Braeburn, Red Delicious or Granny Smith!) at the supermarket. Although these can be lovely apples, the main reason they're commercially grown rather than others is because they're high-yielding varieties. But the truth is that compared to a lot of overlooked varieties they're really quite boring. So when I was planting some orchard trees at home it was an opportunity for me to try to mix things up a bit. If you want to do the same, choose different varieties of apple so you have some for eating and some for cooking and choose ones that ripen at different times, giving you a longer fruiting period. Add some pears, or some stone fruit like plums, greengages, damsons and cherries. Maybe a few unusual ones like quinces, medlars, elderberries or nut trees. Any good garden centre will have small fruit trees for sale.

There are great advantages to planting fruit trees in your garden or outside space. They can give real structure to the plot, they offer shady areas in the summer and, most exciting of all, you'll have a ready supply of quality fresh fruit. If you can't eat all of it and you're a keen cook there's nothing better, because if you have too much of something you have to be resourceful and think of ways to preserve it, like making beautiful jams or chutneys.

When I bought my house it was derelict and nobody had lived in it for years. In the scullery at the back of the kitchen there were two apple storage racks lined with newspaper which was celebrating Margaret Thatcher's election success, so that was the last time any apples had been stored by the previous owners! Eccentric as I might sound, I removed the racks to a safe place before the builders arrived, along with about fifty original kilner jars which I also found, in a little cupboard under the stairs – I now use these for preserving.

It's so nice to be able to go outside and pick your own fruit off the trees. Last year I wanted to make a quick salad for lunch – I had a few salad leaves, a little rocket and mint, some feta cheese all crumbled up, and I wanted to shred some apple into it. So I ran outside, picked an apple and cut it into matchsticks, threw it into the salad and sprinkled on some dressing. It was delicious! I've also just bought myself an old press off the internet, which I'm going to use to make my own apple juice. And I'm going to have a go at making cider as well – I've never done it before, but I'm going to get a kit with instructions. Should be a laugh!

# Sweet pear and apple salad with bitter chicory and a creamy blue cheese dressing

This is an adaptation of an old-school French chicory salad. Chicory, also known as Belgian endive, is quite a bitter leaf, and to contrast the bitterness I've used the sweetness of the fruit, the twang of the vinegar and the creamy silkiness of the cheese. I think it's important to make this with good-quality apples and blue cheese.

Separate the leaves from the chicory, then wash and spin them dry. Core your apples and slice them into matchsticks. Core the pears, slice into eighths and if they're a little underripe, grill them in a screaming hot griddle pan until lightly charred. If they're perfectly ripe, just place in a large bowl with the chicory, apple and most of the herbs.

To make your dressing, place all your dressing ingredients into a liquidizer and blend for just 15 seconds until smooth. Taste to make sure you've got a little extra acidity in there to cut through the bitterness of the leaves, and season if necessary. Pour three-quarters of the dressing over the salad and toss – I usually dress the salad lightly using the tips of my fingers. Divide it between four plates, and finish with a little extra dressing, the remaining herbs and a little extra virgin olive oil. Lovely with some walnuts crumbled over.

serves 4

4 heads of chicory (a
  mixture of red and
  white if possible)
2 good English
  eating apples
2 pears
a handful of fresh soft
  herbs (chervil, tarragon,
  parsley – use any one,
  or a mixture), torn or
  roughly chopped

*for the blue cheese
  dressing*
50g strong blue cheese
50g crème fraîche
5 tablespoons extra virgin
  olive oil, plus a little
  extra for drizzling
4 tablespoons cider vinegar
6 tablespoons water

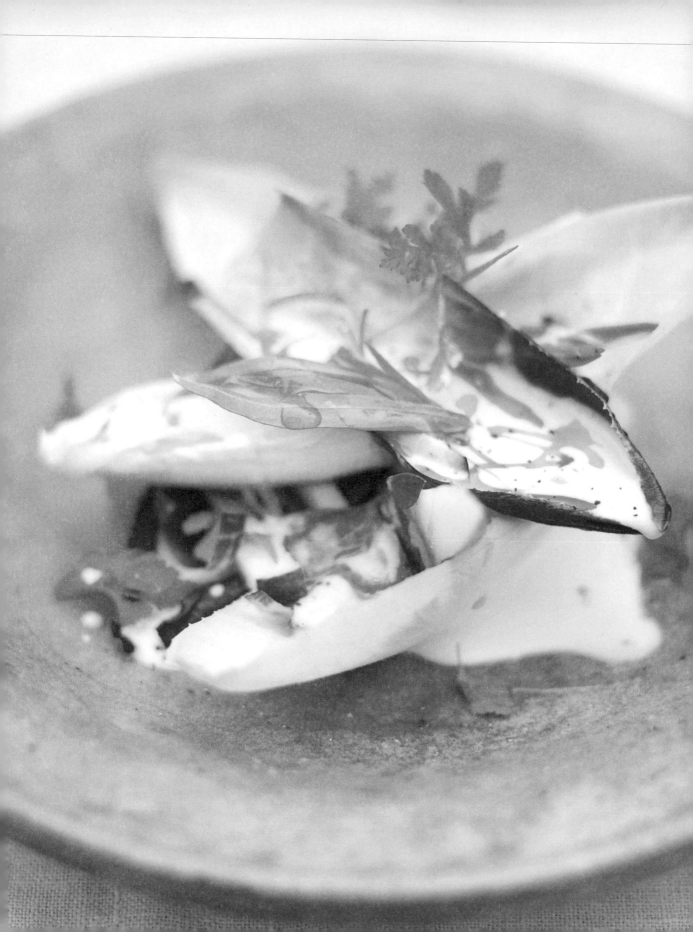

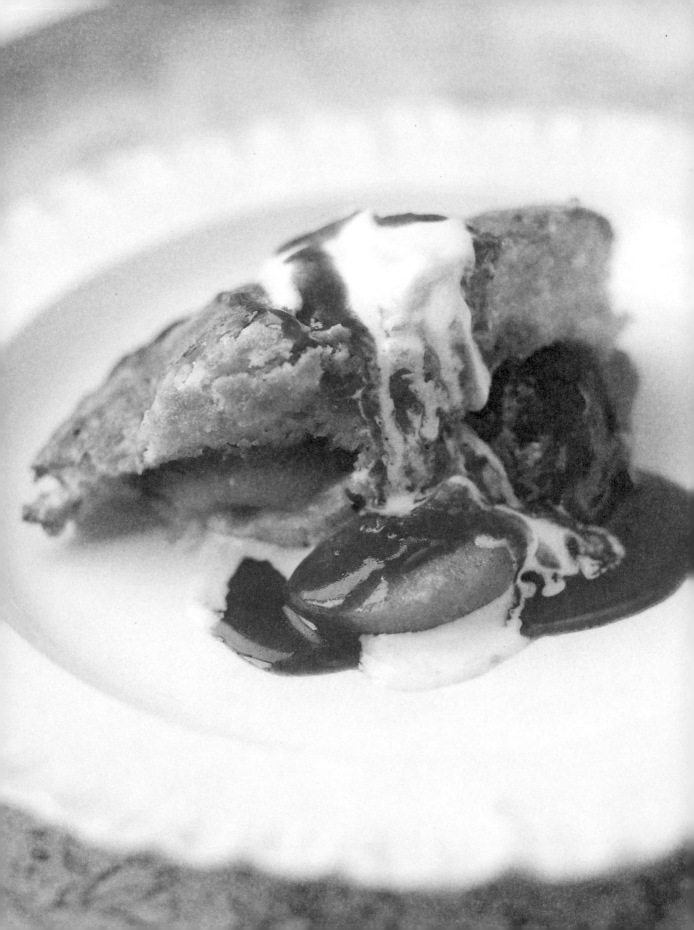

# Orchard Eve's pudding with whisky Jersey cream

This is a classic old English pudding made from lovely stewed fruit with a spongy batter baked around it. Absolutely delicious. If you can't get hold of one of the orchard fruits I've suggested, feel free to use peaches or strawberries (not raspberries, though, as they tend to disappear!). Banana is also delicious, but the end result will be like a banana cake. In the old days this would have been made using tinned pineapple; try it out, but use a nice ripe fresh pineapple instead. Another fruit not to use is kiwi, as it just doesn't work. Jersey cream is one of life's little naughty-but-nice luxuries! You can get it from all good supermarkets. Try lacing it with a little whisky – delicious!

Preheat the oven to 180°C/350°F/gas 4. Peel and core the apples, quinces and pears, and cut them into large wedges. Halve and stone the plums (their skin can be left on). Place in a big saucepan with the butter, brown sugar, spices and bay leaves, give it a stir and stew gently for 20 to 30 minutes with the lid on. When the fruit is soft and cooked, remove the pan from the heat, discard the bay leaves and put to one side.

To make the batter, cream the butter and sugar together with a wooden spoon in a bowl until light and fluffy. Add the eggs one at a time, beating them in well, then fold in the flour. You can make this in a food processor too, it's up to you. Using a slotted spoon, transfer half the cooked fruit (without the juices) into the bottom of a round, 20cm buttered ovenproof baking dish. Top with the batter, then spoon over the remaining fruit, reserving the juices. Bake in the preheated oven for 40 to 45 minutes, or until golden brown and risen. To check whether it's cooked through, stick a skewer or small knife into the middle of the sponge – if it comes out clean, you're in business.

Slice the vanilla pod in half lengthways and scrape the seeds out using the back of your knife. Put them into a bowl with the cream; don't throw the empty pod away – you can use this to make vanilla sugar later. Lightly whisk the cream and vanilla seeds with the icing sugar until it forms soft peaks. Fold in the whisky. Serve straight away with big dollops of the cream and a drizzle of the fruit juices.

**serves 6 to 8**

**1.5kg eating apples, quinces, pears and plums**
**a large knob of butter, plus a little extra for buttering the dish**
**100g brown sugar**
**a pinch of ground cinnamon**
**a pinch of ground nutmeg**
**a pinch of ground ginger**
**3 fresh bay leaves**
**1 vanilla pod**
**1 x 284ml pot of Jersey or double cream**
**1 tablespoon icing sugar**
**a little swig of whisky**

***for the batter***
**200g butter, softened**
**200g golden caster sugar**
**4 large organic or free-range eggs**
**200g self-raising flour**

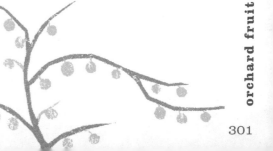

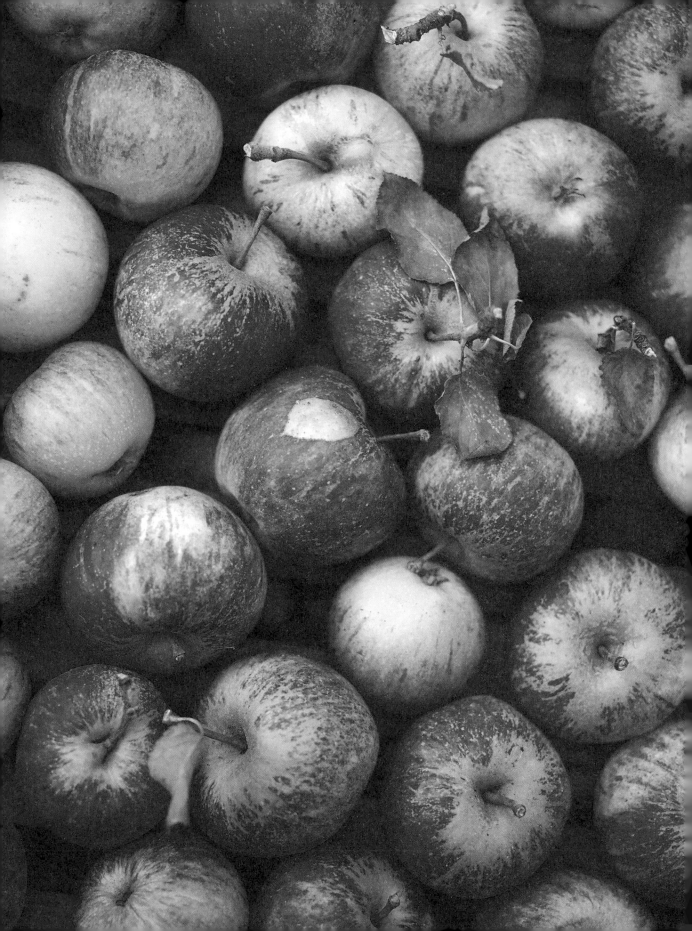

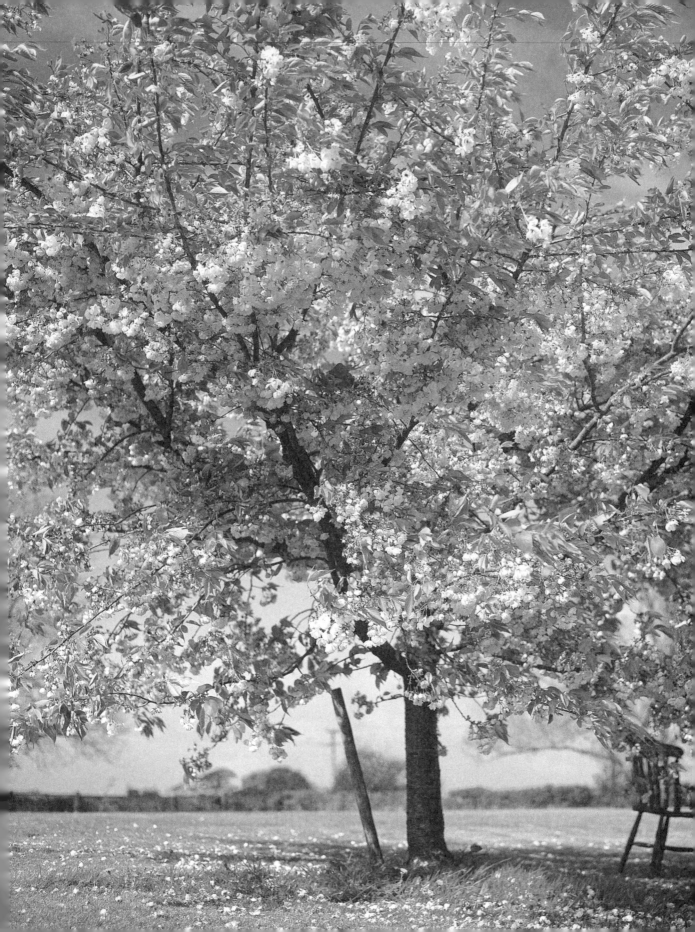

# Quick plum sorbet with sloe gin

When plums are juicy and at their best, they are perfect for turning into a quick sorbet. This recipe is so quick, in fact, that I usually make it from scratch while my guests are at the table! It takes just 2 minutes to whiz up a load of frozen fruit in a food processor with some sugar. You can try different fruit, like strawberries, raspberries or blackcurrants, and experiment with various types of alcohol, rather like making a cocktail. However, you don't have to use alcohol to make this (though a little Champagne with strawberries or red wine with raspberries is really good!). I really got into sloe gin last year and, as sloes are similar to damsons and plums and part of the orchard fruit family, a little swig mixed into this sorbet is brilliant.

PS Sloe gin is easy to buy in the supermarkets now, but if you want to have a go at making your own, here's how to do it. It's so simple! Pick yourself about 600g of sloe berries after the first winter frost (or freeze them to fake it!). When at room temperature, prick them with a fork. Place in a wide-necked jar or bottle, add 300g of granulated sugar and shake the jar a bit. Top with the gin, then close the jar and give it a really good shake. Keep shaking once a day for a month, then once a week for a further two months. Don't open before three months are up.

Cut the plums in half and remove their stones. Place in a freezer bag and put into the freezer for at least 2 hours or until frozen solid. An hour before you want to make your sorbet, put a serving dish into the freezer to get really cold. About 5 to 10 minutes before you start, take the plums out of the freezer. Put them into a food processor with the orange zest, sugar and sloe gin and whiz until smooth (you may have to do this in two batches). Scoop into your frozen serving dish, using a spatula to smooth out the surface. Pop back into the freezer and remove it 5 to 10 minutes before serving, to allow it to soften slightly. Serve in big scoops, with a swig of sloe gin over the top if you like.

**serves 4 to 6**

1kg good-quality mixed plums or other fruit
zest of 1 orange
120g caster sugar or vanilla sugar
50ml sloe gin, plus extra for serving

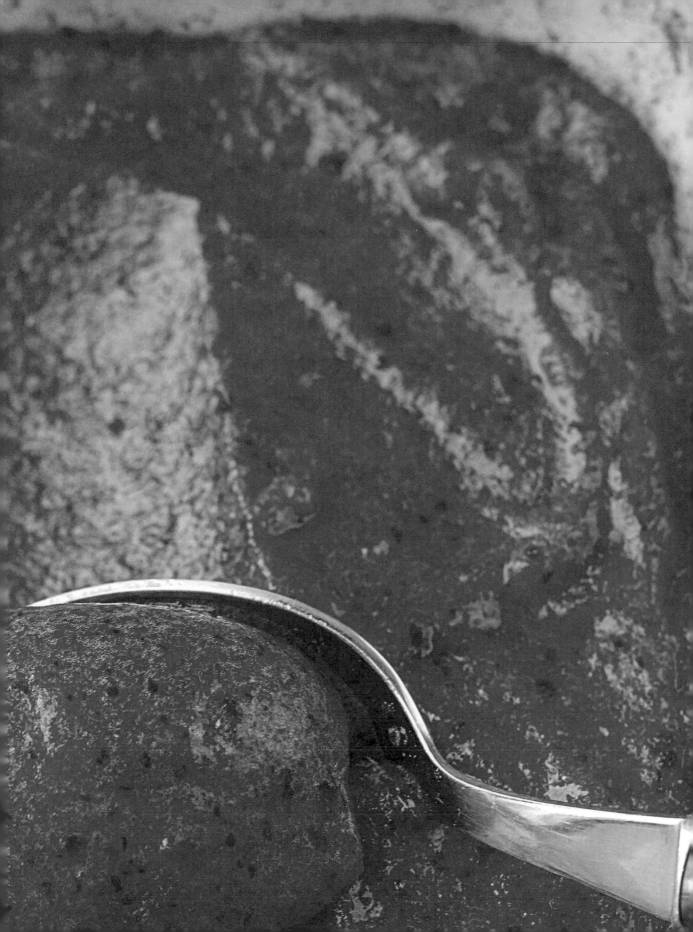

# Plum Bakewell tart

The thing I love about this tart is that it keeps really well, so you can enjoy a nice slice in your lunchbox or with your afternoon tea for a few days! If you think you like Bakewell tart but you've only ever eaten factory versions, have a go at making this. You'll be blown away by a homemade one. Whether your plums are perfectly ripe or slightly sour they'll work a treat in this tart. It will also look a real picture if you use some different coloured ones.

Grease a loose-bottomed 28cm tart tin with a little butter and make your pastry. When you have your ball of dough, wrap it in clingfilm and place it in the fridge to rest for at least half an hour. Then remove it and roll it out on a floured surface. Line the tart tin with your rolled-out pastry, easing it into the ridges at the side. Place in the freezer for an hour.

Meanwhile, make the frangipane. Blitz the blanched whole almonds in a food processor until you have a fine powder and transfer this to a bowl with the flour. Halve your vanilla pod lengthways and scrape out the seeds, using the back of your knife. Now blitz the butter, sugar and vanilla seeds until light and creamy. Put the almond mixture back into the food processor with your lightly beaten eggs and whiz until completely mixed and smooth. Place in the fridge to firm up for at least half an hour.

Preheat the oven to 180°C/350°F/gas 4 and bake the pastry case for around 10 minutes, or until lightly golden. Remove from the oven, leaving the oven on.

Halve the plums and remove the stones. Finely chop *half* of them and place in a saucepan with the vanilla sugar and the mixed spice. Cook gently until softened, with a jammy consistency, then stir in the cornflour and simmer until thickened.

While the plums are cooking, cut the remaining plum halves into quarters and macerate them for 5 minutes by sprinkling them with icing sugar – this will make them juicy, shiny and delicious. Carefully spoon your plum jam into the pastry case and smooth it out across the bottom. Spread the frangipane over the plum jam. Arrange the plums on the surface of the frangipane, pressing them in lightly. Scatter the flaked almonds over the top. Bake the tart in the preheated oven for about an hour, placing a baking tray on the shelf under the tart, just in case it bubbles over. Once cooked through and golden brown on top, remove the tart from the oven and leave it to cool.

I don't always do this, but if you're feeling creative, before serving mix a few tablespoons of icing sugar with a little warm water and drizzle over the top of the cooked tart – Jackson Pollock style! Lovely served with a dollop of crème fraîche.

**makes a 28cm tart**

**a knob of butter**
**½ x sweet shortcrust pastry recipe (see page 352)**
**1kg mixed plums**
**100g vanilla sugar**
**½ teaspoon mixed spice**
**1 teaspoon cornflour, dissolved in 1 tablespoon cold water**
**50g flaked almonds**
**icing sugar**

*for the frangipane*
**285g blanched whole almonds**
**50g plain flour**
**1 vanilla pod**
**250g unsalted butter, cubed**
**250g caster sugar**
**3 large free-range or organic eggs, lightly beaten**

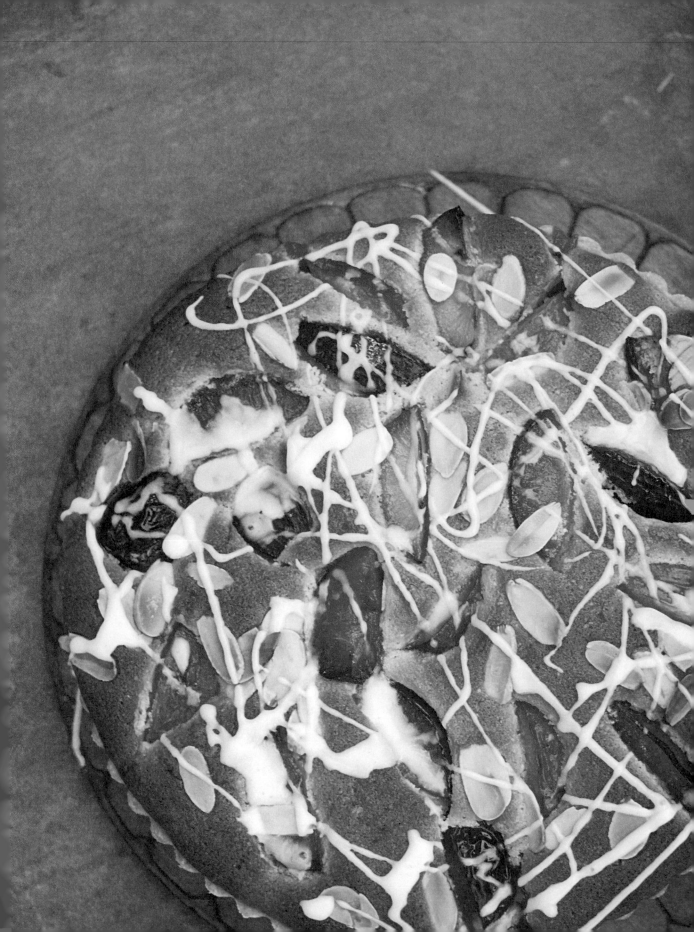

# How I grow orchard fruit

## Soil

Ideally you need deep, well-drained soil, avoiding heavy clay or waterlogged ground. However, the soil in my part of Essex is thick clay that's wet, sticky and cold in winter but in the summer bakes hard and dry. I've found that manure, or good organic compost, improves its texture and fertility. When deciding where to plant fruit trees, bear in mind that they like lots of sunlight and a bit of shelter.

In mid-winter I dug the soil over and mixed in loads of good organic compost. The trees then arrived, all bare-rooted. They were a mixture of 'maiden whips' and 'feathered maidens' (I just love some of these names!). In plain English this means they're one or two years old. Young trees like this grow really quickly, so there's no need to buy bigger, older ones. You can also get pot-grown trees which can be planted at any time of year, but it's usually best done in winter or early spring. Bare-rooted trees should be planted as soon as you get them, but if the ground is frozen or you're busy you can 'heel' them into the ground temporarily for a few weeks. Just dig a trench, place the plants all together at a slight angle, to stop them rocking in the wind, then cover the roots with soil and firm down until you're ready to plant them out properly.

## Planting

Dig a hole about 30 to 50cm across and about the same depth. Get a strong wooden stake 120 to 150cm tall and drive it into the hole just off centre. Chuck in a bit of slow-release organic fertilizer, and position your tree so that it's near, but not rubbing against, the stake. Fill the hole with the soil you dug out, mixing in plenty of organic compost or very well-rotted manure. Firm the soil well, then make a circular ridge round your tree, about 50cm in diameter and 15cm high, and water well. The ridge will help contain water, especially important in the first year or two when you mustn't let the roots dry out. Get a good 'tree-tie' and fix it about 80 to 100cm up the stake. Loosen or tighten it as needed. I planted my trees about 4.5 metres apart.

## Harvesting and storage

I love picking fruit. The secret of when to pick is simply to watch nature at work. The tree will tell you it's time by dropping a few windfalls on to the ground. One of the great things about fruit trees is that the fruit doesn't all come at once. Fruit near the top and on the sunny south side of your tree will usually be ready first, and different varieties will ripen at different times which is really handy.

Softer orchard fruits, like plums, won't store for long, so these are best used straight away or preserved by bottling, making jam or freezing. On the other hand, some varieties of apples and pears can be stored for months. Select undamaged fruits, wrap them individually in tissue or newspaper and lay them out in trays in a cool, dark, frost-free place (like a garage or shed). Inspect them regularly and remove any that show signs of rotting.

## My growing tips

- Many fruit trees and bushes also grow really well in pots, so if you've only got a patio or veranda you can still grow your own mini-orchard!

- My good friend Jekka McVicar helped me select trees and also suggested underplanting with lemon balm, fennel, rosemary, lavender, sorrel, wild garlic, mint, thyme and chamomile – these act as 'companion plants' and they've helped create a lovely natural setting.

- Most people prune their fruit trees immediately after planting and then once a year. This might seem daunting if it's your first time, so if in doubt be gentle rather than over-enthusiastic with your pruners!

- To pick your fruit, simply cradle it in the palm of your hand and lift it gently away from the 'spur' (the short, twiggy bit of tree it's attached to). If it won't come away easily, leave it a little longer. This is important if you want to store your fruit – the longer it hangs on the tree, the better it'll keep. However, early apples and pears should be picked slightly under-ripe and should be eaten within a week or two. Make sure all your fruit is picked before the first autumn frosts, especially late-ripening varieties.

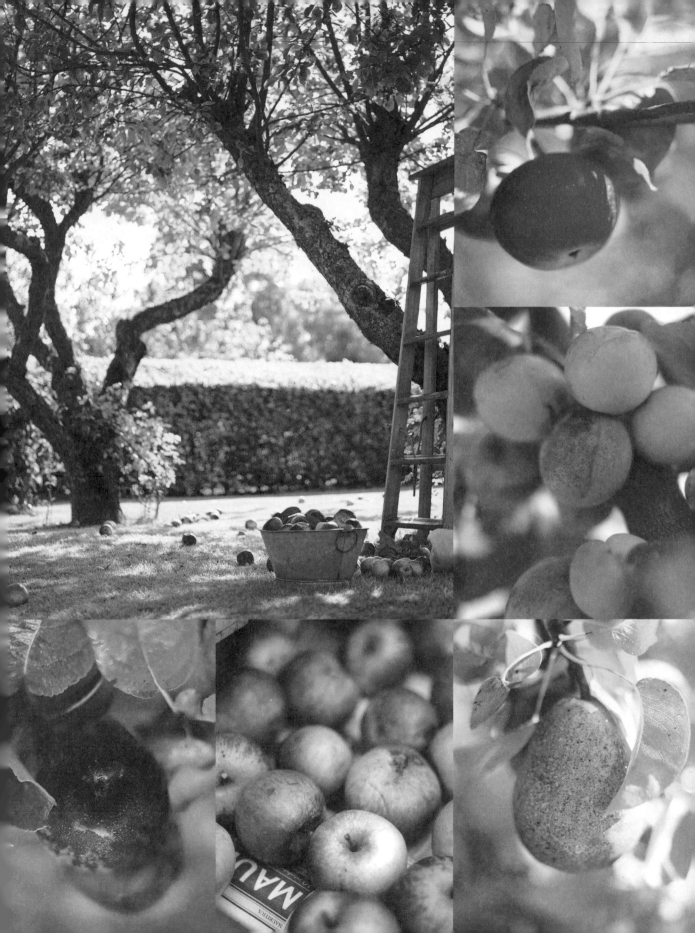

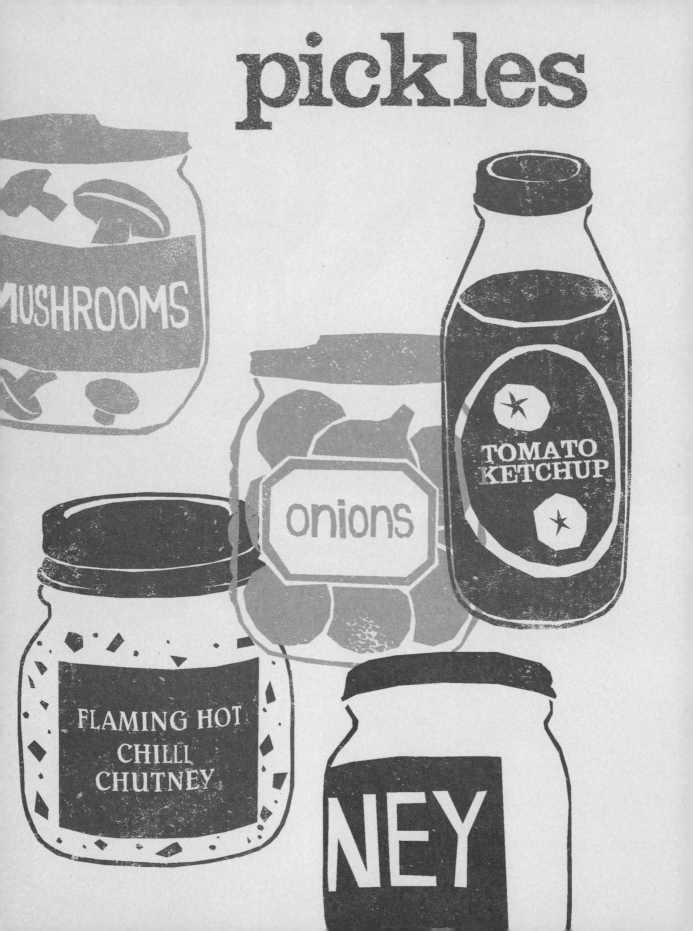

Pickling and preserving are something of a dying art really, because these days preserved food is easily available in our supermarkets. I'm talking about things like jams, pickles, chutneys, salsas, dried mushrooms, sun-dried tomatoes, salted anchovies, smoked products and confit meat in fat.

Most people live by the 'sell by' dates that come stamped on their food: if things go past that date they tend just to get chucked in the bin and new products are bought to take their place. Our ancestors would have needed to understand their food in much greater depth than us – how long it would keep for, how to store it, when best to eat it and, most importantly, how best to preserve it. Fridges weren't invented until the mid nineteenth century, so how was food kept from going off? You know what, when challenged, humans can be incredibly resourceful. In order to survive the colder winter months of the year, people learnt to hoard their food and crops, using different methods of preserving, and stash them away to see them through the winter when there was less food around. It was basically a matter of survival. Imagine your life depending on preserving. Yes, I mean your actual life. It sounds ridiculous to us now, when we can buy whatever we want, but in the old days if you lived out in the wilds and you got it wrong, it would mean that your family might starve to death. So it was an incredibly important skill to learn and get right.

So many of today's dietary or obesity problems stem not from a need of food but from gluttony – getting too much of all the wrong foods. If our lives truly did depend on the food we eat, then we'd probably be a damn sight more knowledgeable about where food comes from and how to make the best of it.

Preserving has continued through the years because we all love the flavour of smoked food, the intensity of dried products, the texture of jams and the zinginess of pickles. These days most of us keep a handful of preserved items in our cupboards, not as food for seeing us through the winter, but because we absolutely adore eating them! For these we need to thank our great-great-great-great ancestors for being so damn clever...

Preserving gives us the opportunity to add some amazing flavours to different foods. And if you're pickling things from your own garden you'll get massive satisfaction from being able to enjoy your own produce in the winter months when it's cold and miserable outside. In this chapter I'm not going to give you recipes covering every way of preserving. Instead I'm focusing on pickling vegetables with different herbs, plus giving you recipes for a chilli chutney and a delicious homemade ketchup. So make sure you have a good old preserving session in the summer when there's a glut of everything – be it from your own garden or when things are cheap down at the market. Have a go, then if you really enjoy it and want to take things further, get hold of an old second-hand pickling book and you can really go to town! Remember, a few hours spent preserving a load of stuff in the summer means you can enjoy it through the rest of the year. Time very well spent ...

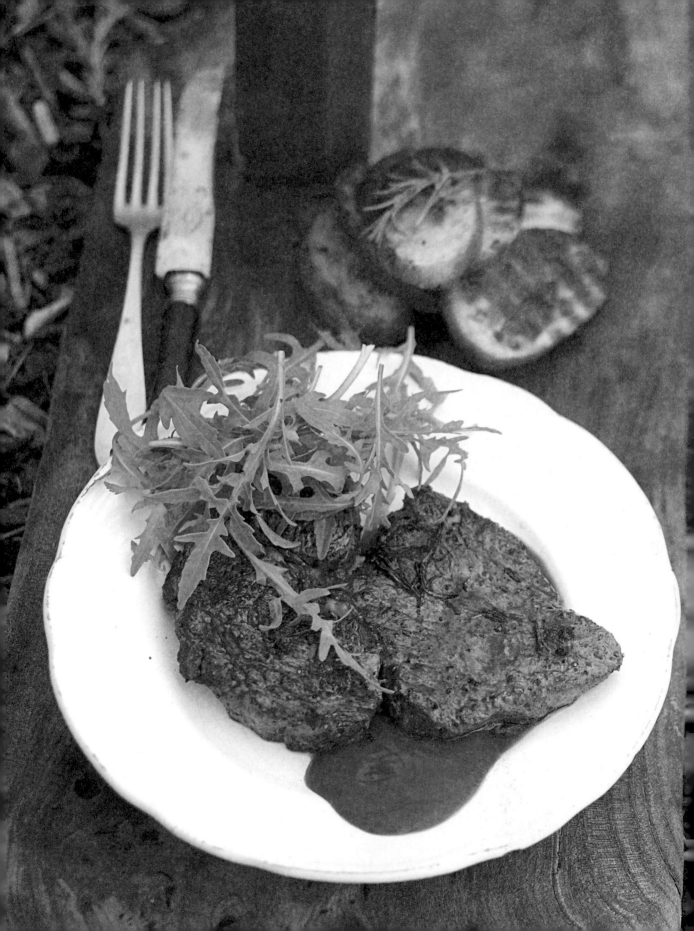

# Homemade ketchup with the best steak and grilled chips ever

When it comes to steak, you should feel free to use the cut you like best, but to my mind ribeye is the daddy! If you've never tried it before, please do. Buy it from a good butcher who has quality meat and, most importantly, try to get beef that has been hung for at least twenty-one days, as this will have much more flavour and tenderness. Even though this is an everyday meal, there are a few little tips and optional extras in this recipe to help make it the best steak you've ever had. And the homemade ketchup goes so well with it.

Either light your barbecue and let it burn down to nice hot glowing coals, or preheat the oven to 180°C/350°F/gas 4 and heat up your griddle pan.

Bring a pan of salted water to the boil and parboil your potato slices for 5 or 6 minutes until tender but still holding their shape, then drain well in a colander. Toss the potatoes with a glug of olive oil, a good pinch of salt and pepper, half the picked rosemary leaves, the sage leaves and the lemon zest.

Look at your steaks – you'll notice there's a big firm piece of white fat right in the middle. Carefully pinch most of it out and then literally push little pieces of it into the steak meat. It may sound a bit mad, but this means you'll distribute the natural fat through the meat, making it tastier and moist in return. Pat the steaks with olive oil. Chop up the rest of the picked rosemary leaves and sprinkle over both sides of your steaks with a good pinch of salt and pepper as well.

To give your steak and potatoes some extra flavour, tie the two remaining rosemary sprigs together and bash them in a pestle and mortar with a little salt, the lemon juice and a glug of olive oil. As you cook and turn your food, brush it with the rosemary branch to flavour it with all the lovely lemony oily juices from the pestle and mortar.

At this point, if you're cooking indoors on a small griddle pan, you need to start griddling your slices of potato, in batches, until they're all nicely charred on both sides. Remove them to a roasting tray, in one layer, and pop them into the oven to crisp a little further. Cook the steaks on the griddle pan to your liking, turning them every minute. It's even better if you're cooking on a barbecue, because you'll have more space so you can do it all at the same time. As the potato slices start to look good, move them over to the edge of the barbecue to keep warm while you cook your steaks, and don't forget to let them rest on a plate before eating.

Great served with a little rocket or watercress salad – and your homemade ketchup, of course!

serves 4

sea salt and freshly
   ground black pepper
16 waxy potatoes
   (use Charlotte or
   Desiree), scrubbed
   and sliced lengthways
   into 1cm slices
extra virgin olive oil
6 sprigs of fresh
   rosemary, leaves picked
   from 4 of them
3 sprigs of fresh sage,
   leaves picked and torn
zest and juice of 1 lemon
4 x 250g ribeye steaks
homemade tomato ketchup
   (see page 314)

# Homemade tomato ketchup

Bizarrely enough for a chef, I really do take my hat off to Heinz, who have become the global brand of quality in the ketchup world. It's such an everyday cupboard product that you've probably never thought to make your own. But if you're growing tomatoes in the garden, or you catch sight of some really beautiful ones at the market in summer, just think how much of a treat it would be to offer your family or guests homemade ketchup. It's great fun to make. And you can make different colours of ketchup using just yellow, orange or green tomatoes – simply exchange the cherry and tinned tomatoes for the same amount of your chosen coloured ones.

Place all the vegetables in a large heavy-bottomed saucepan with a big splash of olive oil and the ginger, garlic, chilli, basil stalks, coriander seeds and cloves. Season with the pepper and a good pinch of salt.

Cook gently over a low heat for 10 to 15 minutes until softened, stirring every so often. Add all the tomatoes and 350ml of cold water. Bring to the boil and simmer gently until the sauce reduces by half.

Add the basil leaves, then whiz the sauce in a food processor or with a hand blender and push it through a sieve twice, to make it smooth and shiny. Put the sauce into a clean pan and add the vinegar and the sugar. Place the sauce on the heat and simmer until it reduces and thickens to the consistency of tomato ketchup. At this point, correct the seasoning to taste.

Spoon the ketchup through a sterilized funnel into sterilized bottles (see page 324 for ways of doing this), then seal tightly and place in a cool dark place or the fridge until needed – it should keep for six months. Great with the steak and chips recipe on page 313.

**makes about 500ml**

1 large red onion, peeled and roughly chopped
½ a bulb of fennel, trimmed and roughly chopped
1 stick of celery, trimmed and roughly chopped
olive oil
a thumb-sized piece of fresh ginger, peeled and roughly chopped
2 cloves of garlic, peeled and sliced
½ a fresh red chilli, deseeded and finely chopped
a bunch of fresh basil, leaves picked, stalks chopped
1 tablespoon coriander seeds
2 cloves
1 teaspoon freshly ground black pepper
sea salt
500g amazing cherry or plum tomatoes, halved *plus* 500g tinned plum tomatoes, chopped
*or*
1kg yellow, orange or green tomatoes, chopped
200ml red wine vinegar
70g soft brown sugar

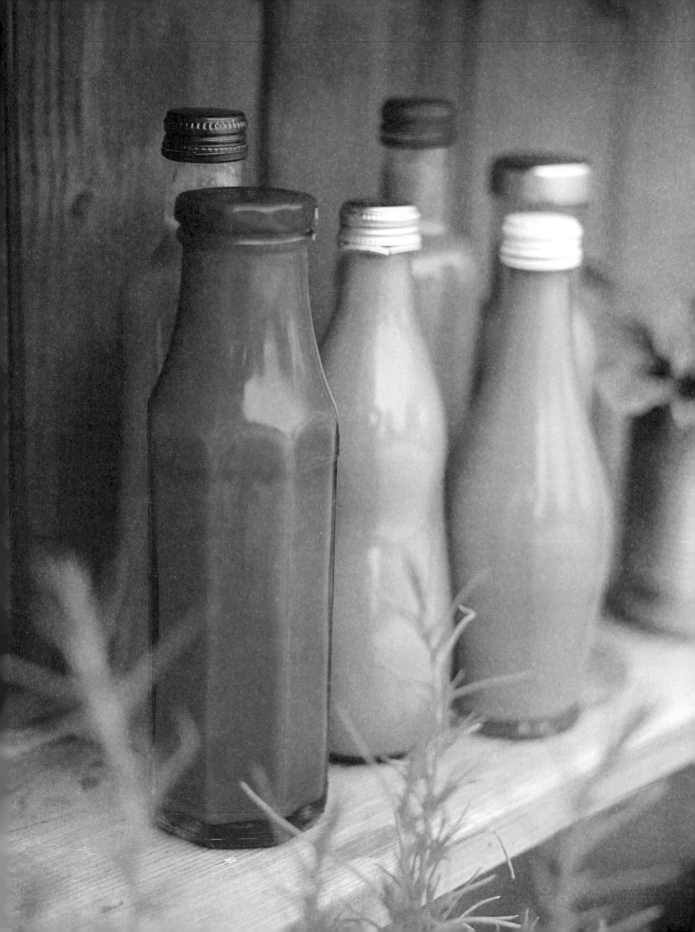

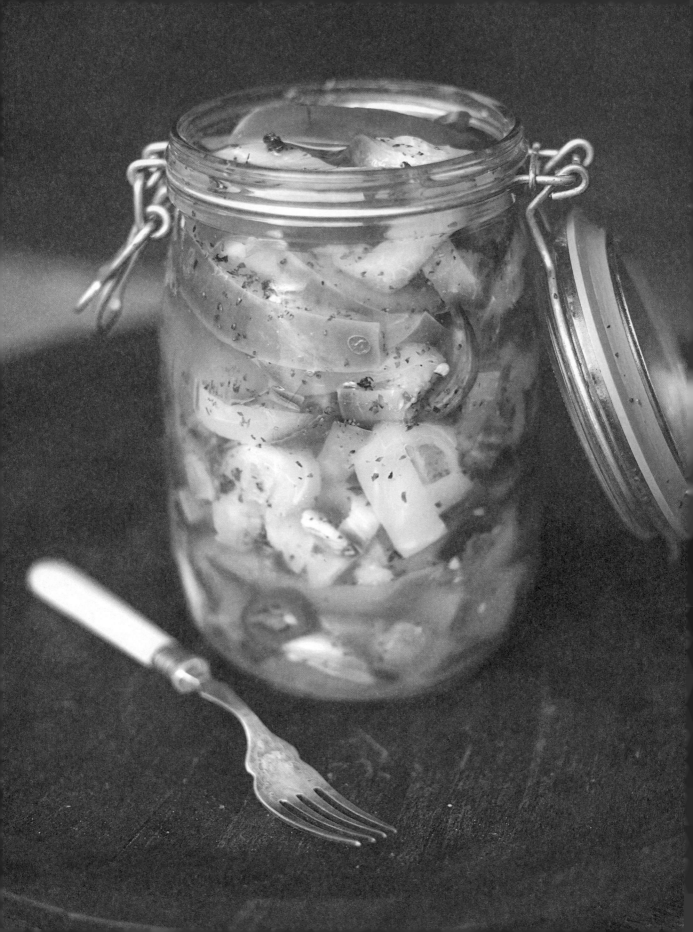

# Amazing pickled and marinated veg

Pickled veg taste totally delicious. I'm going to give you my personal favourite veg and herb combinations – damn simple and they make great presents. Much cooler than turning up with a bottle of wine. Once you've had success with them, have a go at your own variations. You can use one large jar or lots of smaller ones (I prefer smaller ones because once a jar's been opened it will only last for a week or so in the fridge).

Make sure you have some small sterilized jars ready to go (see page 324). Bring the pickling liquid ingredients to the boil in a big pan. Put the pickling marinade ingredients into a large bowl with your chosen herbs and mix well. Slice up your chosen vegetable any way you like, but if it's a larger vegetable try to get the pieces around 1cm in thickness. This way, the flavours and pickling liquid will penetrate sufficiently. Smaller veg, like mushrooms or very small onions, can be left whole.

Place the sliced veg in the boiling pickling liquid and leave for around 3 minutes – they'll probably rise to the surface, so keep pushing them down to ensure they are all immersed. Lift the pieces out with a slotted spoon and place them into your bowl of pickling marinade. Toss together – it will smell fantastic.

Pretty much straight away, put the hot veg and pickling marinade into your sterilized jars, filling them to the very top. Cover the veg completely with the marinade and put the lids on tightly. Put the jars to one side until they're cool. Clean the jars, attach sticky labels and write the date and the contents on them. Store the jars somewhere cool and dark – it's best to leave them for about two weeks before opening so the veg really gets to marinate well, but if you absolutely cannot wait, you can eat them sooner. They'll keep for about three months – but they're so bloody good I'm lucky if the jars last for a couple of weeks in our house!

**makes about 2 litres**

*for the pickling liquid*
1 litre cider or white wine vinegar
1 litre water
2 tablespoons sea salt

*for the pickling marinade*
500ml extra virgin olive oil
5 cloves of garlic, peeled and sliced
1 fresh red chilli, deseeded and chopped

*choose one of the following veg and herb options:*
- 1kg mixed mushrooms and a few sprigs of fresh thyme, rosemary and sage
- 1kg firm aubergines and 2 tablespoons dried oregano
- 1kg firm courgettes and 6 sprigs of fresh mint
- 1kg fennel bulbs and their herby tops
- 1kg small onions and 4 bay leaves
- 1kg red and yellow peppers and a few sprigs of fresh thyme

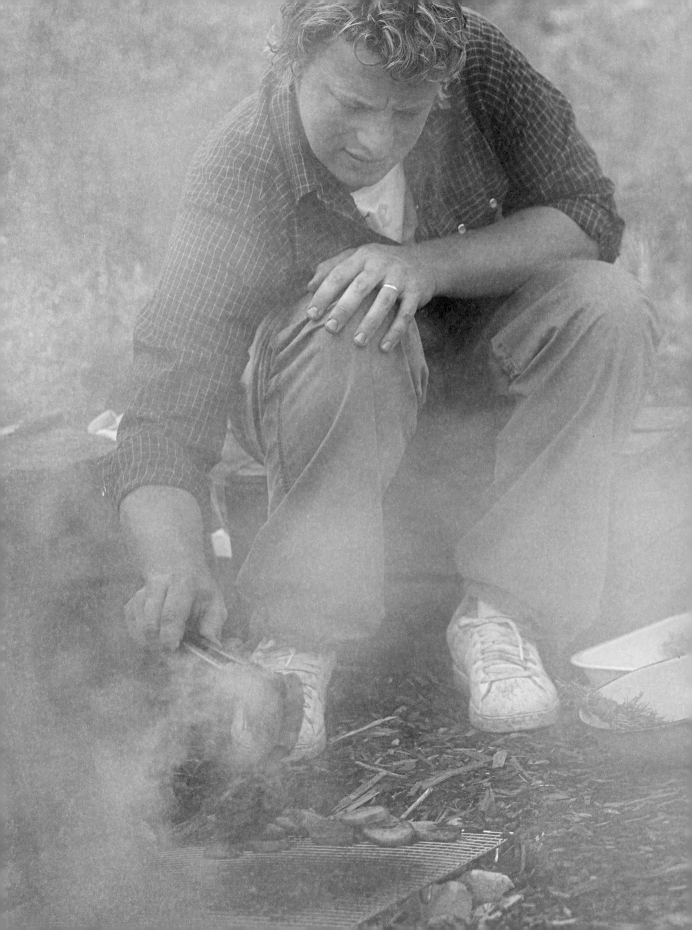

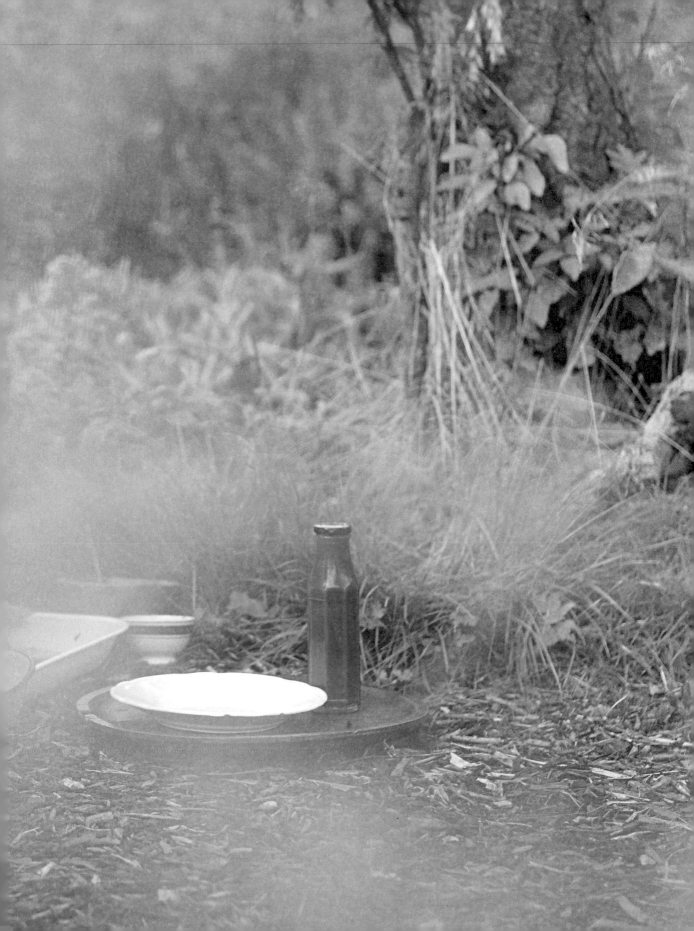

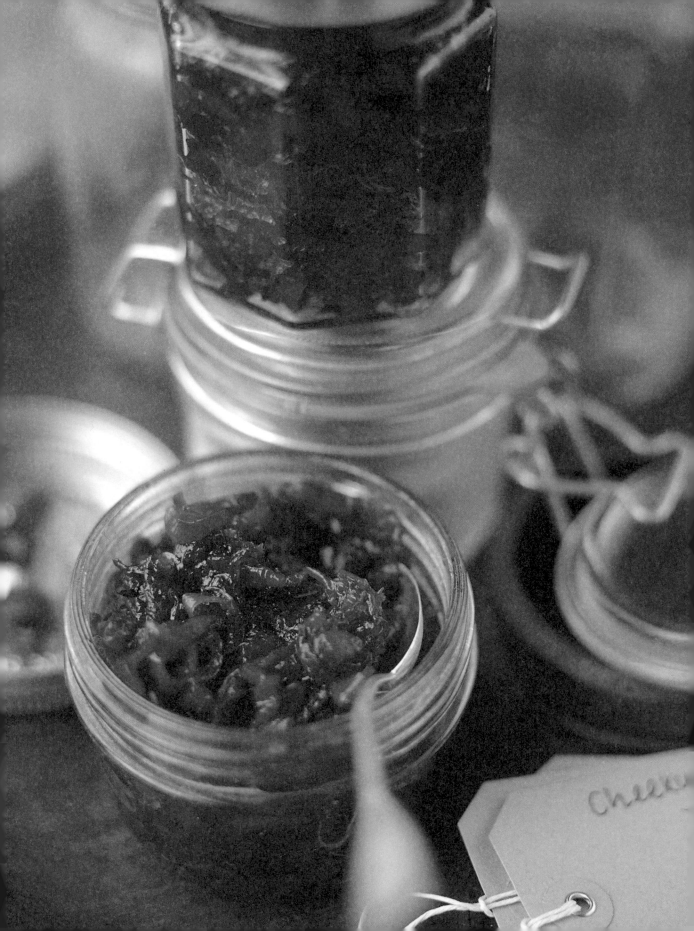

# Cheeky chilli-pepper chutney

This is a great chutney. The sweetness created in the cooking of the peppers calms the heat of the chillies down, giving the chutney a lovely warmth. It's fantastic with crumbly cheese, smeared on toast with melted cheese or with Welsh rarebit (see page 322). Also lovely stirred into gravy with sausages, or with cold leftover meats. Crack on and have a go.

PS You might want to wear a pair of Marigolds when peeling and chopping the chillies or you'll know about it if you rub your eyes afterwards!

If you want your chutney to last for a while, make sure you have some small sterilized jars ready to go (see page 324). Place your chillies and peppers over a hot barbecue, in a griddle pan or on a tray under a hot grill, turning them now and then until blackened and blistered all over. Carefully lift the hot peppers and chillies into a bowl (the smaller chillies won't take as long as the peppers so remove them first) and cover tightly with clingfilm. As they cool down, they'll cook gently in their own steam. By the time they're cool enough to handle, you'll be able to peel the skin off easily.

When you've got rid of most of the skin, trimmed off the stalks and scooped out the seeds, you'll be left with a pile of nice tasty peppers and chillies. Finely chop by hand or put in a food processor and whiz up. Then put to one side.

Heat a saucepan and pour in a splash of olive oil. Add the onions, rosemary, bay leaves and cinnamon and season with a little salt and pepper. Cook very slowly for about 20 minutes or so, until the onions become rich, golden and sticky.

Add the chopped peppers and chillies, the sugar and the vinegar to the onions and keep cooking. When the liquid reduces and you're left with a lovely thick sticky chutney, season well to taste. Remove the cinnamon stick and the bay leaves. Either spoon into the sterilized jars and put them in a cool dark place, or keep in the fridge and use right away. In sterilized jars, the chutney should keep for a couple of months.

**makes about 500g**

8–10 fresh red chillies
8 ripe red peppers
olive oil
2 medium red onions,
  peeled and chopped
a sprig of fresh rosemary,
  leaves picked and chopped
2 fresh bay leaves
a 5cm piece of
  cinnamon stick
sea salt and freshly
  ground black pepper
100g brown sugar
150ml balsamic vinegar

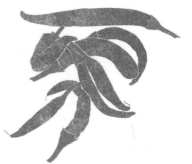

pickles

# Welsh rarebit with attitude

To me this is the most brilliant lunch to have with a good pint of bitter or quality beer. Just the thought of it makes me smile. Let alone being in my favourite pub with the fire going as well. Heaven.

PS My lovely editor, Lindsey, made this for her lunch the other day and decided to leave the eggs out of the mix as she didn't think they'd cook through under the grill. After giving her a hundred lines and various forms of torture, she now knows it's fine to include the eggs. They will cook through in this time. (As I said to Linds, 'Never doubt me, or the chilli jam won't be going on the toast!')

Preheat your grill and get it nice and hot. Whisk the egg yolks with the crème fraîche and mustard powder. Stir in the cheese and season with salt and pepper. Now, I'm rather hoping you've had a go at making the chilli-pepper chutney, but if you haven't then you can cheat by using a good shop-bought version, or simply chop up a little fresh chilli, to your taste.

Lightly toast your slices of bread on both sides. Smear a good tablespoon of your chutney on to each slice, right to the edge, followed by a quarter of your rarebit mixture. By spreading it right to the edge, the crust won't burn. Grill until melted and bubbling. Divide on to plates. With a knife, criss-cross the topping and drizzle with Worcestershire sauce.

**makes 4 slices**

**2 large free-range or organic egg yolks**
**150g crème fraîche**
**1 level teaspoon English mustard powder**
**100g freshly grated Cheddar cheese**
**sea salt and freshly ground black pepper**
**4 tablespoons cheeky chilli-pepper chutney (see page 321) or shop-bought chilli jam, to taste**
**4 x 2cm thick slices of good-quality bread (use sourdough or country style)**
**Worcestershire sauce**

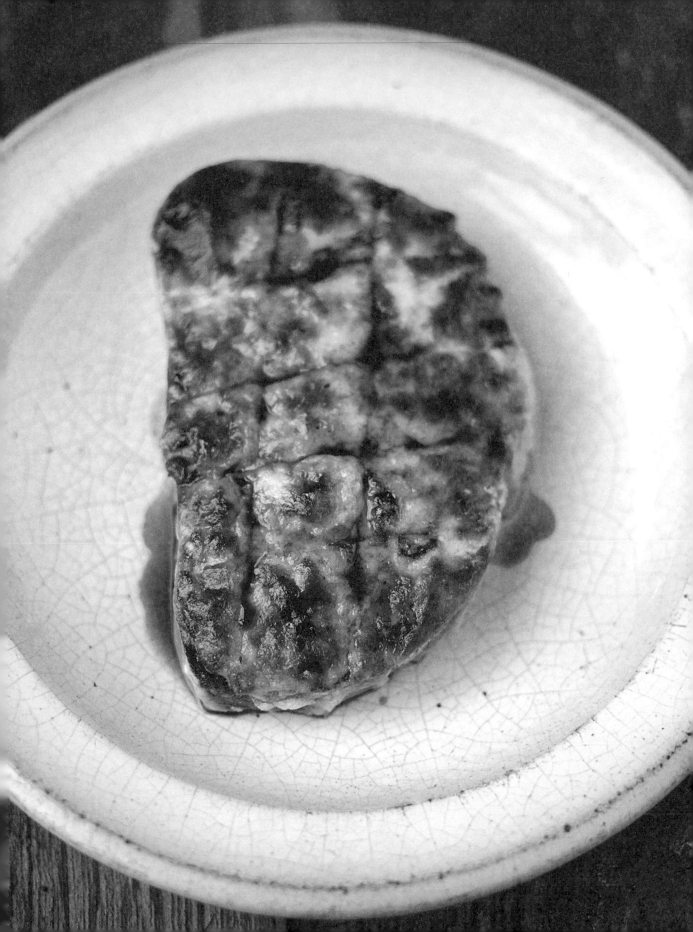

# Pickling

## How to sterilize jars

Before pickling or preserving anything, the one thing you must do is sterilize the jars and their lids to get rid of any bacteria. Either put them in the sink (lids unscrewed from jars) and cover them with boiling hot water from the kettle, filling the jars with the water; or simmer them, completely immersed, in a very large pan of boiling water for 10 minutes; or lay the jars and lids on a baking tray in the oven and heat them at around 100°C/225°F/gas ¼. And if you have a good dishwasher with a very hot cycle you can sterilize them in there as well.

## Some interesting books

- *Jams, Preserves and Chutneys* by Marguerite Patten

- *Preserving* by Oded Schwartz

- *Preserved* by Nick Sandler and Johnny Acton

These three books should be easy to find in good bookshops, but if you fancy it, try having a rummage in some second-hand shops – you might find a lovely pickling book from the old days.

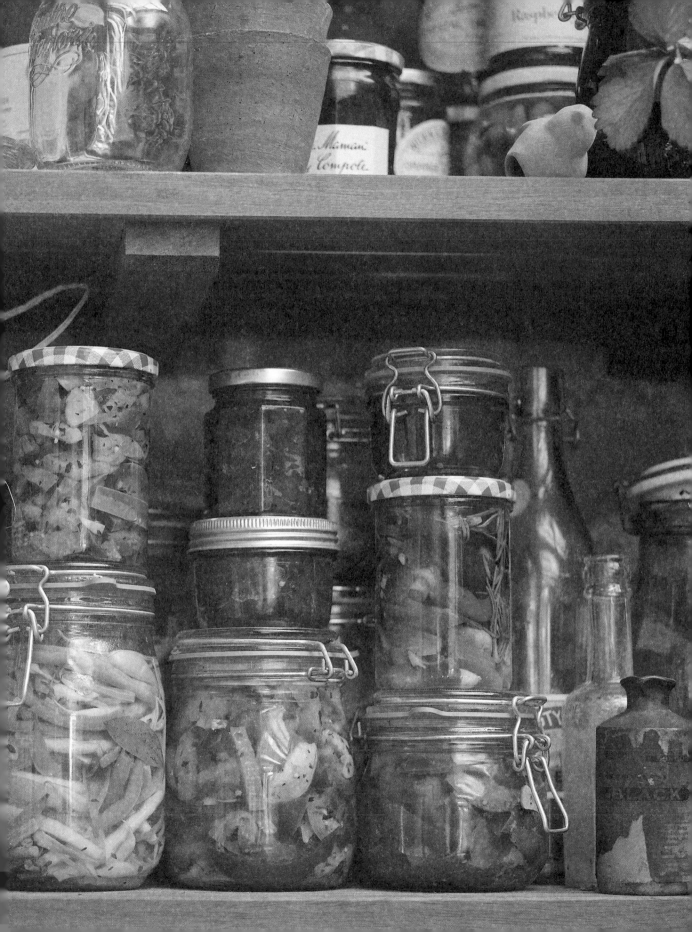

# winter

leeks / pastry / squash / winter salads / winter veg

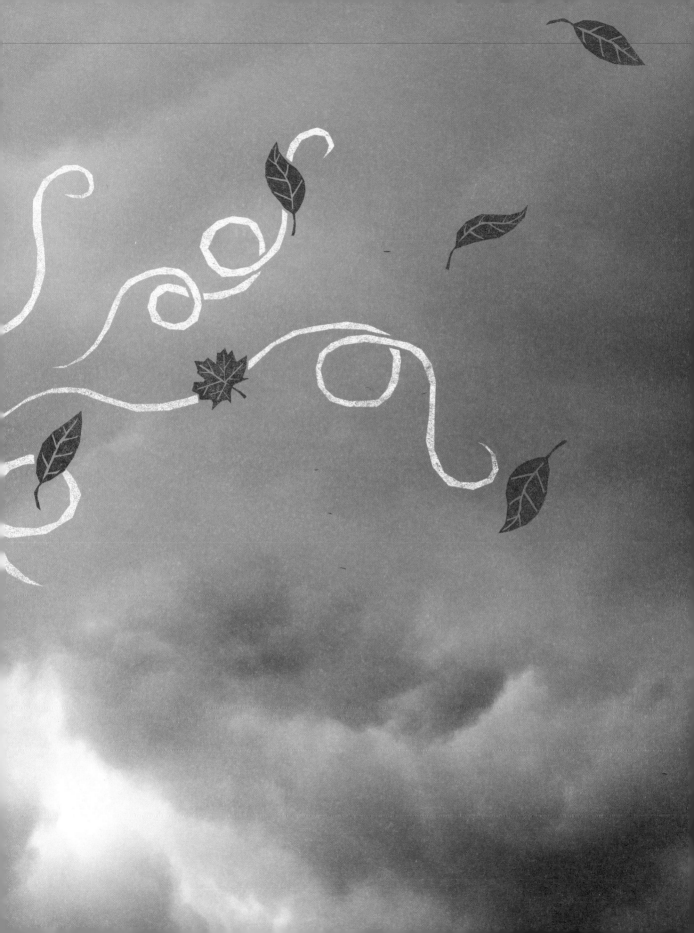

I love leeks, but they are often considered a pretty boring vegetable. Usually sold to us with very little pride or excitement, they end up getting lost in the bases of soups and stews and almost forgotten about. So I want to big them up a bit! Yes, they are a staple vegetable, but to me that just means they're incredibly diverse: they can be used to make chunky or super-smooth soups, added to stews or pot-roasts, served alongside meat or fish as a vegetable dish in their own right, or used in sauces for pasta or risotto. Leeks have an exceptional flavour, especially when cooked slowly and softly, and can add a sweetness to a dish in a similar way to their cousin,

the onion. For me, a good baby leek can be as delicious as a spear of asparagus. One of my favourite things to do with baby leeks is cook them quickly in boiling water for a couple of minutes to soften them and then drain and toss them in chopped herbs, olive oil and a squeeze of lemon juice before grilling them very quickly on both sides or roasting them in the oven. Absolutely delicious.

Nutritionally, leeks are very good for you. Most importantly, like the rest of the allium family, they're really good at lowering bad cholesterol and raising good cholesterol. Doctors reckon that eating two or three portions of leeks,

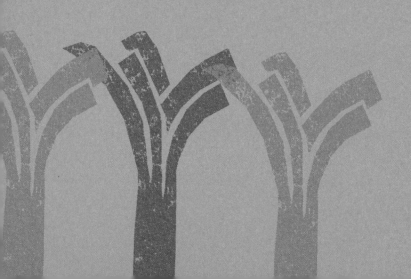

or other alliums, a week can drastically reduce your chances of getting many types of cancer.

When I was a child I always associated leeks with Welsh people, and now I know where the association came from. St David's Day on 1 March celebrates a victory in AD 640 by the Welsh, under King Cadwallader, against the invading Saxons. The Welsh decided to wear leeks in their hats to distinguish themselves from the enemy! Now, war and fighting is bad enough, but imagine having to do it with a massive leek strapped to your head. I've got to hand it to Cadwallader though – his boys definitely stuck out from the crowd!

When it comes to growing them, whether in a window box or in a scraggy corner of the garden, a growing leek is the most beautiful thing. For me, a veg garden isn't a veg garden without leeks in it. You can pick them when they're small and the thickness of a pen, or you can leave them to grow and harvest them when they're massive triffids! All you need to remember is that the smaller they are, the less cooking they need.

In this chapter I want to show you a few different techniques for how I get the most flavour out of leeks. Have a go at these recipes and you'll become known for the best leeks in town!

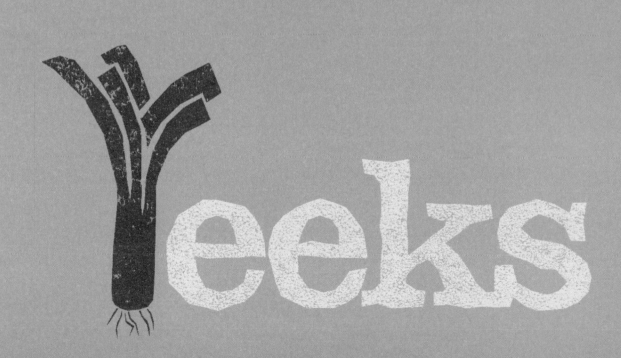

# Roasted concertina squid with grilled leeks and a warm chorizo dressing

I think this is a great, robust, spicy, exciting dish. The flavours from the chorizo dressing along with the grilled leeks and fennel are just incredible.

To achieve the beautiful concertina effect, take a squid and place a large chef's knife flat inside it. Using a second knife, slice the squid across at 1cm intervals, as if you're cutting it into rings. You won't be able to cut all the way because of the other knife.

Light your barbecue or preheat a griddle pan to hot. Preheat your oven to maximum. Parboil the baby leeks for 3 minutes in a pan of boiling salted water, drain in a colander and let them steam dry. Dress them with some olive oil and a pinch of salt. Cook the leeks on the barbecue or in the griddle pan on both sides until nicely marked, then add the fennel wedges and chargrill these dry on both sides until they are also marked. Add the radicchio leaves and dry grill these on both sides to wilt them – 30 seconds on each side should do. Put the leeks, fennel and radicchio into a large bowl – they might look a bit sad, but don't worry because you're going to pep them up!

For the chorizo dressing, heat a frying pan with a couple of glugs of olive oil. Fry the chorizo until the fat renders out, add the rosemary and garlic, toss and take off the heat after 30 seconds. Add the balsamic vinegar and half the lemon juice to the pan, mix and put to one side.

Drizzle some olive oil over each squid, sprinkle with salt and pepper and toss well. Preheat an ovenproof pan on the hob, pour in some olive oil and toss the reserved tentacles in the oil for 1 minute. Add all 4 squid and whack the pan in the preheated oven for a few minutes or until cooked and lightly browned.

Pour the chorizo dressing over your chargrilled veggies and add a good squeeze of lemon juice. Take the squid out of the oven. Serve each of your guests a nice pile of the dressed veggies, a concertina squid, some tentacles and half a lemon. Sprinkle over some of the reserved herby fennel tops and tuck in!

serves 4

4 medium-sized squid, skinned, cleaned and prepared (tentacles removed but reserved)
8 baby leeks, outer leaves trimmed back, washed
olive oil
sea salt and freshly ground black pepper
1 bulb of fennel, cut into thin wedges, herby tops reserved
1 radicchio, leaves separated, washed and spun dry
2 lemons, halved

**for the chorizo dressing**
olive oil
100g chorizo sausage, chopped into small pieces
a sprig of fresh rosemary, leaves picked and chopped
2 cloves of garlic, peeled and finely grated
extra virgin olive oil
3 tablespoons balsamic vinegar
juice of 1 lemon

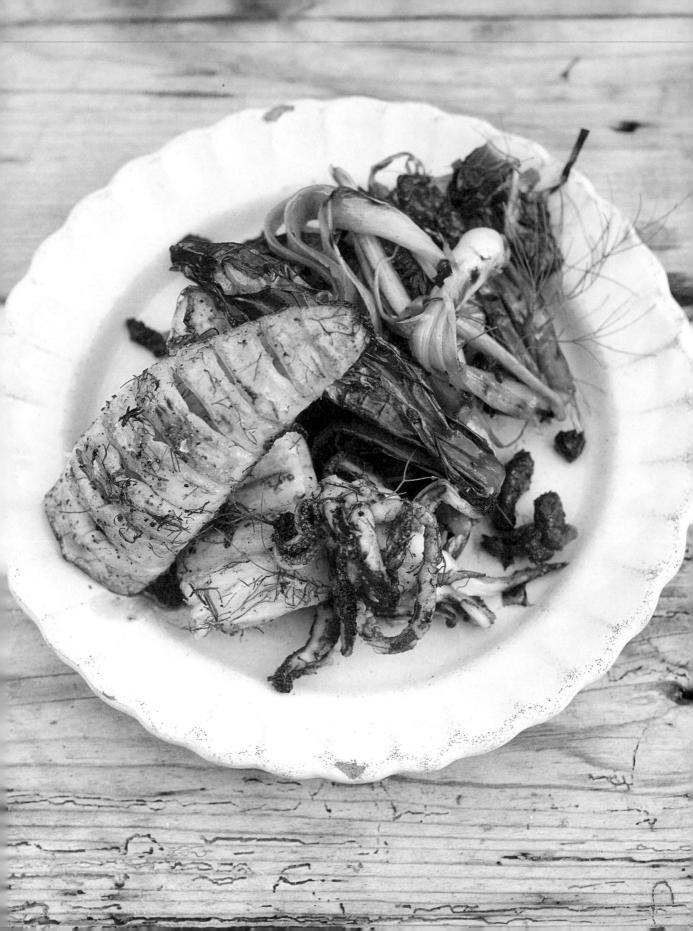

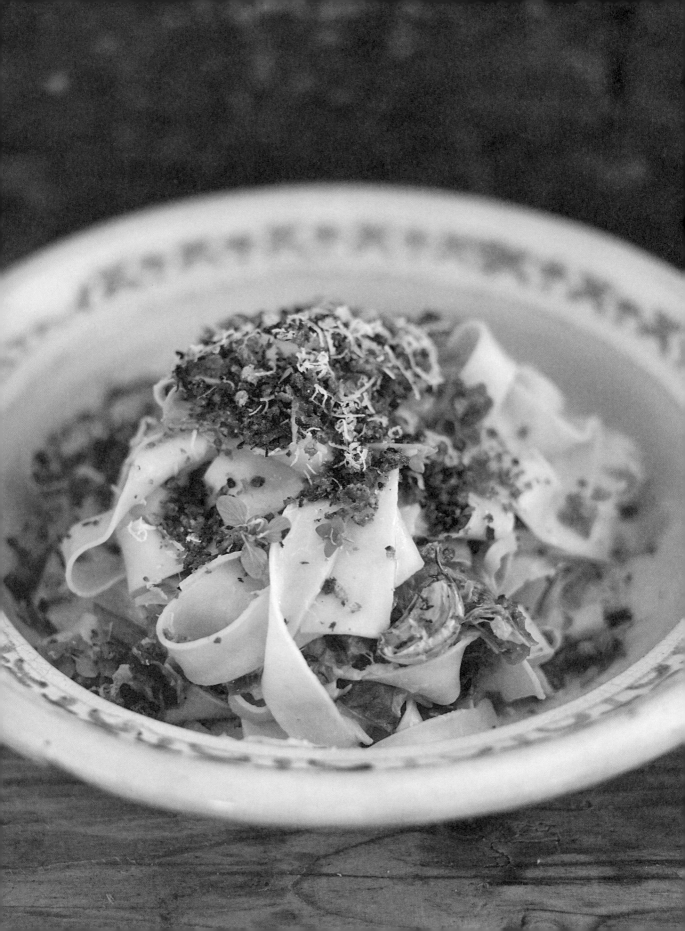

# Cheat's pappardelle with slow-braised leeks and crispy porcini pangrattato

I've called this great dish, with its slap-you-round-the-face flavours, 'cheat's pappardelle', as you can cheat by cutting your own pappardelle from ready-made fresh lasagne sheets. Pangrattato is a rich breadcrumb mixture originally used by poor people in Italy for giving their food extra flavour when they had no Parmesan cheese.

Halve the leeks lengthways and cut at an angle into 1cm slices. Heat a wide saucepan, add a splash of oil and a knob of butter, and when you hear a gentle sizzling add the sliced garlic, thyme leaves and leeks. Move the leeks around so every piece gets coated. Pour in the wine, season with pepper and stir in the stock. Cover the leeks with the slices of Parma ham, place a lid on the pan and cook gently for 25 to 30 minutes. Once the leeks are tender, take the pan off the heat.

To make the pangrattato, whiz the mushrooms and bread with a pinch of salt and pepper in a food processor until the mixture looks like breadcrumbs. Heat a generous glug of olive oil in a frying pan. Add the garlic cloves and the rosemary and cook for a minute, then fry the breadcrumbs in the oil until golden and crisp. Put your garlic cloves on a chopping board and give them a quick bash with the bottom of a pan to crush them. Keep shaking the pan – don't let the breadcrumbs catch on the bottom. Drain on kitchen paper, discard the rosemary, and allow the breadcrumbs to cool.

Bring a big pan of salted water to the boil. Lay the lasagne sheets on a clean working surface and sprinkle with a little flour. Place the sheets on top of each other and slice into 1cm strips. Toss through your fingers to shake out the pappardelle, then cook in the boiling water 2 minutes or until al dente.

Remove the Parma ham from the saucepan, slice up and stir back into the leeks. Season to taste with salt and pepper, then stir in the Parmesan and the rest of the butter. Drain the pasta, reserving a little of the cooking water, and add the pasta to the leeks. Add a little of the cooking water if need be, to give you a silky, smooth sauce. Serve quickly, sprinkled with some pangrattato, extra Parmesan and any leftover thyme tips. Serve the rest of the pangrattato in a bowl on the side.

serves 4 to 6

5 big leeks, outer leaves
   trimmed back, washed
olive oil
3 good knobs of butter
3 cloves of garlic, peeled
   and finely sliced
a few sprigs of fresh
   thyme, leaves picked
a small wineglass
   of white wine
sea salt and freshly
   ground black pepper
500ml good-quality
   vegetable or chicken
   stock
12 slices of Parma ham
2 x 250g packets of
   fresh lasagne sheets
flour, for dusting
2 handfuls of freshly
   grated Parmesan cheese,
   plus extra for serving

*for the pangrattato*
a small handful of dried
   porcini mushrooms
½ a ciabatta bread,
   preferably stale,
   cut into chunks
olive oil
2 cloves of garlic
a sprig of fresh rosemary

leeks

# Roasted white fish and leeks

This is a beautiful dinner. Try to get some lovely sustainable fresh white fish fillets off the bone, like North Atlantic cod, haddock, brill, turbot or pollock. Just ask your fishmonger what's sustainable and he should be able to advise you. The marinade we're going to make is fantastic with white fish.

Preheat the oven to 200°C/400°F/gas 6 and place a baking tray in the oven to warm up.

To make your marinade, bash up the thyme, rosemary and bay leaves with a pinch of salt in a pestle and mortar until the salt turns green. Pour in 2 glugs of olive oil, add a pinch of pepper and the lemon juice and give it a stir.

Bring a pan of salted water to the boil and parboil the leeks for about 3 minutes. Drain in a colander and let them steam dry.

Put the fish, lemon, rosemary sprigs and leeks into a bowl. Pour in the marinade and toss to cover everything in the lovely marinade flavours. Place the fish, skin side down, into the preheated tray. Scoop the lemon, rosemary, leeks and marinade out of the bowl and place over and around the fish. Place 2 rashers of bacon over each piece of fish and roast in the oven for around 15 minutes until the fish is just cooked and the bacon is lovely and crisp. If, after 15 minutes, your fish and bacon are perfect but your leeks could do with a bit more colour, keep the fish and bacon in a warm place while you put your leeks back in the oven to colour up.

Take the tray out of the oven and pile the leeks on to a serving plate. Place the fish and bacon on top and drizzle with the cooking juices – delicious! Also great served with some smooth mashed potato.

serves 4

16 baby leeks, trimmed
    and washed
4 x 200g fillets of lovely
    white fish, off the
    bone, scaled, skin on
1 large lemon, cut into
    8 thin wedges
4 sprigs of fresh rosemary
8 rashers of smoked
    streaky bacon

*for the marinade*
a couple of sprigs each of
    fresh thyme, rosemary
    and bay, leaves picked
sea salt and freshly
    ground black pepper
olive oil
juice of ½ a lemon

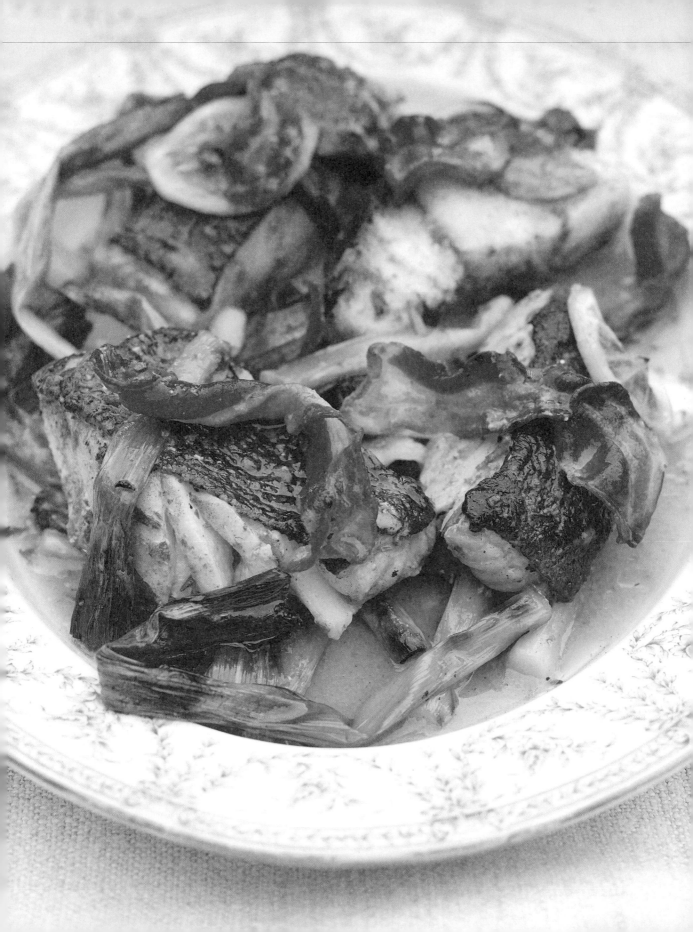

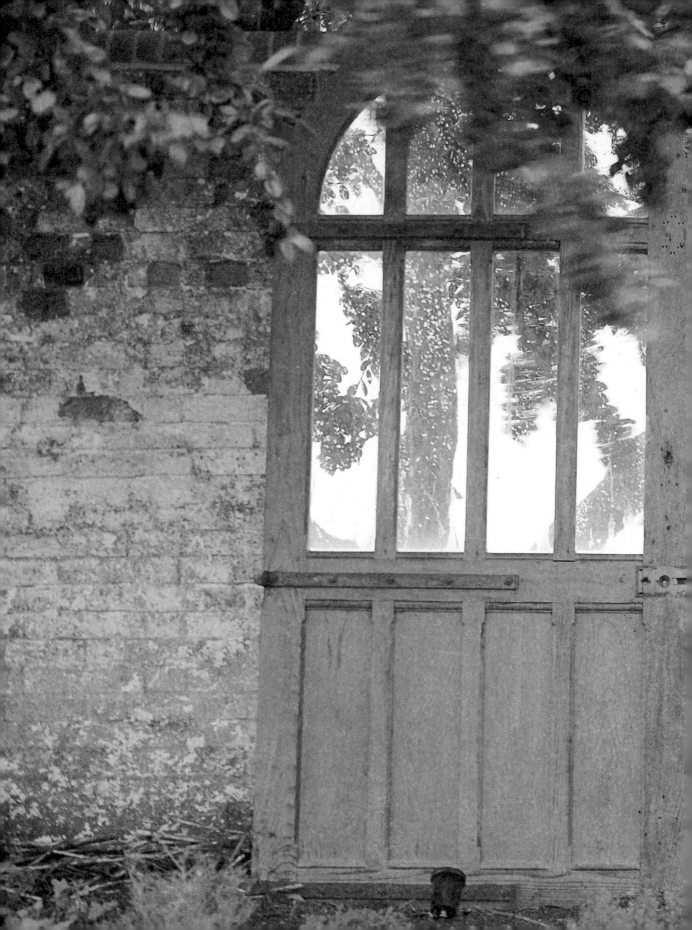

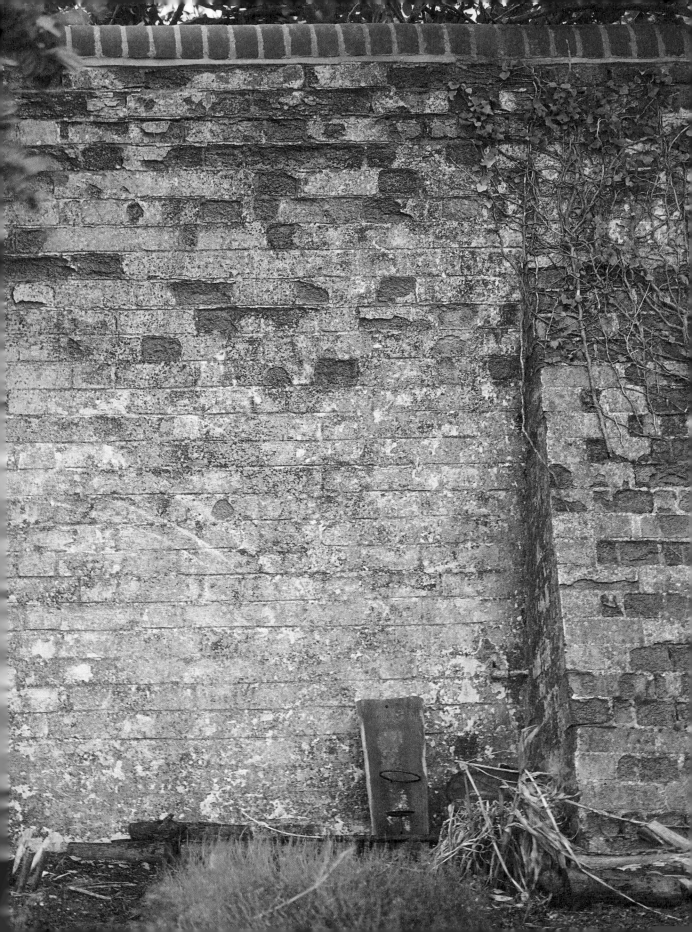

# How I grow leeks

## Soil

Leeks prefer a sunny position in light, well-drained, fairly rich soil, but will grow well in almost any ordinary garden soil, even in heavy clay. They like to be watered well, but don't like to sit in waterlogged ground.

## Planting

I start my leeks off by sowing them indoors in modules or pots during late February or early March. Fill the modules or pots with a good organic potting compost, then sow three to five seeds 0.5cm deep in each one and water them carefully. After ten to twelve weeks, about the end of May, beginning of June, the seedlings will be ready to be planted outside.

To get two different sizes of leek, I usually plant the seedlings in two different ways. First, I plant some of the modules in the soil about 15cm apart – this will give you loads of tasty baby leeks, as they won't have too much room to grow in. If you have space to work with, split some of the remaining modules up carefully and plant the seedlings singly, again about 15cm apart. The extra space means they'll grow to a really good size.

## Harvesting and storing

In November, after a few frosts, the fibres in your leeks will have broken down a bit, making them more tender. A freshly picked leek looks quite robust, but peel away a layer or two and you get these incredible, pale, beautiful colours. The white bits, which haven't seen the sun, are tender and delicious, and absolutely buttery to eat. The greener bits, nearer the top, you can use in many types of cooking; you just need to cook them a bit longer.

Most varieties of leek can remain in the ground throughout the winter until needed – if you're lucky you'll be able to harvest them for up to eight months of the year. You should be able to start harvesting in late summer, with your larger ones coming out of the ground in the autumn. The great thing about leeks is that you can pick them when they're different sizes – from pencil-thin babies to monstrously giant ones! Never pull leeks out of the ground by force as they will probably break in two, leaving you with just a handful of leaves. Instead, lever them out with a spade or a fork. Once picked, you can store them in the fridge for about ten days.

## My growing tips

- Don't grow leeks in the same place year after year as there will be an increased risk of pests and diseases.

- Water young plants generously, especially in hot, dry conditions, until they're well established. Mulching with well-rotted compost in summer can really help to keep the moisture in.

- If you want your plants to have nice long white shanks, you have to pull the soil up around the stems as they grow taller. This is called 'earthing up' or 'blanching'.

- Once you've picked your leeks, dig some gulleys with a spade and pop in the leeks, with their roots still attached. Keep them upright – cram a load into a small area as they've already done their growing. Just pat the soil back over the leeks when you're done. This is called 'heeling' and will not only give you some garden space back, but it will keep your leeks alive, healthy and fresh. You can pull them out as and when you need them, for months to come.

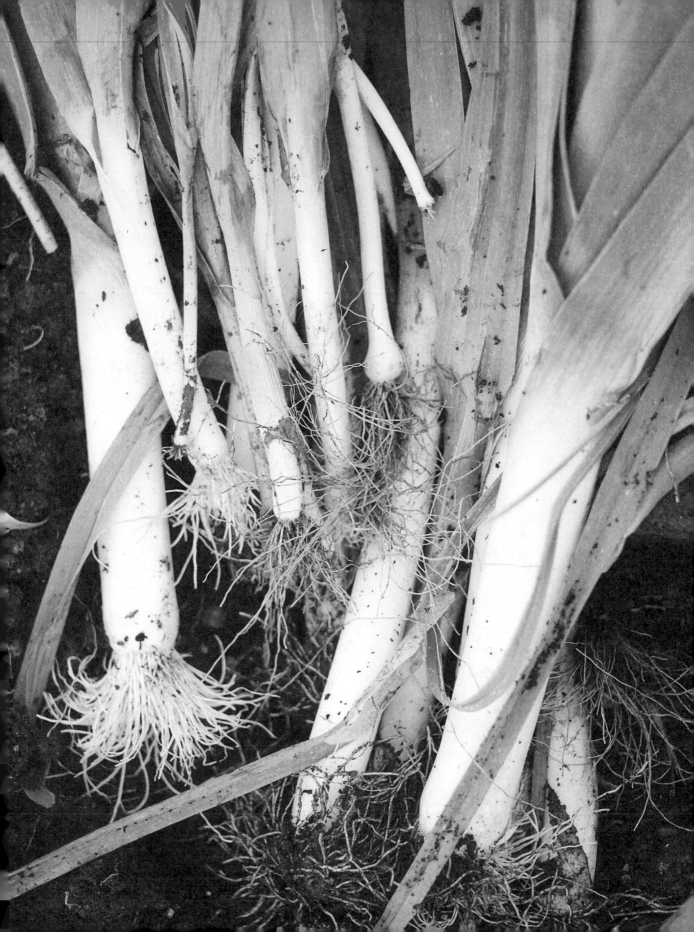

Pastry must be one of the best-loved foods around, not just in the UK but all over the world. Whether it's used in a dessert, or to make a breakfast pastry, or simply as the crust on top of a stew, pastry is incredibly versatile. It can be used in nearly all aspects of cooking, and it's culturally diverse as well. Every country has its own version. The Egyptians were the first people we know of that made it – they used coarsely ground grains, presumably brought together and bound with a little water, while honey, spices and fruit were used as flavourings.

Over the last few thousand years, with migrations, wars, the influence of different religions and, most importantly, lots of trading routes opening up – Greece, Italy, the Far East, Africa, Spain, Portugal, the Middle East – pastry has been embraced by just about every culture I can think of. We Brits love to use it to make sweet and savoury pies; in China and Japan it's made using rice or sesame-based doughs and filled with fruit or bean curd; the eastern Mediterranean countries are famous for baklava – a delicacy made from layers and layers of filo pastry and sweet filling. As you can imagine, I can't possibly include everything there is to know about pastry, so for this chapter I'm going to show you how to make the most widely used versions of shortcrust: sweet and savoury.

The basic recipe for sweet or savoury shortcrust is one you can learn for life. Regardless of what recipe you're going to use it for, or how you tweak it, you'll know that it will give you pretty much the same results every time. I'll also give you two methods for making shortcrust – one by hand and one in a food processor.

The steak, Guinness and cheese pie recipe in this chapter uses the popular and well-loved puff pastry. Now, much as I would love to give you the tedious recipe for puff pastry I was taught when I was learning to be a chef, I feel it doesn't have any relevance to this book. Apart from it being a total palaver to make, you can buy really good-quality all-butter puff pastry in your local supermarket. A wonderful way to cheat, and also, like shop-bought filo, a massive asset to have in your freezer should you need to make something delicious for dinner or dessert.

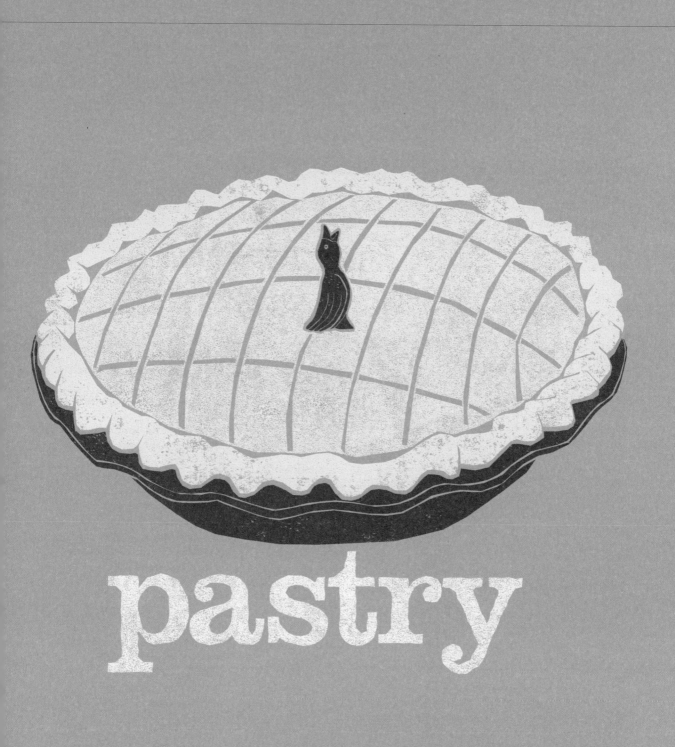

pastry

# Steak, Guinness and cheese pie with a puff pastry lid

This pie is a real winner – damn fine comfort food for a cold evening! As it uses bought puff pastry, it's quick to prepare, and you can make the filling the day before if you want.

Preheat the oven to 190°C/375°F/gas 5. In a large ovenproof pan, heat a glug of olive oil on a low heat. Add the onions and fry gently for about 10 minutes – try not to colour them too much. Turn the heat up, add the garlic, butter, carrots and celery and scatter in the mushrooms. Mix everything together before stirring in the beef, rosemary, a pinch of salt and a level teaspoon of pepper.

Fry fast for 3 or 4 minutes, then pour in the Guinness, stir in the flour and add just enough water to cover. Bring to a simmer, cover the pan with a lid and place in the preheated oven for about 1½ hours. Remove the pan from the oven and give the stew a stir. Put it back into the oven and continue to cook it for another hour, or until the meat is very tender and the stew is rich, dark and thick. A perfect pie filling needs to be robust, so if it's still quite liquidy, place the pan on the hob and reduce until the sauce thickens. Remove from the heat and stir in half the cheese, then season carefully and leave to cool slightly.

Cut about a third of the pastry off the block. Dust a clean work surface with flour and roll both pieces of pastry out evenly with a floured rolling pin to the thickness of a pound coin. Butter an appropriately sized pie dish, then line with the larger sheet, leaving the edges dangling over the side. Tip the stew into your lined dish and even it out before sprinkling over the remaining cheese. Brush the edges of the pastry with a little beaten egg.

Cut the other rolled sheet of pastry to fit the top of the pie dish and criss-cross it lightly with a sharp knife. Place it over the top of the pie and fold the overhanging pastry on to the pastry lid to make it look nice and rustic. Brush the top with beaten egg, then bake the pie directly on the bottom of the oven for 45 minutes, until the pastry is cooked, puffed and golden. Delicious served simply with peas.

serves 4 to 6

olive oil
3 medium red onions, peeled and chopped
3 cloves of garlic, peeled and chopped
30g butter, plus extra for greasing
2 carrots, peeled and chopped
2 sticks of celery, trimmed and chopped
4 field mushrooms, peeled and sliced
1kg brisket of beef or stewing beef, cut into 2cm cubes
a few sprigs of fresh rosemary, leaves picked and chopped
sea salt and freshly ground black pepper
1 x 440ml can of Guinness (no lager, please!)
2 heaped tablespoons plain flour
200g freshly grated Cheddar cheese
500g best-quality ready-made all-butter puff pastry
1 large free-range or organic egg, beaten

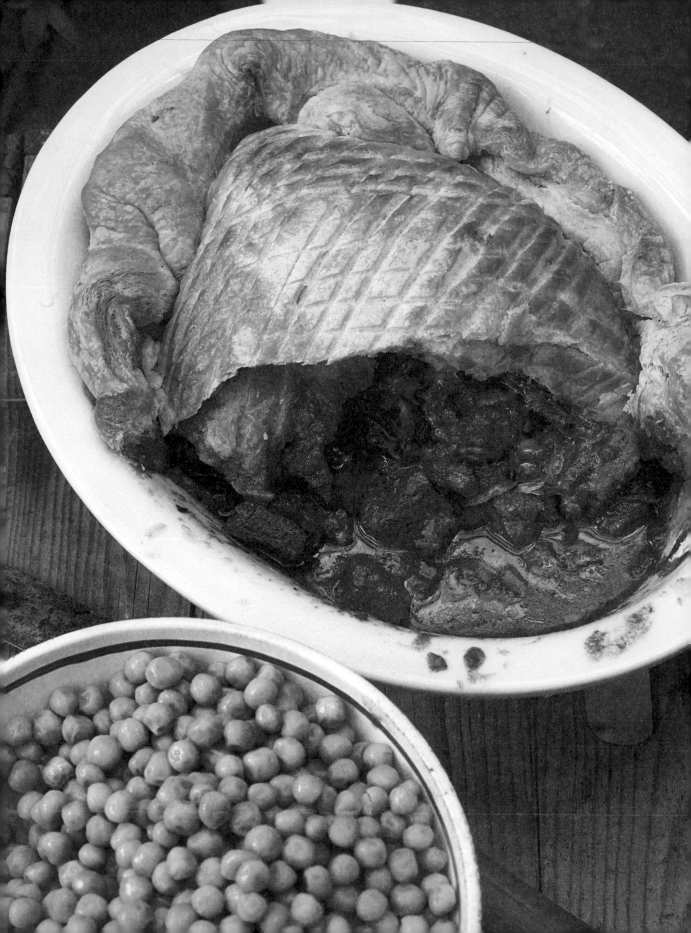

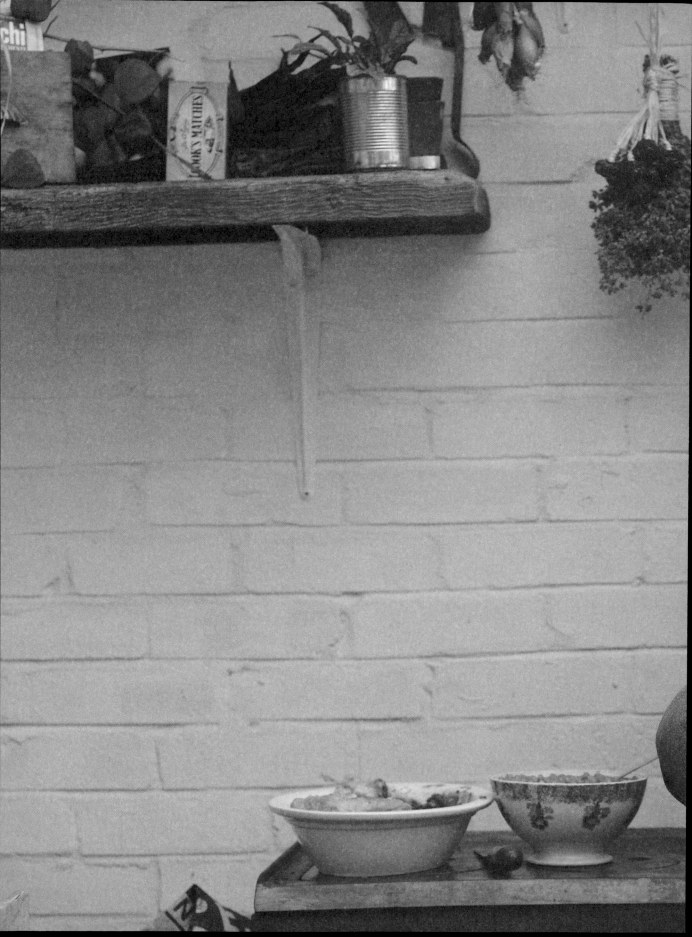

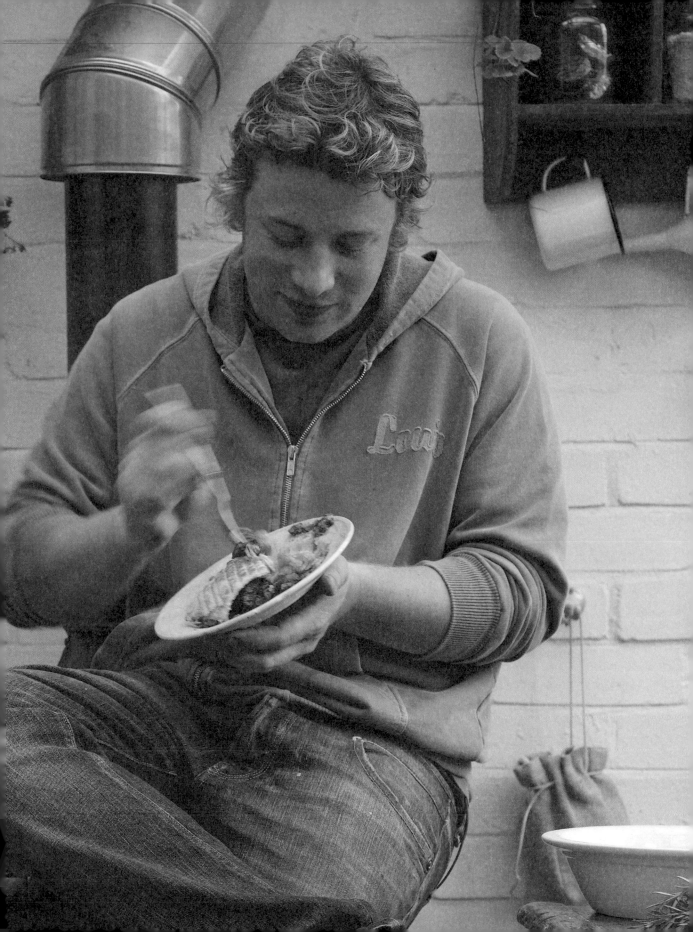

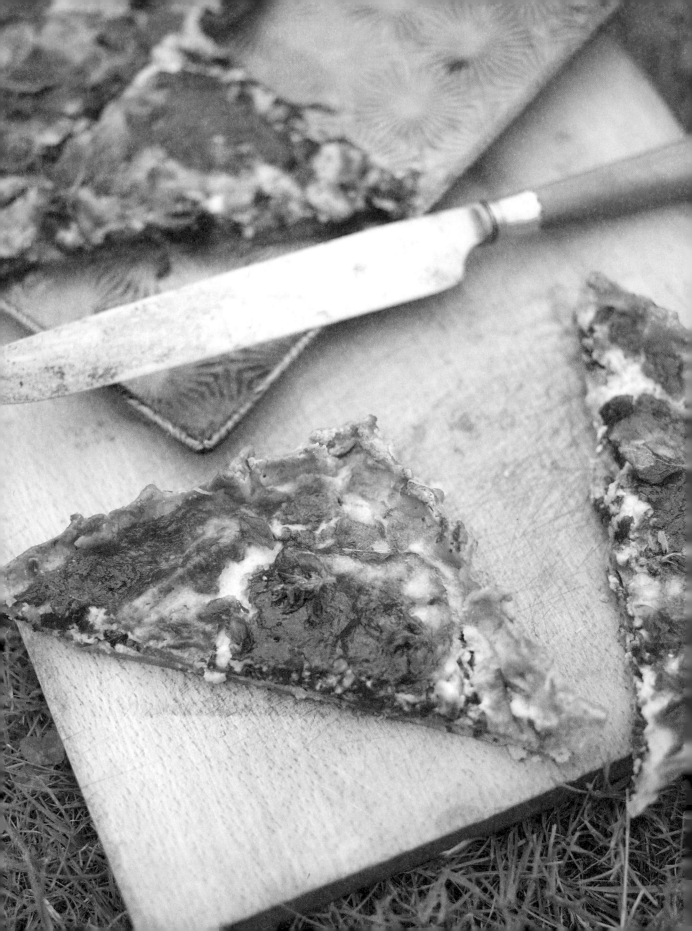

# Italian ham and spinach tart

This Italian-style quiche reminds me of the food my mum used to cook for me when I was a child. I just love it. For the filling, feel free to add a few stoned olives, torn-up sun-dried tomatoes, different cheeses or anchovies.

First, make your pastry dough, wrap it in clingfilm and rest it in the fridge for at least half an hour. Dust a clean work surface with flour, get the pastry out and roll it with a floured rolling pin into a rectangular shape about 0.5cm thick and big enough to line a shallow baking tray about 30 x 40cm.

Grease the tray with butter and line it with the pastry. Trim any excess off the edges of the tray, leaving a 1cm overhang. Pinch this overhanging dough up to give a little rim. This not only gives it a rustic edge but also stops the pastry from shrinking and it means there's no need to fill the pastry case with beans or rice before baking it blind. Prick the pastry all over with a fork and chill in the freezer for another 30 minutes.

Preheat the oven to 190°C/375°F/gas 5. Remove the tray from the fridge and bake your pastry case in the preheated oven for 6 to 8 minutes, until lightly golden. This is called baking it blind, and it stops the pastry from going soggy when you add the filling. Next, heat a glug of olive oil in a large frying pan and gently fry the onions on a low heat for 10 minutes until they're soft and sweet, but don't let them colour. Turn up the heat, add the garlic, the spinach (in batches if your pan isn't big enough) and most of the marjoram. Season lightly and give it a good stir. Take the pan off the heat when the spinach has wilted – this will only take a couple of minutes.

To make the filling mixture, put the crème fraîche into a bowl, stir in the Parmesan, eggs and a pinch of salt and pepper, mix together and set aside. Now spread the spinach mixture over your pastry case. Sprinkle over the ham, and spoon the mixture evenly over the top, smoothing it out with the back of the spoon. Grate over a generous helping of Parmesan, sprinkle over the rest of the marjoram and drizzle with some olive oil.

Bake in the preheated oven for about 15 to 20 minutes, or until the top is golden and bubbling and the filling has set. Lovely served with a little salad of watercress, dressed with olive oil, a squeeze of lemon juice and some salt and pepper.

serves 6 to 8

½ x savoury shortcrust
   pastry recipe (see
   page 353)
a knob of butter
olive oil
3 red onions, peeled and
   finely sliced
1 clove of garlic, peeled
   and sliced
350g spinach (you can
   also use nettles, Swiss
   chard or borage), washed,
   thick stems removed
a few sprigs of fresh
   marjoram or oregano,
   leaves picked and chopped
sea salt and freshly
   ground black pepper
500g crème fraîche
150g freshly grated
   Parmesan cheese, plus
   extra for grating
3 large free-range or
   organic eggs
200g cooked smoked ham,
   torn into shreds or
   chopped

# Blackberry and apple pie

This is the best apple pie in the world. You can't go wrong with Bramley cooking apples, delicious blackberries and stem ginger. The cooking time can depend on how freshly picked the apples are, so the best thing is to cook them until they're softened first. And I don't know if you've noticed this, but blackberries in shops never seem to taste of anything these days unless they've just been picked from a local grower – so do try to get fresh ones if you can, or pick your own straight from the bush!

First, make your pastry dough, wrap it in clingfilm and rest it in the fridge for at least half an hour. Then preheat the oven to 180°C/350°F/gas 4. Put the butter and sugar into a saucepan and, when the butter has melted, add the apples, stem ginger and a tablespoon of the ginger syrup. Slowly cook for 15 minutes with a lid on, then add the blackberries, stir and cook for 5 more minutes with the lid off.

Meanwhile, remove your pastry from the fridge. Dust your work surface with flour, cut the pastry in half and, using a floured rolling pin, roll one of the pieces out until it's just under 1cm thick. (Rolling the dough between two layers of greaseproof paper will also stop it sticking to your rolling pin.) Butter a shallow 26cm pie dish and line with the pastry, trimming off any excess round the edges using a sharp knife.

Tip the cooled apples and blackberries into a sieve, reserving all the juices, then put the fruit into the lined pie dish so you have a mound in the middle. Spoon over half the reserved juices. Brush the edge of the pastry with beaten egg. Roll out the second piece of pastry, just as you did the first, and lay it over the top of the pie. Trim the edges as before and crimp them together with your fingers. Brush the top of the pie with the rest of the beaten egg, sprinkle generously with sugar and the cinnamon, and make a couple of slashes in the top of the pastry.

Place the pie on a baking tray and then put it directly on the bottom of the preheated oven for 55 to 60 minutes, until golden brown and crisp. Slice the pie into portions and serve with a generous dollop of custard.

**serves 6 to 8**

1 x sweet shortcrust pastry recipe (see page 352)
50g butter, plus extra for greasing
100g golden caster sugar, plus extra for sprinkling
2 large Bramley apples, cored, peeled and each cut into 16 wedges
4 Cox's apples, cored, peeled and each cut into 8 wedges
1 heaped tablespoon chopped stem ginger, in syrup
150g blackberries
1 large free-range or organic egg, beaten
½ teaspoon ground cinnamon

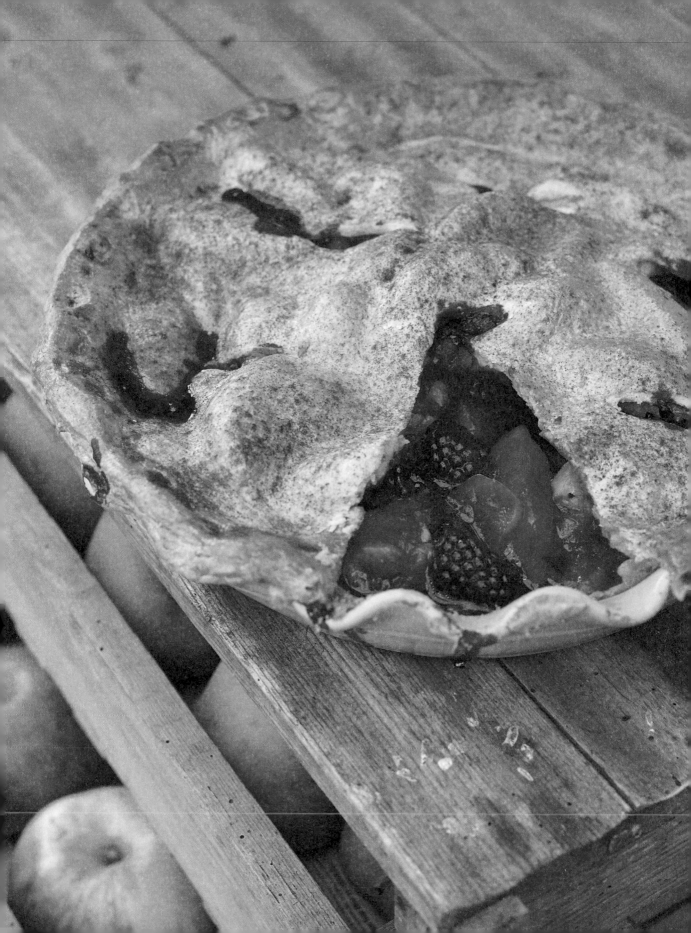

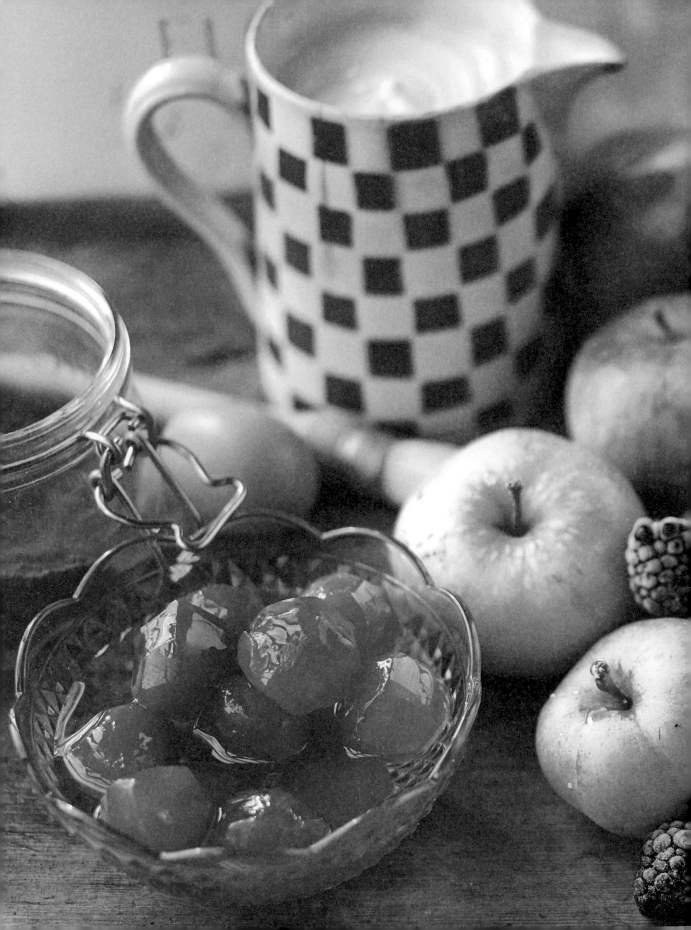

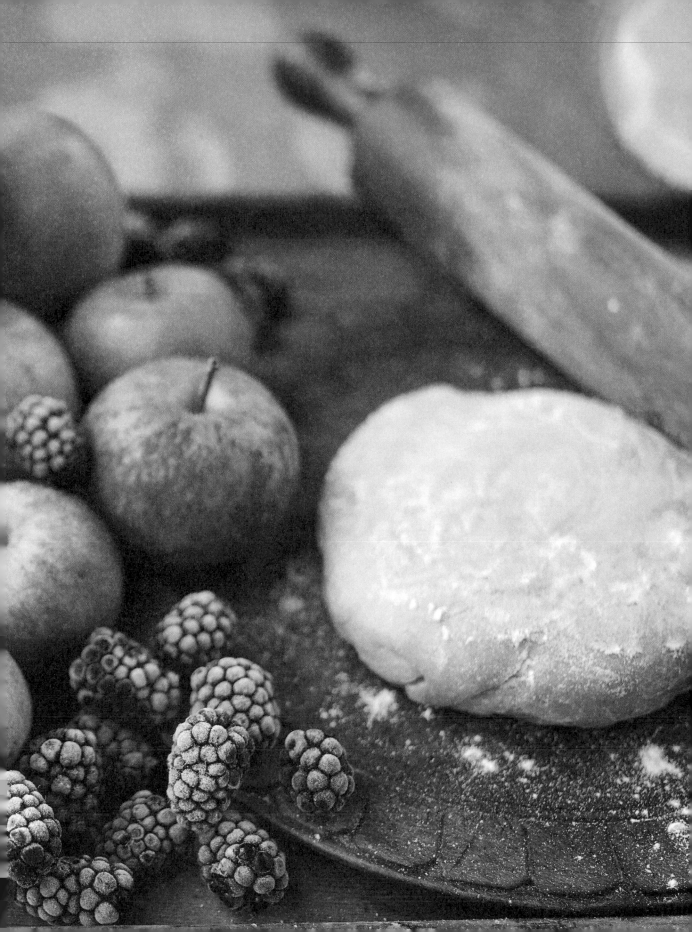

# Old-fashioned sweet shortcrust pastry

This pastry is perfect for making apple and other sweet pies. Even if you've never made pastry before, as long as you stick to the correct measurements for the ingredients and you follow the method exactly, you'll be laughing. The one place where you can experiment is with flavouring. If you don't fancy using lemon zest, try another dry ingredient like orange zest instead. Or a pinch of cinnamon, nutmeg or cocoa powder. Vanilla seeds are great too. Just remember to be subtle and don't go overboard with any of these flavours!

Try to be confident and bring the pastry together as quickly as you can – don't knead it too much or the heat from your hands will melt the butter. A good tip is to hold your hands under cold running water beforehand to make them as cold as possible. That way you'll end up with a delicate, flaky pastry every time.

PS You can also make this pastry using a food processor (see the method opposite).

Sieve the flour from a height on to a clean work surface and sieve the icing sugar over the top. Using your hands, work the cubes of butter into the flour and sugar by rubbing your thumbs against your fingers until you end up with a fine, crumbly mixture. This is the point where you can spike the mixture with interesting flavours, so mix in your lemon zest.

Add the eggs and milk to the mixture and gently work it together till you have a ball of dough. Flour it lightly. Don't work the pastry too much at this stage or it will become elastic and chewy, not crumbly and short. Flour your work surface and place the dough on top. Pat it into a flat round, flour it lightly, wrap it in clingfilm and put it into the fridge to rest for at least half an hour.

**makes about 1kg**

500g organic plain flour, plus extra for dusting
100g icing sugar, sifted
250g good-quality cold butter, cut into small cubes
zest of 1 lemon
2 large free-range or organic eggs, beaten
a splash of milk

# The best savoury shortcrust pastry

This savoury pastry is good for making tarts, quiches and the like. The two main principles behind making it are the same as for a sweet pastry: stick to a ratio of half fat to flour, and bring the pastry together as quickly as possible without pulsing the dough too much. Like the sweet pastry, you can flavour this savoury one in different ways. Try things like paprika, black pepper, nutmeg or mace instead of the rosemary and thyme.

In my opinion, an exceptional savoury pastry is made with suet or lard, rather than butter. This gives the pastry a great flavour, a slightly richer texture and a delicious caramelized crust when it comes out of the oven. Feel free to use butter instead, if you're at all concerned about the fat intake of lard, but if you're eating this only once in a while, why not spoil yourself and do it properly? There's nothing better!

PS You can also make this pastry the old-fashioned way (by hand!) if you're feeling nostalgic (see the method opposite).

Put the flour, lard, cheese and a generous pinch of sea salt into a food processor and pulse for 20 to 30 seconds or until the mixture is crumbly and fine. Add the rosemary and thyme leaves or your chosen flavouring.

Pour in the eggs and add the milk. Pulse for a few more seconds until the mixture comes together. Scoop your dough out of the food processor on to a clean floured work surface and pat it a few times to make it more compact – don't be tempted to knead it. When you have a flat round, wrap the dough in clingfilm and place it in the fridge to rest for at least half an hour.

**makes just under 1kg**

**500g organic plain flour,
  plus extra for dusting**
**200g lard, cut into cubes**
**50g freshly grated
  Cheddar cheese**
**sea salt**
**a sprig of fresh rosemary,
  leaves picked**
**a few sprigs of fresh
  thyme, leaves picked**
**2 large free-range or
  organic eggs, beaten**
**a splash of milk**

pastry

# squash

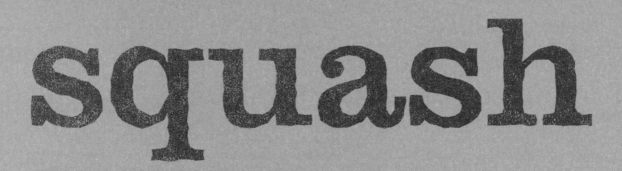

For me the world of squash is an exciting and mysterious one. I love all the different shapes, sizes and colours and the way the plants sprawl around and grow over things – I find it absolutely fascinating! They're brilliant to grow at home.

Historically, squash and pumpkins are pretty intertwined, as they're part of the same family, and in botanical terms they're actually classified as fruit, not vegetables. They've been grown and eaten for the last 10,000 years in the area between Guatemala and Mexico in South America, and became a big favourite of the Native Americans. Although you can't always generalize, summer squashes, like courgettes and pattypans, are very fast-growing and can be cooked and consumed very quickly, sometimes even eaten raw. Winter squashes, such as butternut and acorn, are normally ready by the end of the summer and can be stored successfully for many months. They need to be cooked to get the best flavour out of them.

When it comes to cooking squash, I try to avoid the more cellular, stringy, watery varieties and go for those with denser flesh, as they have better flavour and hold their shape better. The supermarkets tend to sell favourite varieties like butternut squash, but I'd love you to try some different types – it's great to experiment. However, bearing in mind its popularity, I've given you a handful of recipes in this chapter mainly using the good old butternut.

Squash can be made into incredible soups, with flavours like rosemary, sage and smoky bacon, and they're fantastic when tossed in spices like fennel seeds, chilli and cinnamon, then roasted and torn into really interesting winter salads of rocket and radicchio, drizzled with balsamic vinegar. They can be flavoured subtly, but I much prefer them with a confident use of spices and herbs as they're a wonderful carrier of flavours. They're also very good for you, as they contain loads of vitamin A, B, C and E along with a bit of potassium for healthy blood pressure. A general rule is that the more orange they are, the better they are for you. The seeds are also great when roasted and tossed into salads or stir-fries.

One of the first squash dishes I ever enjoyed was an Italian dish called agro dolce (which means 'sweet and sour'), using vinegar for sourness and raisins and dried grapes for sweetness, cooked like a little stew – delicious. Another great thing to do with squash is to include it as part of an antipasti plate – great at the end of the summer. Simply cut the squash into chunks about 3mm thick, chargrill them for 3 or 4 minutes, then season with a little chopped fresh chilli, drizzle over some good extra virgin olive oil and serve with a handful of rocket. In culinary terms, the things you can do with squash are endless . . .

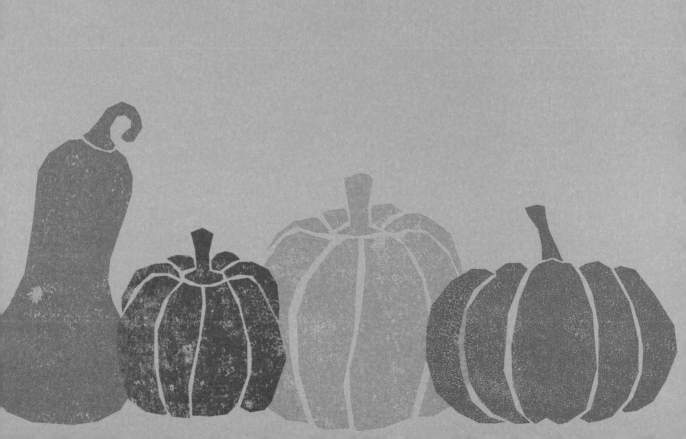

# Whole roasted cricket ball squash

I love this recipe – it's damn simple, looks quirky and there's something special about having your own individual natural pot of incredible flavour! This works well as a snack or a starter. (My old boss Rose Gray, from the River Café, used to call these little gem squash 'cricket ball squash' because of their size.)

Preheat your oven to 180°C/350°F/gas 4. Slice off the top part of the squash, where the stalk comes out, leaving you with a lid for each (like taking the top off a boiled egg). Please do this carefully – no slipping! Scoop out the seeds and discard them. Crush up all the herbs and spices in a pestle and mortar or Flavour Shaker until ground to a powder. Drain the sun-dried tomatoes, reserving the oil. Drizzle a little of the oil into each of the squash and use your fingers to smear it round the insides. Season the inside of each squash with salt and pepper, followed by a sprinkling of the spice mixture. Finely chop up the sun-dried tomatoes and add these to the squash, giving each one a little mix around. Place the lid on top of each squash. Place in a baking dish and roast in the preheated oven for around 45 minutes to an hour, until the flesh inside is soft.

Take your squash out of the oven. I like to let them cool down for a little while I simply dress the rocket with a pinch of salt and pepper, a drizzle of good extra virgin olive oil and a squeeze of lemon juice. Place a whole squash on to each of your four serving plates. Cut up the goat's cheese and place some on each plate. Serve with the dressed rocket and a teaspoon for scooping out the incredible flavours.

PS I like the fact that there's something lovely and simple about the recipe above, but there are lots of variations that can be introduced to it – you could try stuffing the squash with sautéd mushrooms, cheese or smoky bacon.

serves 4

4 gem squash
1 teaspoon dried oregano
1 level teaspoon coriander seeds
1–2 dried red chillies, chopped, to taste
a pinch of ground cinnamon
8 sun-dried tomatoes in oil
sea salt and freshly ground black pepper
a large handful of rocket, washed and spun dry
extra virgin olive oil
½ a lemon
250g tasty crumbly goat's cheese or feta cheese

squash

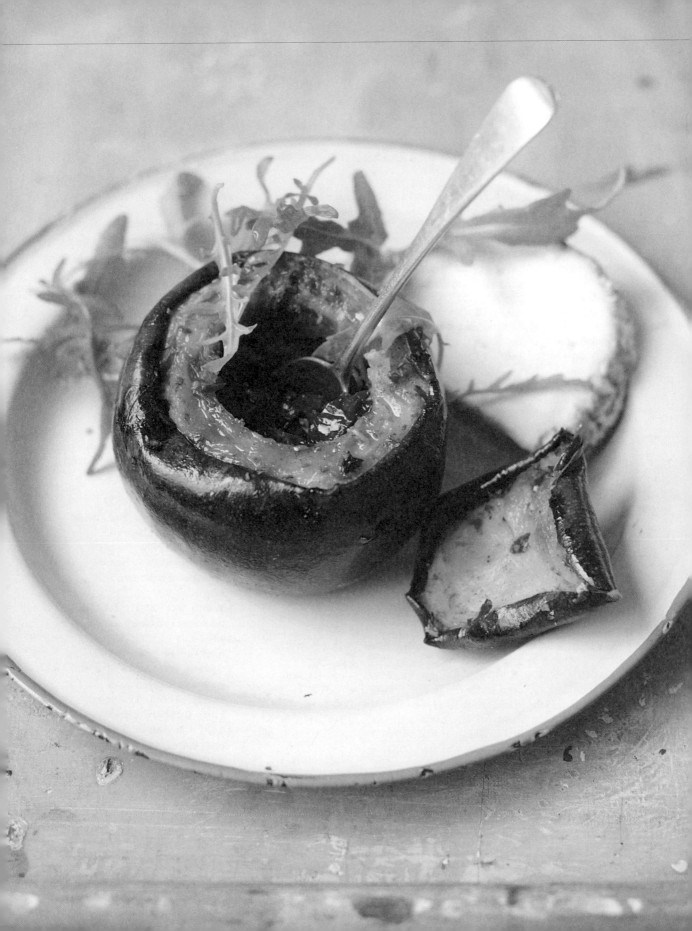

# Asian squash salad with crispy duck

This warm salad with rich, tender duck meat and crispy skin is perfect to big up incredible spiced roasted squash. I love it served on a big platter and dressed at the very last minute.

Preheat the oven to 180°C/350°F/gas 4. Wash the duck and pat it dry, inside and out, with kitchen paper, then rub it all over, inside as well, with salt and pepper. Place it in a tray and roast in the preheated oven for around 2 hours, turning it every now and then. Halfway through, you'll probably need to drain away a lot of the fat from the bird. Don't throw it away, though! Sieve it and keep the fat (but no meat juices) in a jar in the fridge for a couple of months and use it to roast potatoes.

In a pestle and mortar or a Flavour Shaker, bash up the dried chillies and coriander seeds and add the ground cinnamon and a good pinch of salt and pepper. Scoop the seeds out of your squash and put them to one side. Cut the squash into wedges, place them in a roasting tray, and drizzle over enough olive oil just to coat. Sprinkle over the ground spices and give the squash a good toss, spreading the pieces out in one layer. Once the duck has been in the oven for 1 hour and 15 minutes, add the tray of squash to the oven and roast for about 45 minutes.

Meanwhile, rinse the squash seeds after removing any fibres. Season with salt and pepper and drizzle with olive oil. Toast them in a dry frying pan until they're golden and crisp, and put aside. To make the dressing, put the lime juice and zest into a bowl and add the same amount of extra virgin olive oil, plus the sesame oil and the soy sauce. Stir in the sugar, chilli, garlic, the green spring onion ends and coriander stalks. Taste and adjust the sweet-and-sourness and the seasoning. You want it to be a little limey, to contrast with the rich duck.

After 2 hours, if the duck is nice and crispy, and the squash soft and sticky, take both trays out of the oven. If they need more time, leave them in until perfectly done. Using two forks, shred the duck meat off the bone and put into a large bowl. While the duck and squash are still warm, toss with the toasted seeds, half the coriander leaves, half the mint and half the white spring onion slices. Pour on the dressing and toss together. Serve sprinkled with the rest of the coriander, mint and white spring onion slices.

serves 4 to 6

1 x 2kg Gressingham duck
sea salt and freshly
  ground black pepper
a small bunch of fresh
  mint, leaves picked
  and chopped

*for the roasted squash*
1–2 dried red chillies,
  crumbled
1 teaspoon coriander seeds
½ teaspoon ground
  cinnamon
sea salt and freshly
  ground black pepper
1 large butternut squash or
  2 onion squash, quartered
olive oil

*for the dressing*
zest and juice of 1–2 limes
extra virgin olive oil
1 teaspoon sesame oil
1 tablespoon soy sauce
1 teaspoon soft brown
  sugar
1 fresh red chilli, deseeded
  and finely chopped
1 clove of garlic, peeled
  and finely grated
5 spring onions, white
  parts trimmed and
  finely sliced, green
  ends finely chopped
a large bunch of fresh
  coriander, leaves picked
  and stalks finely chopped

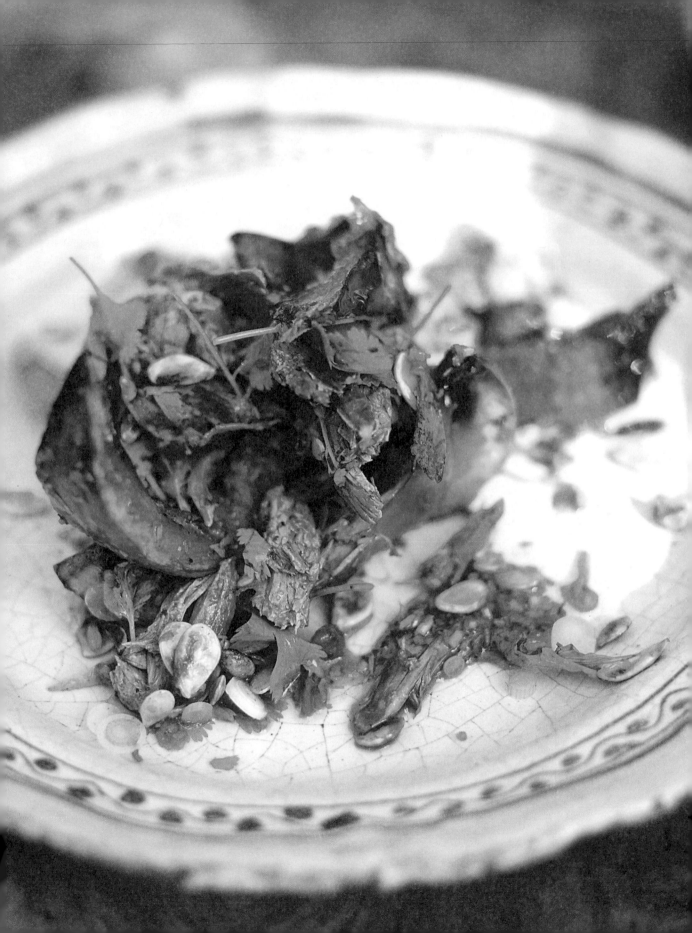

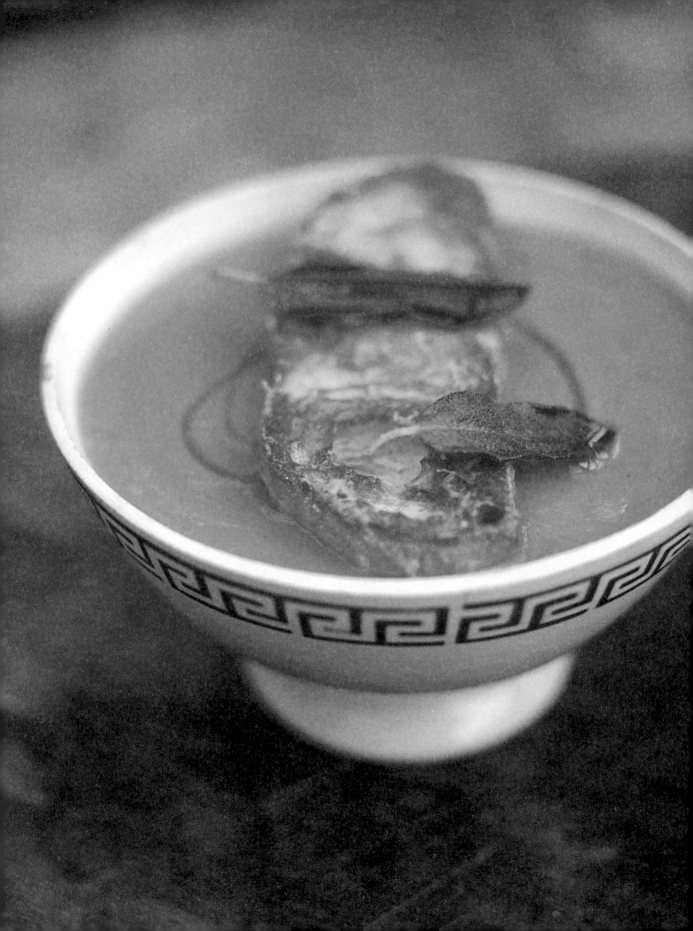

# Superb squash soup with the best Parmesan croutons

This fantastic soup is best made with varieties of squash that have dense, orange flesh, such as butternut or onion squash. It's important to use good chicken stock and season the soup well to bring out the nutty, sweet flavour of the squash. Once you've mastered this recipe, you can take the soup in different ways by adding pearl barley, dried pasta, or some chopped smoked bacon. Even the smallest amount of dried porcini.

PS I made this in my pressure cooker the other day, with really great results – it's so quick!

Put a very large saucepan on a medium heat and pour in a couple of glugs of olive oil. Add the sage leaves and fry for around 30 seconds or until dark green and crisp. Quickly remove them with a slotted spoon to a bowl lined with kitchen paper – you'll use these for sprinkling over at the end. In the pan you'll be left with a beautifully flavoured oil, so put it back on the heat and throw in your onion, celery, carrot, garlic, rosemary leaves, chilli and a good pinch of salt and pepper. Cook gently for about 10 minutes until the vegetables are sweet and soft. Add the squash and the stock to the pan, bring to the boil and simmer for around half an hour.

While the soup is cooking, make your croutons. Drizzle a little olive oil over the ciabatta slices, pat it in and press some grated Parmesan on to each side. Place in a non-stick pan without any oil and fry until golden on both sides.

When the squash is soft and cooked through, whiz the soup with a hand blender or pour it into a liquidizer and pulse until you have a smooth purée (but you can leave it slightly chunky if you like). Most importantly, remember to taste and season it until it's perfect. Divide the soup between your bowls, placing 2 croutons on top of each. Sprinkle with a few of your crispy sage leaves and drizzle with a swirl of good-quality extra virgin olive oil.

serves 8

olive oil
16 fresh sage leaves
2 red onions, peeled and chopped
2 sticks of celery, trimmed and chopped
2 carrots, peeled and chopped
4 cloves of garlic, peeled and chopped
2 sprigs of fresh rosemary, leaves picked
½–1 fresh red chilli, to taste, deseeded and finely chopped
sea salt and freshly ground black pepper
2kg butternut squash, onion squash, or musque de Provence, halved, deseeded and cut into chunks
2 litres good-quality chicken or vegetable stock
extra virgin olive oil

*for the croutons*
extra virgin olive oil
16 slices of ciabatta bread
a block of Parmesan cheese, for grating

squash

361

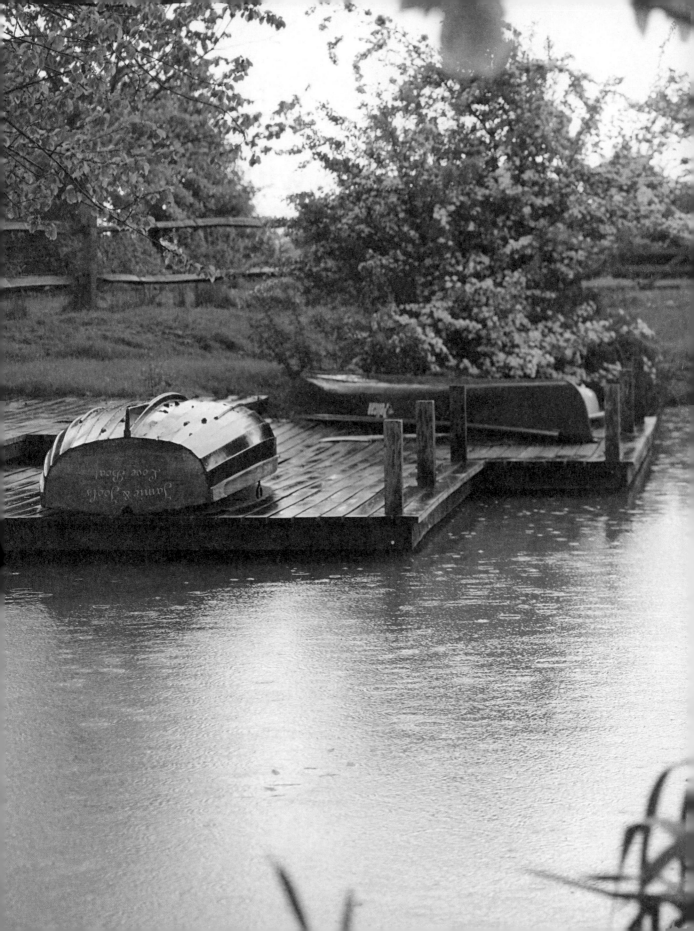

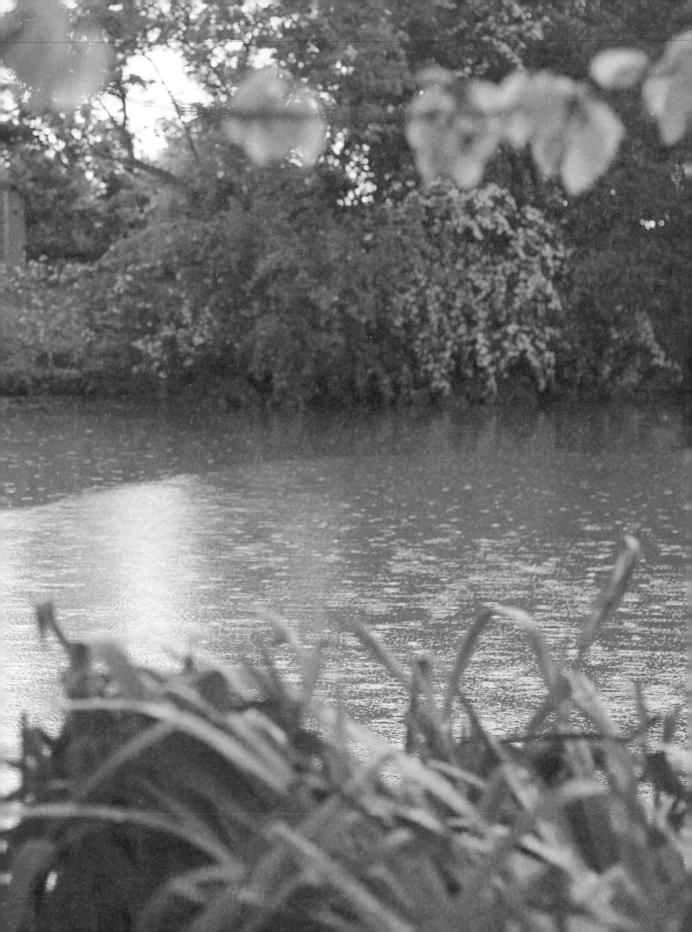

# Butternut squash muffins with a frosty top

My kids love these squash muffins. They taste a bit like carrot cake, as the two vegetables are very similar – I've simply swapped carrots for squash. Both of them are wonderful carriers of flavours like cinnamon, cloves and vanilla. The skin of a butternut squash goes deliciously chewy and soft when cooked, so there's no need to peel it off. Give these little cakes a go – they're a perfect naughty-but-nice treat. And a great way of getting your kids to eat squash!

Preheat the oven to 180°C/350°F/gas 4. Line your muffin tins with paper cases.

Whiz the squash in a food processor until finely chopped. Add the sugar, and crack in the eggs. Add a pinch of salt, the flour, baking powder, walnuts, cinnamon and olive oil and whiz together until well beaten. You may need to pause the machine at some point to scrape the mix down the sides with a rubber spatula. Try not to overdo it with the mixing – you want to just combine everything and no more.

Fill the paper cases with the cake mixture. Bake in the preheated oven for 20 to 25 minutes. Check to see whether they are cooked properly by sticking a wooden skewer or a knife right into one of the cakes – if it comes out clean, they're done. If it's a bit sticky, pop them back into the oven for a little longer. Remove from the oven and leave the cakes to cool on a wire rack.

As soon as the muffins are in the oven, make your runny frosted topping. Place most of the clementine zest, all the lemon zest and the lemon juice in a bowl. Add the soured cream, icing sugar and vanilla seeds and mix well. Taste and have a think about it – adjust the amount of lemon juice or icing sugar to balance the sweet and sour. Put into the fridge until your cakes have cooled down, then spoon the topping on to the cakes.

Serve on a lovely plate (on a cake stand if you're feeling elegant, or on a rustic slab if you're more of a hunter-gatherer type!), with the rest of the clementine zest sprinkled over. For an interesting flavour and look, a few dried lavender flowers or rose petals are fantastic.

**makes 12 muffins**

400g butternut squash, skin on, deseeded and roughly chopped
350g light soft brown sugar
4 large free-range or organic eggs
sea salt
300g plain flour, unsifted
2 heaped teaspoons baking powder
a handful of walnuts
1 teaspoon ground cinnamon
175ml extra virgin olive oil

*for the frosted cream topping*
zest of 1 clementine
zest of 1 lemon and juice of ½ a lemon
140ml soured cream
2 heaped tablespoons icing sugar, sifted
1 vanilla pod, split lengthways and seeds scraped out
optional: lavender flowers or rose petals

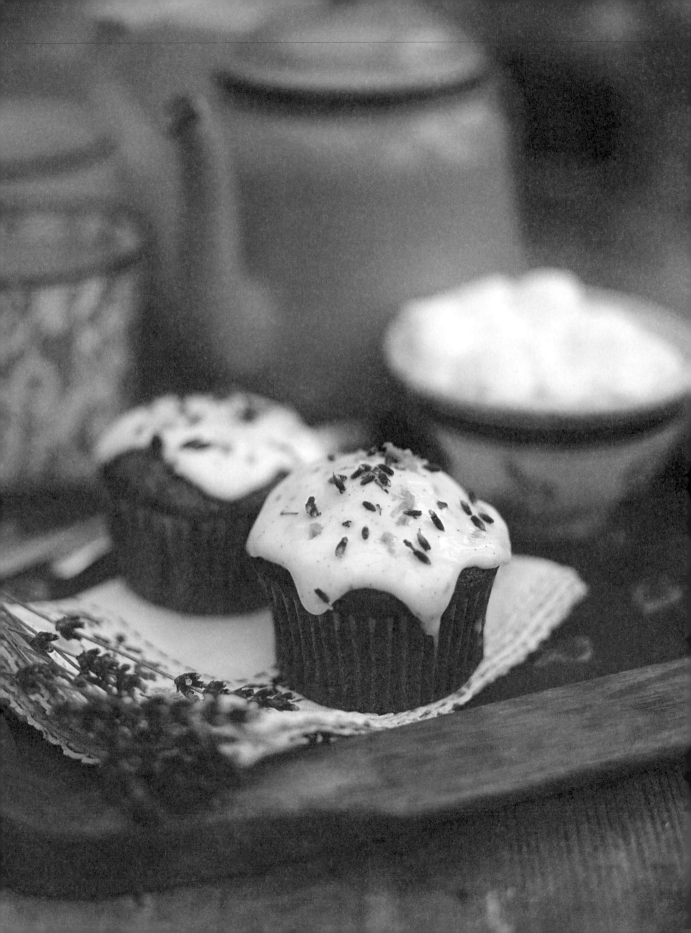

# How I grow squash

### Soil

Squash are greedy plants and they love to grow in a good, rich soil in a sunny spot of the garden, so aim to add lots of well-rotted manure to the soil before planting. The best place to grow them can actually be on an old compost heap!

### Planting

I like to sow my squash seeds in pots (usually two seeds per 6 to 8cm pot) towards the end of April, and keep them in the greenhouse or indoors on a light windowsill until the last frosts have passed, around mid-May, and they can be moved outside.

I've found that if I put my squash plants into a slightly raised mound of well-rotted manure on top of the soil, it really gets them going! All you need to do is space them about 1 to 2m apart and remember to keep them well fed and watered.

### Harvesting and storing

Summer squash can be picked during the growing season, through the summer, as they are at their best when small. Winter squash will generally be ready for harvesting from early September to early November. You'll be able to tell that they're ready when the stalks start to dry out and wither, and the skin hardens, becoming deeper and richer in colour. After picking them, leave them out in the sun to ripen for as long as possible. There is a reason for this – sun-ripened squash store for longer, so let them have a good old sunbathing session!

Squash can be stored in a cool, dry frost-free place like a shed or garage. However, don't stack them too high. The air needs to circulate round them, or they'll end up rotting quite quickly.

### My growing tips

- Chickens love pecking at young squash shoots, so cover them up if you keep hens.

- If it looks like it will freeze and you have just planted out your baby plants, cover them overnight. You can do this by using some special gardening fleece or simply whacking a big plant pot over the top.

- Once your squash have formed, slip a tile or slate underneath them to keep the bases dry and prevent them from rotting.

- If you want to grow bigger fruit, you can stop the plants growing further by pinching out the ends of the growing shoots when about four squash have formed on the plant. By doing this, all the plant's energy will go into enlarging these, rather than into growing lots of smaller ones.

- Squash flowers are delicious and can be used in just the same way as courgette flowers. They are very delicate and will wilt quickly after picking – you won't see them in supermarkets very often because of this. If you want good flowers, you'll need to go to a supplier, or simply grow your own.

- Keep some gardening fleece handy to protect any late-ripening fruit from early frosts in the autumn.

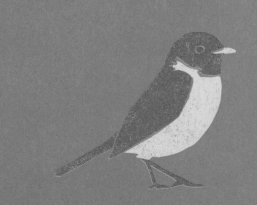

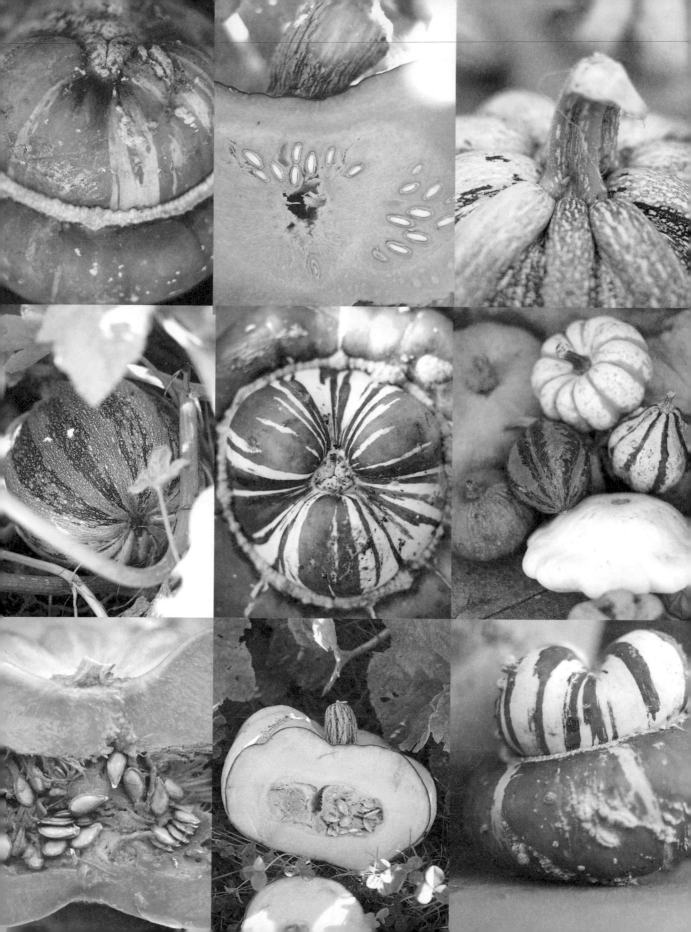

You may be thinking that winter and salads don't go together, but let me tell you … they do! There's no reason why winter salads can't be exciting. Recently I found myself in my garden on a very rainy, windy day, with floods happening just down the road and trees getting blown over (including one of mine). I didn't expect to see much that I could use in a salad, but when I stopped to have a little look at what was in the ground ready to be eaten there was actually quite a lot of good stuff there! Normally, in the UK, we'd be having cold winters and regular frosts, but as it's been fairly warm over the past few years, the changes have really shown up in the garden in terms of which plants have benefited and continued growing.

If you want to brighten up your garden a bit in the winter and keep it ticking along, there are loads of different things you can plant. Funnily enough, the exciting things that do really well in colder weather are those plants from Mediterranean or Asian climates. Things like Italian rocket and radicchio, dandelions and chicories, through to Asian mustards and cresses, moulis and radishes. All very exciting stuff. There are also some British-style leaves like sprouting cabbage and baby broccoli shoots, yellow celery leaves and chervil that will all be there in some shape or form on the plants during winter. Even though some of these little shoots and leaves may come from the cabbage family, if used when small enough they're delicious in salads because they taste more like a salad leaf than a vegetable. If you have any of these things in your garden during

the winter you won't need to venture near a shop for salad ingredients. I've even picked rocket in the snow and it was good as gold!

I think salads during winter should be about mixing things up a bit. You could delicately slice up some root vegetables that you stored away in the summer, and serve them with the big, bold, unconventional and exciting sauce on page 373 (an absolute show-stopper!). Or buy whatever's in season and simply dress your winter leaves. It's all good! Winter leaves can often be bitter – things like dandelion, Treviso, chicory – and this has to be balanced with thick balsamic vinegar, crispy smoked bacon, a garlicky dressing or a creamy one. Another recipe in this chapter is a roast carrot and avocado salad with winter leaves – admittedly, avocados aren't grown in the UK, but they are two a penny in the shops. To serve them alongside roast carrots with lovely dressed winter leaves and nutty seeds is a delight, and it will put a bit of spice back into those dark winter evenings!

I know it's sometimes easy to get stuck in a rut, making the same old salad and never feeling inspired to try something new, no matter what time of year. If that's how you feel, and if you only ever eat salad in summer, you're probably reading this thinking there's no point in trying to grow any winter salad leaves. But when it's as easy as snipping open a £1 packet of seeds and quickly sowing them in a pot and leaving it on your windowsill, you'll find it's addictive and you'll get right into growing some leaves, no matter

# winter salads

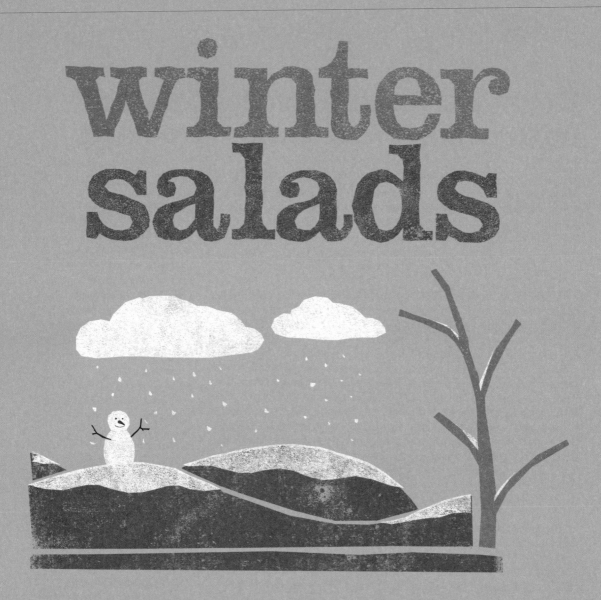

how old you are or how stuck in a rut you might be! When I first moved to London I was living in a studio flat and my windowboxes were filled with herbs. As I didn't have any room for salad leaves as well, I'd go and sprinkle salad seeds, rocket and wild fennel in a quiet spot in my local park, then I'd keep an eye on them and go back and pick them when they were ready!

There's a very fine line between salad leaves and weeds. For instance, rocket is essentially a weed. Sometimes it will flower and go to seed but to be honest, if I went back to that spot in the park today there would still be some rocket growing there. Fennel seeds itself year after year as well. So go and have a little sprinkle and you'll be knocking up some lovely salads in no time!

# Roast carrot and avocado salad with orange and lemon dressing

If you're going to use cooked carrots in a salad you've got to make it with some attitude! This fantastic Moroccan-style salad combines roast carrots with avocados – and because they have the same texture in your mouth, I thought I'd add the chargrilled flavour and crunch of toasted ciabatta to round things off. With spices, seeds, soured cream and a delicious citrus dressing, you've got a winner.

Preheat the oven to 180°C/350°F/gas 4. Parboil your carrots in boiling, salted water for 10 minutes, until they are very nearly cooked, then drain and put them into a roasting tray. You should flavour them while they're steaming hot, so while the carrots are cooking get a pestle and mortar and smash up the cumin seeds, chillies, salt and pepper. Add the garlic and thyme leaves and smash up again until you have a kind of paste. The idea here is to build up the flavours. Add enough extra virgin olive oil to generously cover the paste, and a good swig of vinegar. This will be like a marinade, a rub and a dressing all in one! Stir together, then pour over the carrots in the tray, coating them well. Add the orange and lemon halves, cut-side down. These will roast along with the carrots, and their juice can be used as the basis of the dressing. Place in the preheated oven for 25 to 30 minutes, or until golden.

While the carrots are roasting, halve and peel your avocados, discarding the stones, then cut them into wedges lengthways and place in a big bowl. Remove the carrots from the oven and add them to the avocados. Carefully, using some tongs, squeeze the roasted orange and lemon juice into a bowl and add the same amount of extra virgin olive oil and a little swig of red wine vinegar. Season, and pour this dressing over the carrots and avocados. Mix together, have a taste and correct the seasoning. Call your gang round the table while you toast or griddle your ciabatta slices.

Tear the toasted bread into little pieces and add to the dressed carrot and avocado. Mix together, toss in the salad leaves and cress and transfer to a big platter or divide between individual plates. Spoon over a nice dollop of soured cream, sprinkle over your toasted seeds and drizzle over some extra virgin olive oil.

serves 4

500g medium differently coloured carrots, with their leafy tops
2 level teaspoons whole cumin seeds
1 or 2 small dried chillies, crumbled
sea salt and freshly ground black pepper
2 cloves of garlic, peeled
4 sprigs of fresh thyme, leaves picked
extra virgin olive oil
red or white wine vinegar
1 orange, halved
1 lemon, halved
3 ripe avocados
red wine vinegar
4 x 1cm thick slices of ciabatta or other good-quality bread
2 handfuls of interesting mixed winter salad leaves (like Treviso, rocket, radicchio or cavolo nero tops), washed and spun dry
2 punnets of cress
1 x 142ml pot of soured cream
4 tablespoons mixed seeds, toasted

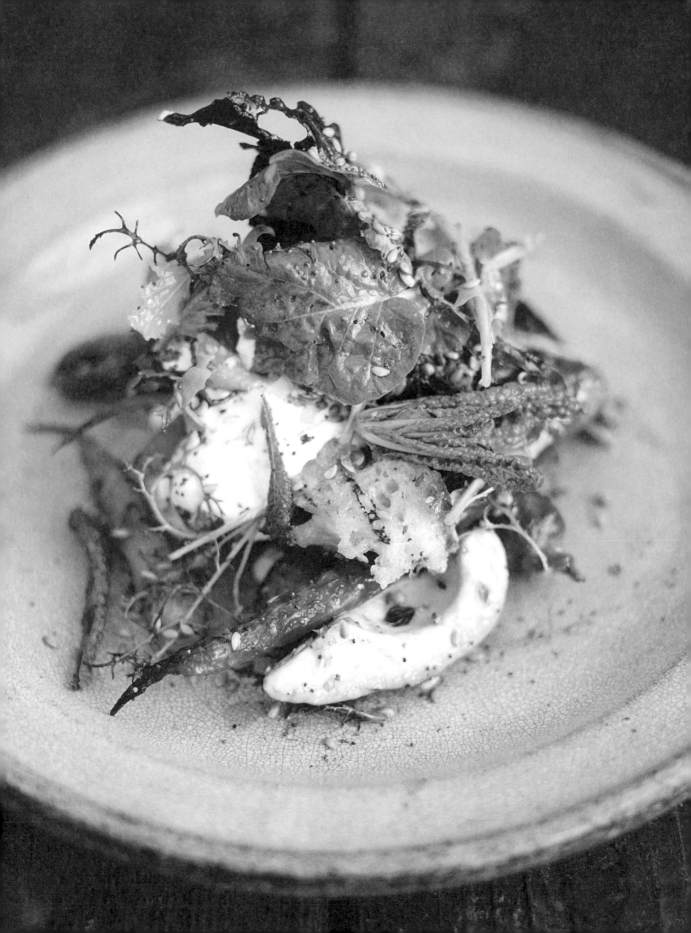

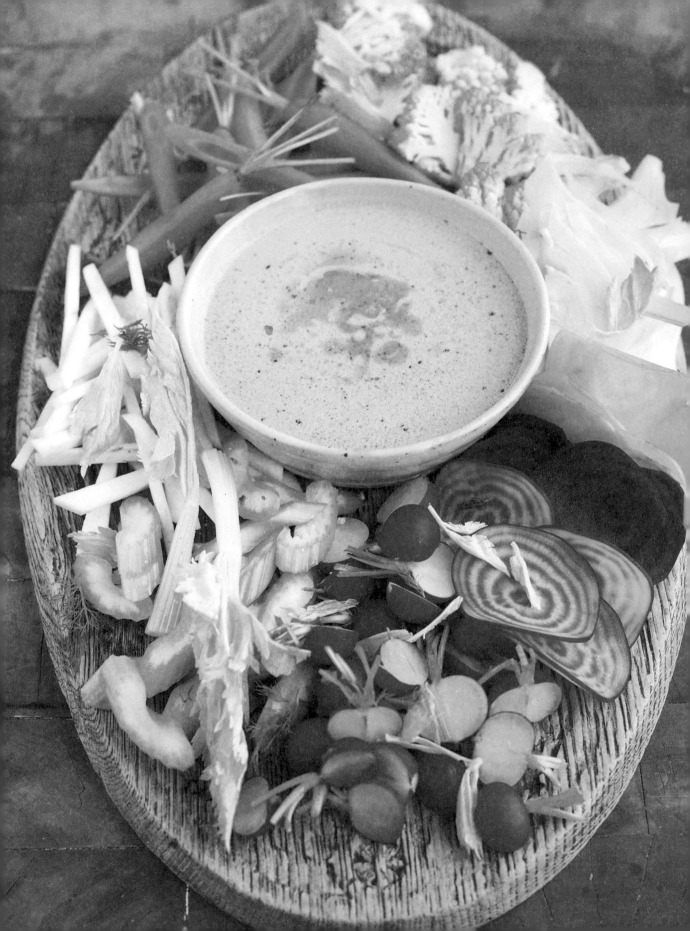

# Winter crunch salad with a mind-blowing sauce

This is a really interesting, delicious winter salad dish which is a great way of using up all the crunchy winter veg that's available. Its proper name is bagna cauda, which basically means 'hot bath' in Italian, and the idea is that you have a load of raw or just cooked pieces of vegetable which you dip into a delicious, warm sauce. You may like your sauce to be thick and oozy but I prefer mine to be quite thin and delicate, like the texture of thin custard, with a lovely sheen to it.

You can use any vegetables you want, and depending on the season you can do a light summer version or a more root-veg-based winter one. I actually prefer my veg to be raw, as I love the crunch you get from them, but if you want to boil them briefly until they're al dente, feel free.

First, prepare all your veg, because once the sauce is done you'll be ready to serve! To make your sauce, put the garlic cloves, milk and anchovies into a saucepan and bring to the boil. Simmer slowly for 10 minutes, or until the garlic is soft and tender, keeping a close eye on the pan to make sure the milk doesn't boil over. Don't worry if it splits and looks a little lumpy – simply remove from the heat and whiz the sauce up with a hand blender. Gently blend in the extra virgin olive oil and the vinegar a little at a time – you're in control of the consistency at this point. If you like it thick, like mayonnaise, keep blending. Now taste it and adjust the seasoning. Make sure there's enough acidity from the vinegar to act like a dressing. It should be an incredible, pungent warm sauce.

There are two ways you can serve this – with both you need the sauce to be warm. Either pour the sauce into a bowl and place this on a plate, with the veg arranged around the bowl, or serve the veg in a big bowl and drizzle the sauce over the top. Sprinkle over the reserved herby fennel tops and celery leaves and finish with a drizzle of extra virgin olive oil.

serves 4

**for the sauce**
6 cloves of garlic, peeled
300ml milk
10 anchovy fillets in oil
180ml good extra
    virgin olive oil, plus
    extra for drizzling
2 or 3 tablespoons good
    white wine vinegar

**for the vegetables**
a few young carrots,
    peeled and finely sliced
a few small raw beetroots,
    peeled and finely sliced
a few sticks of celery,
    trimmed and thinly
    sliced, yellow
    leaves reserved
½ a small Romanesco
    or white cauliflower,
    broken into florets
a bulb of fennel, trimmed
    and finely sliced,
    herby tops reserved
a handful of small
    beetroot leaves, if
    available, washed
a bunch of radishes,
    trimmed and washed
½ a celeriac, peeled
    and finely sliced

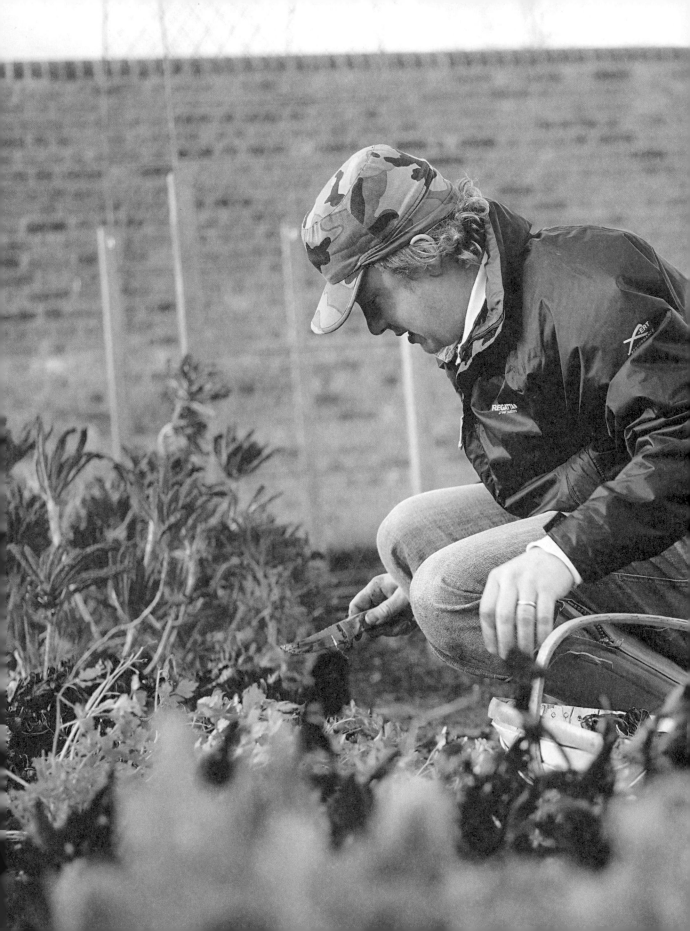

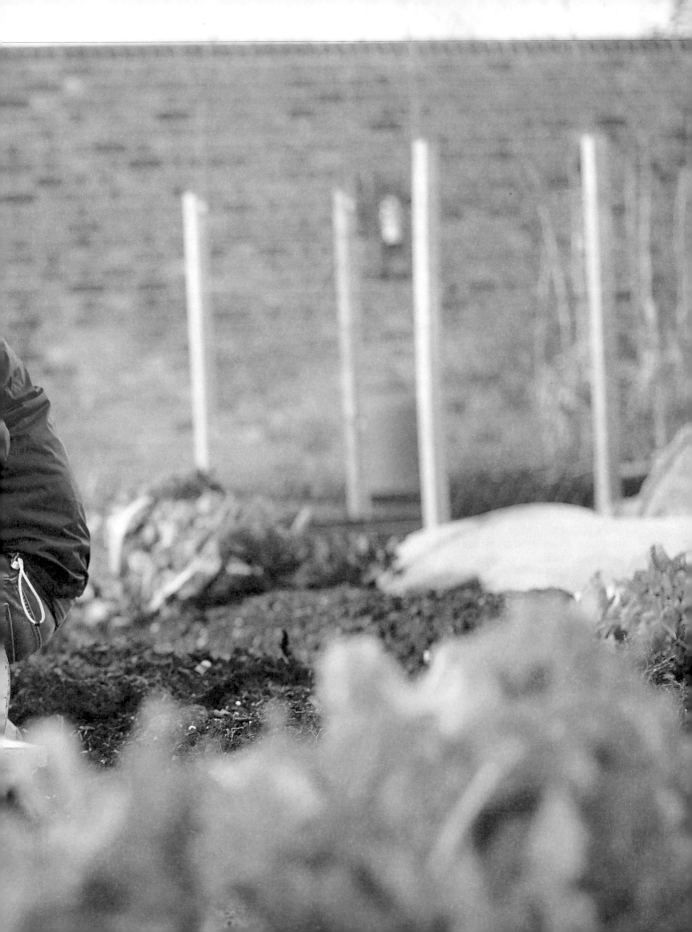

# Tuna ceviche with salad shoots, herb cresses and a kinda yuzu dressing

Herb cresses and shoots are great fun to grow, but you can also find them in supermarkets, farmers' markets and health food shops. They're crunchy, sweet and nutritious and can really transform a salad. You can use salmon or white fish instead of tuna, but make sure it's good quality. And look for deep cherry-red tuna, not grey. Ask your fishmonger to remove the skin and trim any dark meat or sinews off your tuna loin.

In Japan I came across an incredible fruit called a yuzu, which has a tangeriney/grapefruity/lemony flavour. It's almost impossible to get hold of in the UK, so I've blended three citrus juices together. It's surprisingly close to the real thing.

To make your dressing, mix the citrus juices and zests together, add a pinch of salt and put to one side. Next, heat 2 to 3cm of vegetable oil in a small, deep saucepan. As a temperature guide, you can put a little piece of potato in the oil; when it turns golden and floats to the surface, the oil is hot enough, so remove the potato and put all the garlic in the pan. Move the slices around, keeping a close eye on them, and as soon as they start to turn golden remove them quickly and carefully with a slotted spoon. Wait too long and they'll burn! Drain on kitchen paper. Add all the ginger slices to the pan and fry until golden – again, don't let them burn – then remove to drain on kitchen paper.

Get a sharp knife and cut the tuna in half lengthways; place flat and slice into 0.5cm-ish thick slices – be careful! Lay the slices out on a big platter or on individual plates and sprinkle with a little salt, the garlic and the ginger. In a bowl, mix the shoots and cresses, giving them a little scrunch together, then place them on top of the tuna either on the platter or on the individual plates.

Drizzle your kinda yuzu dressing over the top of the shoots and tuna, followed by a few tiny glugs of soy sauce and sesame oil. What a mad-looking dish, made up of completely different colours and textures – I love it!

serves 4

vegetable oil
a piece of potato, peeled
6 cloves of garlic, peeled and very finely sliced
a thumb-sized piece of root ginger, peeled and very finely sliced
1 x 400g piece of fresh tuna loin, skin and sinews removed
sea salt
2 big handfuls of interesting mixed shoots, sprouts or cresses (try any combo of peanut and bean shoots, shiso, basil, coriander and mustard cresses, winter cabbage, beetroot and chard shoots)
soy sauce
sesame oil

for your kinda yuzu dressing
zest and juice of 1 lime
juice of ¼ of a grapefruit
zest and juice of 1½ tangerines or clementines
sea salt

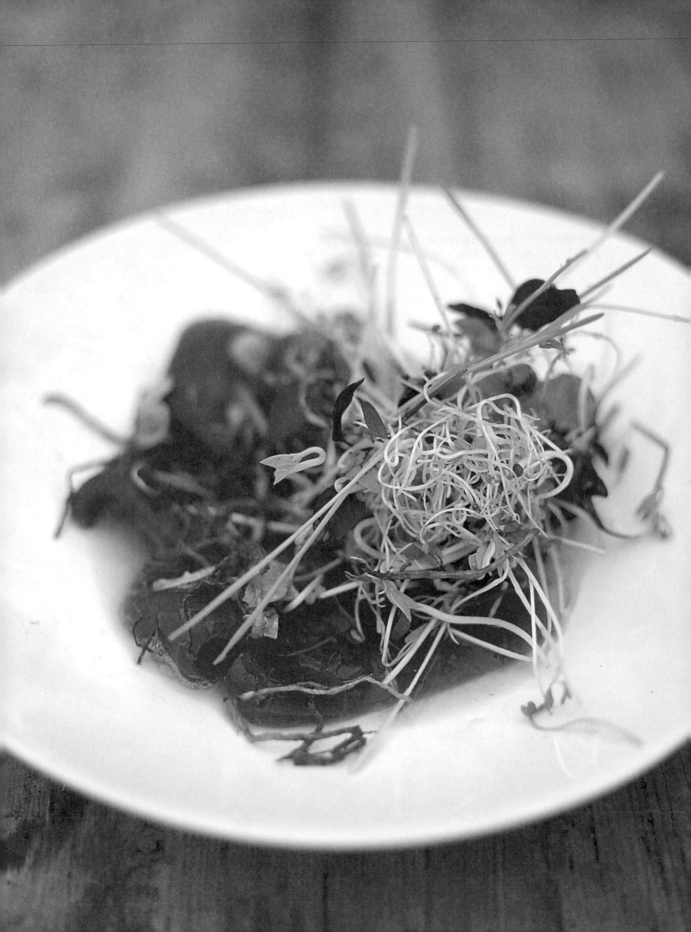

# How I grow
# winter salads

### Soil
Most winter salads can be sown directly into the soil from mid-summer to early autumn. This gives them some warm weather to grow before things slow down for the winter. Pick a well-drained spot in the garden that's sheltered and sunny. The soil needs to be prepared by adding a little well-rotted organic compost and a few handfuls of an organic fertilizer per square metre. Mix well and rake out any lumpy bits.

### Planting and sowing
Although winter salads can be sown directly outside, there are a few types – radicchio and winter radish in particular – that I normally start off indoors in little pots or module trays. This method gives me big, strong plants that I can either cut or pull up whole. I normally sow them in July and plant them outside during August and September. After that it will take them about three months to grow to full size.

To sow outside all you need to do is smooth over the surface of your prepared soil and make little furrows about 2cm deep. Space the furrows about 15 to 20cm apart. Sprinkle your salad seeds into each furrow, cover with 1 to 2cm of soil and carefully water them. Don't forget to label each variety!

### Harvesting
Many winter salads can be harvested a little at a time by simply cutting a few leaves from each plant. This will enable you to 'cut and come again' without weakening individual plants too much. Large heads of radicchio, however, can be cut completely and they will grow new baby shoots again. Only harvest what you need each time. Winter salads usually store best by leaving them growing outside ... saves room in your fridge too!

### My growing tips
- Give winter salad leaves a better chance of surviving cold weather by protecting them with cloches or garden fleece.

- Winter salad leaves can be easily grown in pots or growbags. Put them in the warmest, sunniest spot in the garden. If you have a greenhouse or polytunnel, even if it's unheated, you'll be amazed at how well they'll crop.

- A lot of winter salad leaves look very ornamental and are great planted in tubs as a bit of a feature. It's a bonus that you can eat them!

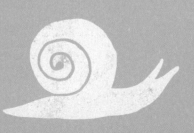

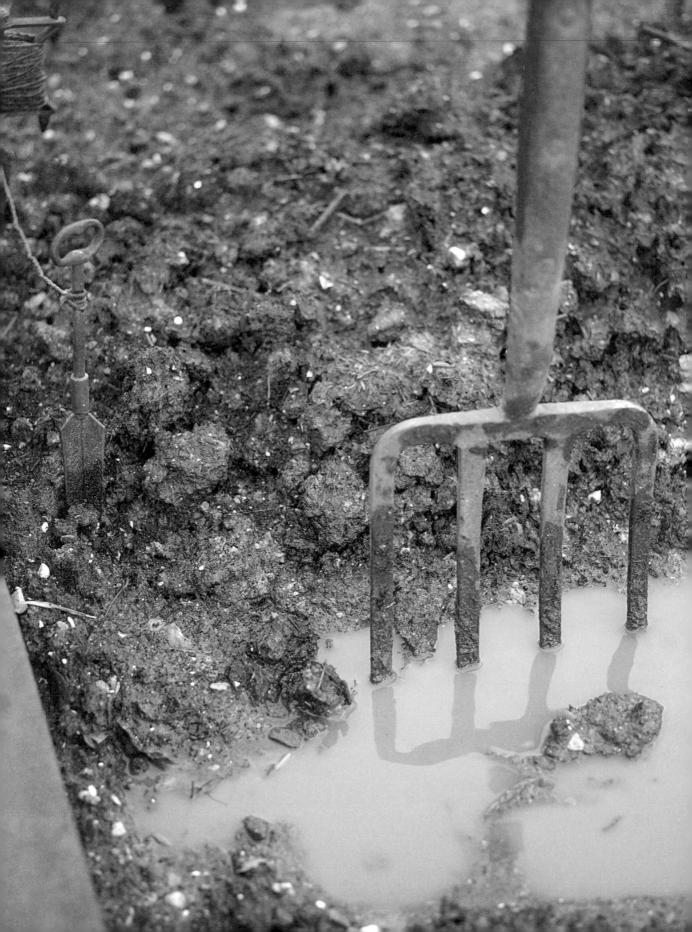

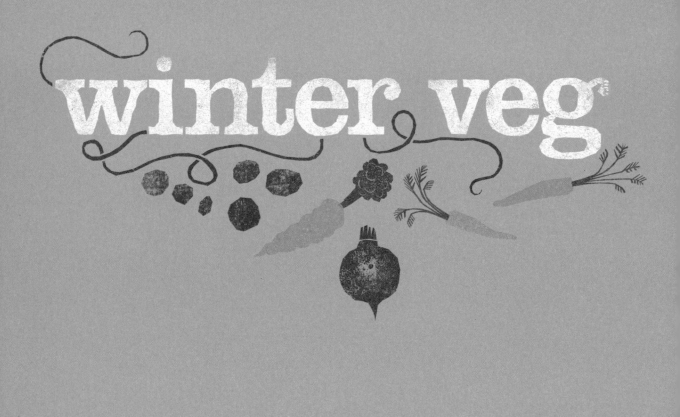

winter veg

I used to find winter a bit depressing because of the miserable weather. But it's gone doolally recently – in the last few months we've had flash floods, snowdrifts one day, warm sunshine the next, dark mornings, dark evenings, trees getting blown down all over the place, and the garden looking as naked and boring as it can. But over the last few years, since I started to fall in love with the idea of growing stuff in my garden, I've come to understand how utterly exciting this miserable weather can be! And it's all thanks to the Yoda of gardening, Walter Revell.

Walter was a professional arable and pig farmer who used to prop himself up against the bar in my parents' pub every day. He was a big man, strong as an ox, with hands like shovels. (He once ate the eyeballs from a spit-roasted pig at the local village fête and offered some to me with the tendons hanging from the fork – I had nightmares for weeks!) When he heard customers in the pub whingeing about winter being an awful time of year he would say, 'My friend, this is a time to feed your beds with manure, let the rain, wind and frost help to break it all down into the soil, and make the worms happy. Then sit back and look at your garden – look at the gaps in your naked beds to see where your problems are. Then you can correct them for next year.'

Walter used to enthuse about the different seasons because he saw the advantages each one brought with it. The colder months of winter can help kill off some of the pests and fungi that may have damaged your plants during the previous summer. Cold weather also helps improve the flavour of a whole host of veggies. The entire brassica family, for instance – cabbages, Brussels sprouts, broccoli and kohlrabi – develop a better flavour during cold winter weather. Frosts help to break down their structure so they become less stringy and not only taste better, but are far more tender.

I've obviously reached the age where I've started to sound like my old man, and like good old Walter Revell. Now, when a good day gets rained off, and the cold weather kicks in, I always think, 'Well, the garden's going to love it.' And I've learnt that if you plan ahead and plant an assortment of winter veg in the summer you can reap the rewards from your garden every day of the year. Things I've got growing in my garden at this time of year that I get excited about are cabbages and kale, good old Brussels sprouts, carrots, swedes, turnips, celeriac, parsnips, beetroot, winter radishes and Jerusalem artichokes.

There are so many brilliant things you can do with these vegetables, so embrace the cold times and enjoy stews, thick soups, pot-roasts and slow-cooks. Or think about using them thinly sliced in beautiful colourful salads, to make some light, fresh food in the middle of winter. Either way, whether you're growing or buying from your local farmers' market, stay optimistic and I think you'll be surprised by what you see.

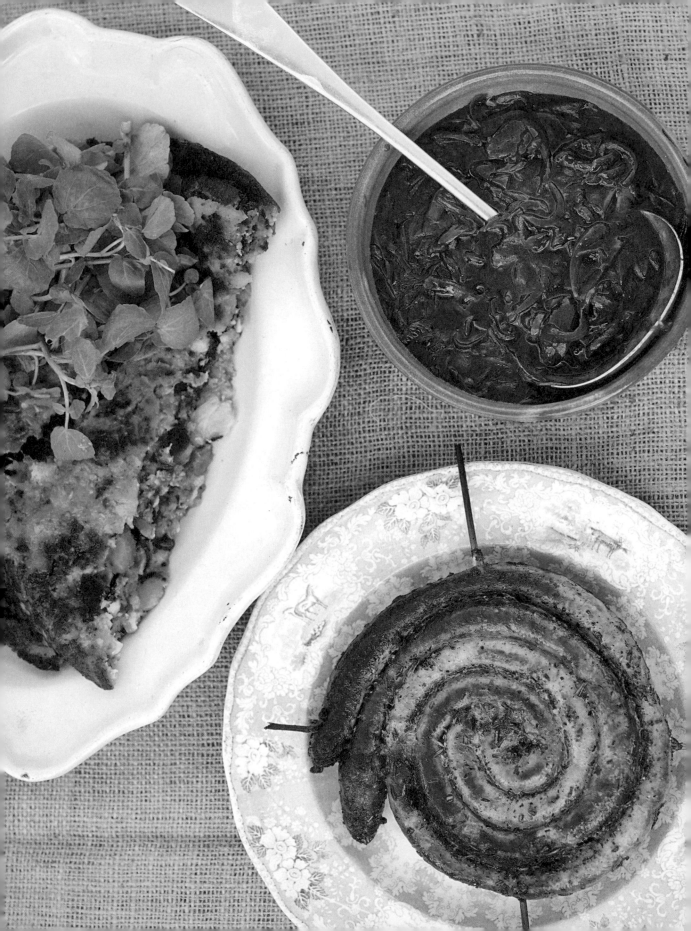

# Bubble and squeak with sausages and onion gravy

Bubble and squeak is a classic British dish of smashed-up winter veg, traditionally made from the Sunday roast leftovers. Use about 60 per cent potato to get the right consistency, then whatever veg you like – carrots, Brussels, swedes, turnips, onions, leeks or Savoy cabbage.

Cook the potatoes and mixed veg in a pan of boiling water for 15 to 20 minutes. When they're cooked right through, drain and put to one side. Heat a glug of olive oil and half the butter in a large frying pan and add the chestnuts. When they start to sizzle, add your potatoes and veg. Mash the veg up in the pan, then pat the mixture into a thick pancake shape. Fry on a medium heat for about half an hour, checking it every 5 minutes. When the bottom turns golden, flip it over bit by bit and mash it back into itself. Pat it out flat again and continue cooking until really crisp all over.

Preheat the oven and a roasting tray to 220°C/425°F/gas 7. Unravel the pork sausage links and squeeze the filling between them until all 6 sausages are joined together. Do the same to your venison or beef sausages. Pat them to flatten them a bit. Drizzle with olive oil and massage this into your 2 long sausages. Sprinkle over a pinch of pepper, the rosemary and some nutmeg. Put one sausage on top of the other and roll them up like a liquorice wheel! Poke two skewers through, in a cross shape, to hold the sausages together.

Take the preheated tray from the oven. Drizzle in some olive oil and add the onions. Season, add the remaining butter and stir. Place the sausage wheel on the onions and stick the bay leaves between the sausages. Drizzle with some more oil and roast in the preheated oven for around 40 minutes or until golden and crisp. When your sausages and onions are done, your bubble and squeak should be ready too. If it still hasn't browned, put it under a hot grill for 5 minutes.

Remove the sausages to a plate and place the tray with the onions on the hob. Whack the heat up to full and stir in the flour, balsamic vinegar and stock. Bring to the boil and leave to thicken to a nice gravy consistency, stirring every now and then, and season to taste. Remove the skewers and cut the sausages into wedges. Serve the bubble and squeak with a good portion of sausage, a spoonful of onion gravy and perhaps some lovely dressed watercress.

serves 6

750g floury potatoes, peeled and cut into chunks
600g mixed winter vegetables (see the introduction), peeled or trimmed and chopped into equal-sized chunks
olive oil
2 knobs of butter
1 x 200g vacuum pack of chestnuts
6 good-quality pork sausages, linked together
6 good-quality venison or beef sausages, linked together
sea salt and freshly ground black pepper
a small bunch of fresh rosemary, leaves picked and finely chopped
nutmeg, for grating
3 red onions, peeled and finely sliced
a few bay leaves
1 tablespoon flour
125ml balsamic vinegar
300ml good-quality vegetable or chicken stock

winter veg

# The best winter veg coleslaw

Coleslaw is something most of us have grown up eating, yet a lot of the time it must have been made so badly! With this in mind, I want to bring it back with a vengeance. I've used yoghurt instead of mayonnaise to bind the vegetables because it not only tastes better, in my opinion, but it's also healthier. If you're struggling to find radishes or fennel, don't worry. Just do what you can, but remember that the more interesting crunchy vegetables you can get shredded into this baby, the better!

PS If you haven't got round to getting yourself a food processor yet, and you're serious about cooking, do go and buy one. It won't be a waste of money – unlike most kitchen gadgets you'll use it all the time, especially for recipes like this one.

Shred the carrots, fennel, and your choice of radishes, beetroot, turnip or celeriac on a mandoline, or use the julienne slicer in your food processor. Put the veg into a mixing bowl. Slice the cabbage, onion and shallot as finely as you can and add to the bowl. In a separate bowl, mix half the lemon juice, a glug of extra virgin olive oil, the chopped herbs, yoghurt and mustard. Pour this dressing over the veg and mix well to coat everything. Season to taste with salt and pepper and the rest of the lemon juice if you like.

Really delicious served with thinly sliced leftover roast lamb, pork or rare roast beef, drizzled with extra virgin olive oil.

serves 6

2 carrots, different
   colours if you can
   find them, peeled
1 bulb of fennel, trimmed
use at least 2 of the
   following: 3–4 radishes;
   1 light-coloured beetroot,
   peeled; 1 turnip, peeled;
   ½ a small celeriac, peeled
400g red and white
   cabbage, outer
   leaves removed
½ a red onion, peeled
1 shallot, peeled
1 lemon
extra virgin olive oil
a handful of fresh soft
   herbs (use mint, fennel,
   dill, parsley and chervil),
   leaves picked and chopped
250ml yoghurt
2 tablespoons mustard
sea salt and freshly
   ground black pepper

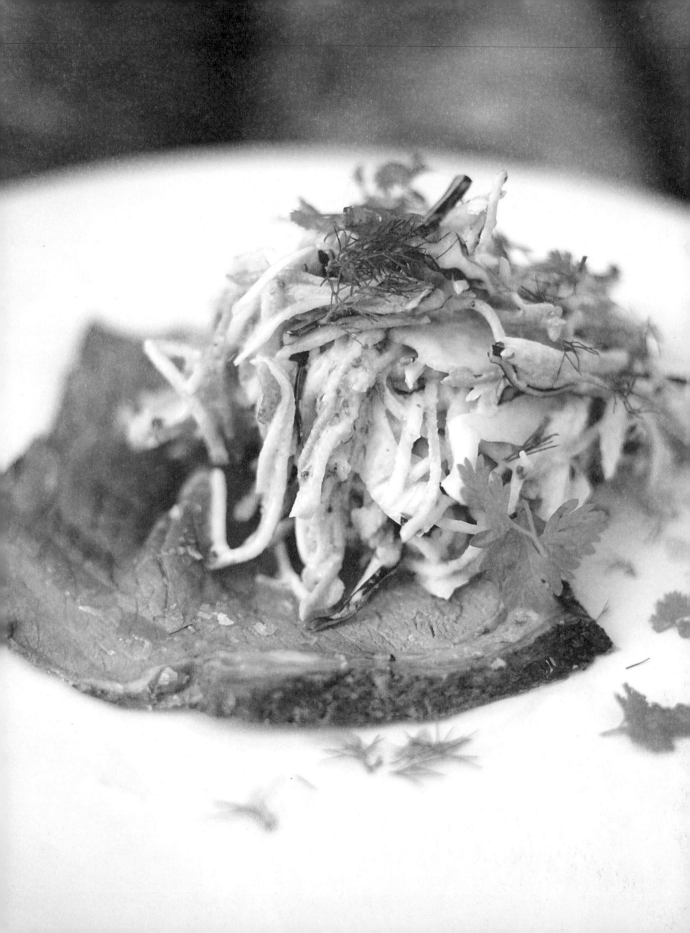

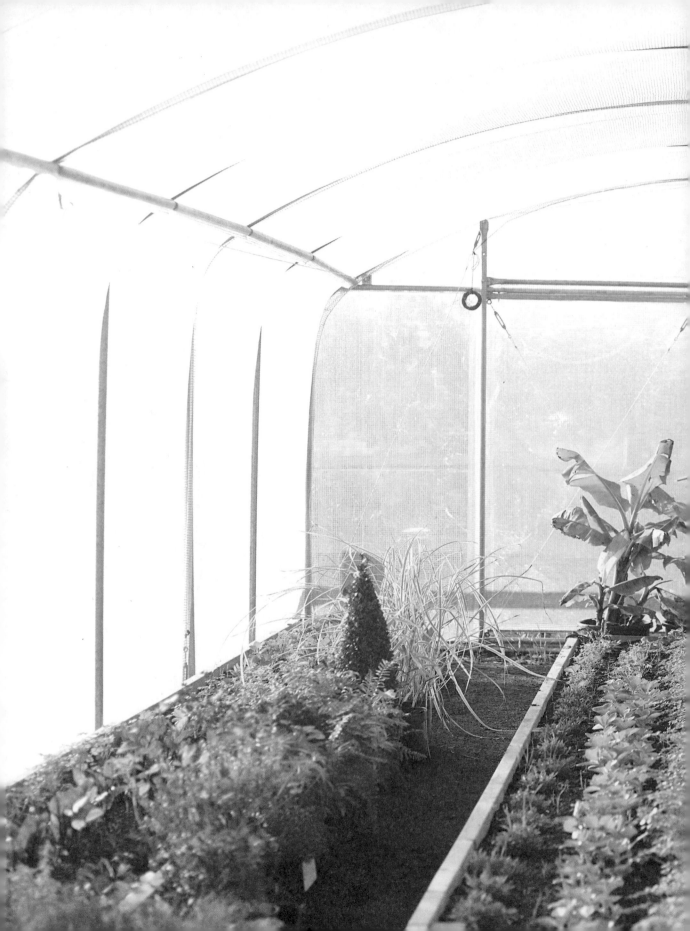

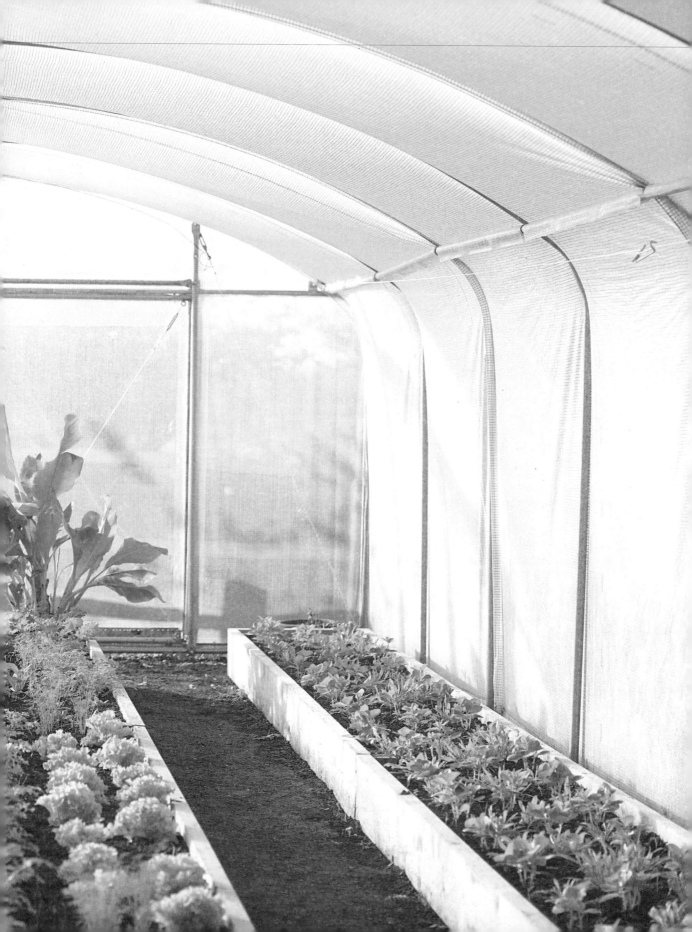

# Italian bread and cabbage soup with sage butter

This scrumptious, thick bread soup is about bigging up the cabbage family – the king of winter veg. It's layered like a lasagne, with grilled bread and cabbage in stock, and as it cooks it plumps up a bit like bread and butter pudding. Fontina cheese is available in good supermarkets or cheese shops, but you can substitute good-quality Cheddar or Gruyère.

Preheat your oven to 180°C/350°F/gas 4. Bring the stock to the boil in a large saucepan and add the cabbage, cavolo nero and/or kale. Cook for a few minutes until softened (you may have to do this in two batches). Remove the cabbage to a large bowl, leaving the stock in the pan.

Toast all but 5 of the bread slices on a hot griddle pan or in a toaster, then rub them on one side with the garlic halves, and put to one side. Next, heat a large 10cm deep ovenproof casserole-type pan on the hob, pour in a couple of glugs of olive oil and add your pancetta and anchovies. When the pancetta's golden brown and sizzling, add the rosemary and cooked cabbage and toss to coat the greens in all the lovely flavours. Put the mixture and all the juices back into the large bowl.

Place 4 of the toasted slices in the casserole-type pan, in one layer. Spread over one third of the cabbage leaves, sprinkle over a quarter of the grated fontina and Parmesan, and add a drizzle of olive oil. Repeat this twice, but don't stress if your pan's only big enough to take two layers – that's fine. Just pour in all the juices remaining in the bowl and end with a layer of untoasted bread on top. Push down on the layers with your hands.

Pour the stock gently over the top till it just comes up to the top layer. Push down again and sprinkle over the remaining fontina and Parmesan. Add a good pinch of pepper and drizzle over some good-quality olive oil. Bake in the preheated oven for around 30 minutes or until crispy and golden on top.

When the soup is ready, divide it between your bowls. Melt the butter in a frying pan and quickly fry the sage leaves until they're just crisp and the butter is lightly golden (not burnt!). Spoon a bit of the flavoured butter and sage leaves over the soup and add another grating of Parmesan. Such a great combo!

serves 8

3 litres good-quality chicken or vegetable stock
1 Savoy cabbage, stalks removed, outer leaves separated, washed and roughly chopped
2 big handfuls of cavolo nero and/or kale, stalks removed, leaves washed and roughly chopped
about 16 slices of stale country-style or sourdough bread
1 clove of garlic, unpeeled. cut in half
olive oil
12–14 slices of pancetta or smoked streaky bacon
1 x 100g tin of anchovy fillets in oil
3 sprigs of fresh rosemary, leaves picked
200g fontina cheese, grated
150g freshly grated Parmesan cheese, plus a little for serving
sea salt and freshly ground black pepper
a couple of large knobs of butter
a small bunch of fresh sage, leaves picked

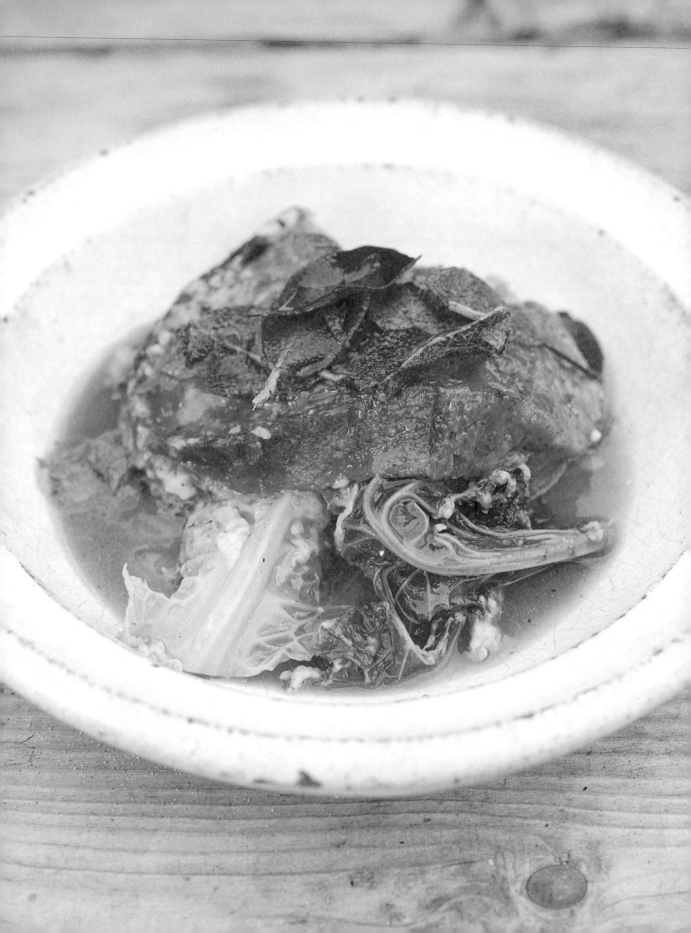

# How I grow winter veg

## Soil

Winter is the best time of the year to enrich your soil. Compost, or well-rotted manure, should be spread all over your veg plot (except where carrots or parsnips are going to be grown). You can leave it on the surface, to protect and warm your soil, and worms and other creatures will slowly dig it in for you. Traditionally all the old dead and finished crops are tidied away in winter. Plants that have suffered from pests or diseases should definitely be cleared up too, but remember that if you're too tidy you could accidentally kill good bugs like hibernating ladybirds and lacewings. So try to leave piles of sticks or logs and dried-up stalks around the garden – perhaps even buy some 'bug boxes' and give your friendly bugs a ready-made winter hotel!

## Planting

There are loads of different types of winter veg, and many ways of growing them. I usually sow most of my varieties in modules or pots which I leave in a greenhouse or on a sunny windowsill until they have germinated and grown big enough to face life outside. While still in their pots, the seedlings can go outside in a sheltered spot to toughen up a bit more.

Some gardeners use 'seed beds' in a spare corner of the garden instead of pots and transplant the seedlings into their final positions. Parsnips and carrots must be sown directly into the soil, though, and not transplanted.

**Cabbage** can be started indoors or sown directly into the soil. For winter use, sow from late March to mid May.

**Celeriac** is grown as a root vegetable for its large and well-developed taproot rather than for its stems and leaves. It has good keeping properties, and should last three to four months if clamped.

**Parsnips** can be sown directly into the soil from March to April, 1 to 2cm deep and in rows about 30cm apart. Picking can start from October.

**Radicchio** is easy to grow and matures after about three months. If left any longer, the leaves become bitter. Once picked, the leaves will keep in the fridge for up to a week. New leaves often grow from the roots after the first cut, even in winter, so don't pull the plant up until spring.

**Swedes** can be sown from June to mid July into pots or modules for planting out when ready. Sow two seeds in each pot or module and leave the strongest seedling to grow on.

**Turnips** can be sown from mid July to mid August in pots or modules and planted out when ready. Alternatively, sow directly into the soil leaving 10 to 15cm between plants.

## Harvesting and storing

The ideal way to store any type of root vegetable is by the old-fashioned method of 'clamping'. In the old days, before fridges and freezers, everyone used to store their hardy root vegetables this way (see page 114).

## My growing tips

- If I have space in my vegetable garden for, say, twelve cabbages, I sow about eighteen into the module tray and choose the best ones for planting outside.

- Most winter veg need plenty of water through the summer and autumn and appreciate a mulching with well-rotted compost in early autumn. This aids water conservation and feeds the soil at the same time.

- If your garden is exposed, you can help your winter veg to grow by protecting them from harsh weather with temporary windbreaks, or a bit of warmth with garden fleece or cloches.

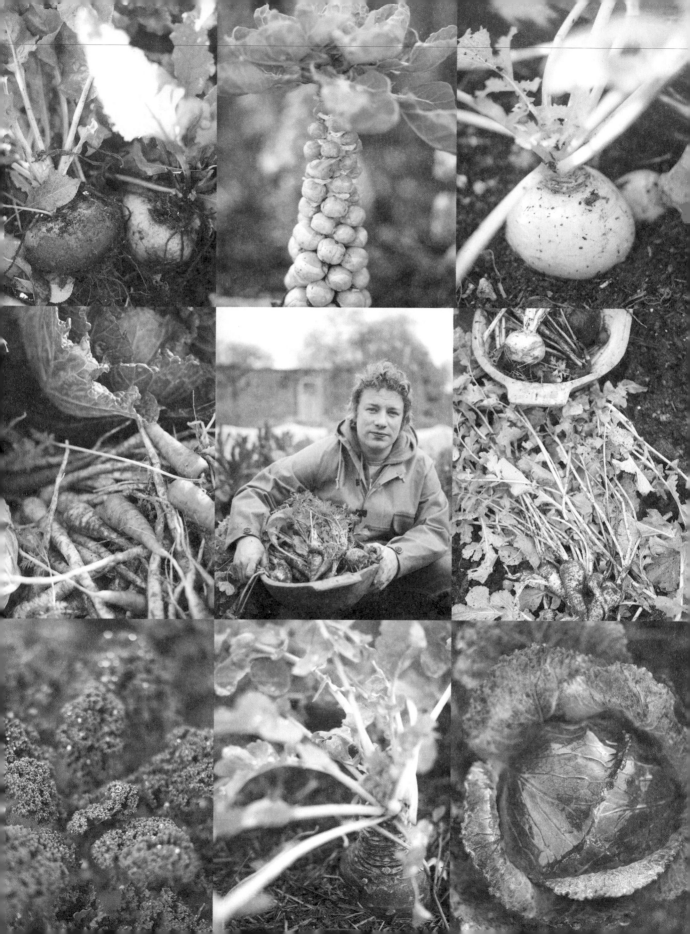

# useful stuff

## My favourite seed and plant varieties

## Vegetables

### Asparagus

**Connovers Colossal:** easy and cheap to grow from seed; sometimes seeds itself around the garden too.

**Crimson Pacific F1:** amazing purple spears with sweet taste; keeps colour if steamed gently.

**Jersey Knight F1:** an all-male hybrid producing huge quantities of big butch spears with a purplish tinge.

**Scaber Montina (wild asparagus):** the tastiest ever! A real connoisseur's variety; thin spears, easy to grow from seed.

### Beans

**Dwarf beans**
**Hildora:** a lovely yellow waxpod; easy to grow, easy to pick, very tasty.

**Purple Queen:** the best-tasting purple bean; turns green when cooked.

**Runner beans**
**Painted Lady:** an old variety; great taste, pretty red and white flowers.

**Scarlet Emperor:** another old variety; probably the best true runner bean flavour.

**Borlotti beans**
**Borlotto Lingua di Fuoco:** a fantastic Tuscan bean; beautiful to look at, even more beautiful to eat!

### Beets

**Bull's Blood:** grown for its amazing deep red-purple edible leaves.

**Burpee's Golden:** orange flesh.

**Chioggia:** beautiful old Italian variety; pinky-red and white striped flesh.

**Pablo:** good for baby beetroots.

### Broad beans

**Aqua Dulce:** hardy, reliable, for early sowing.

**Grando Violetto:** Italian variety, purple pods.

**Masterpiece Green Longpod:** green-seeded, sweet, loads of beans.

**Red Epicure:** unusual variety, wonderful deep pinkish seeds.

**Witkiem Manita:** reliable, fast-growing, white-seeded bean for late sowing.

### Broccoli

**Purple Early:** crops from February.

**Purple Late:** crops from March to April.

**Rudolph:** very early, crops from January.

### Brussels sprouts

**Evesham Special:** traditional variety, perfect for Christmas.

**Maximus:** modern long-cropping variety.

**Red Bull:** amazing purple sprouts, great taste.

**Rubine:** purple sprouts, variable but looks very pretty.

### Cabbage

**Cantassa:** a type of Savoy.

**Golden Acre, Pyramid:** spring.

**Hispi, Winningstadt:** summer/autumn.

**January King, Holland Winter White:** winter.

**Red Flare, Kalibos, Buscaro:** lovely red varieties.

### Calabrese

**Pacifica:** summer-heading, makes loads of smaller spears after main head is cut.

**Tiara:** very early.

### Carrots

**Orange**
**Amsterdam Forcing:** very quick-growing; small tender roots.

**Autumn King:** really hardy, crops well into winter.

**Nantes:** typical-looking, good taste.

**St Valery:** long roots, good taste.

**Coloured**
**Kinbi:** bright yellow, great taste.

**Purple Haze:** gorgeous-looking, even more amazing when sliced.

**Rainbow Mix:** all the best colours and tastes in one mix.

**Samurai:** red-skinned, pink-fleshed, long narrow roots.

**White Belgium:** easy to grow, mild flavour.

### Cauliflower

**Graffiti:** amazing purple heads, great for dips.

**Snowball:** white head, great taste.

**Veronica:** the best Italian Romanesco cauliflower, wonderful flavour.

### Chillies

**Dorset Naga:** one of the hottest chillies in the world!

**Habanero:** very hot but more versatile.

**Jalapeño:** a milder chilli, good for Mexican cooking.

### Courgettes

**Costa Romanesque:** probably the best-tasting courgette; nutty tender flesh, unusual ridged pale green fruit.

**Nero di Milano:** dark green; easy to grow.

**Rondo di Nizza:** unusual round variety, great for stuffing.

**Soleil:** bright yellow; tasty and disease-resistant.

### Garlic

**Elephant Garlic:** a real showstopper; massive mild-tasting bulbs that roast well.

**Lautrec:** classic French garlic, amazing curly flower stems.

**Printanor, Thermidrome:** reliable varieties bred for the British climate.

**Purple Wight:** big white purple-splashed bulbs.

### Kale

**Dwarf Green Curled:** wonderful convoluted frilly green leaves, easy to grow.

**Nero di Toscana:** cavolo nero, classic Italian kale; one of the easiest veg to grow, edible from baby seedling leaves in spring right through the year.

**Redbor:** ornamental frilly deep red/purple leaves.

**Red Russian:** pretty, wavy red/blue leaves.

## Kohlrabi

**Azur Star:** round purple stems, mild flavour.

**Superschmelz:** grows huge but stays tender.

## Leeks

**Autumn Mammoth:** the name says it all.

**Giant Winter, Musselburgh, St Victor:** these crop through winter and spring; dependable, tasty and very hardy. St Victor turns a spectacular deep purple after cold weather.

**Lyon:** reliable early leek.

## Onions

### Brown onions
**Borettana:** an Italian variety, small and sweet, perfect for pickling.

**Sturon:** large onion, stores really well.

### Red onions
**Long Red Florence:** distinctive torpedo shape, great for slicing.

**Red Baron:** a popular variety to grow from sets.

**Tropea Rossa:** a Calabrian classic, rumoured to boost virility!

### White onions
**Musona:** attractive Spanish-type cooking onion, good-sized bulbs.

### Spring onions (or scallions)
**Purplette:** a gorgeous little round onion with a purply-red bulb.

**Rossa Lunga di Firenze:** bright red flesh that really stands out in salads.

**White Lisbon:** white flesh, reliable and hardy.

### Shallots
**Longor:** the classic French variety, with elongated bulbs and copper-colour skin; mild flavour.

**Red Sun:** large round bulbs with red-brown skin.

## Parsnips

**White Gem, Tender and True:** reliable old favourites.

## Peas

**Carouby de Mausanne:** purple-flowered, green-podded, tasty mangetout.

**Ezetha's Krombek Blauwschok:** violet-flowered, purple-podded; eat young as a mangetout, or leave to mature.

**Kelvedon Wonder:** the Essex pea; easy to grow.

**Waverex:** petit pois type, small, sweet peas.

## Peppers

**Atris, Corno di Toro Rosso:** good sweet Italian peppers.

**Bell Boy:** your everyday bell pepper.

**Californian Wonder:** mild sweet flavour; pick green or leave till red.

## Potatoes

### Earlies
**Accent:** a waxy-textured, fine-flavoured new potato.

**Epicure:** a great-tasting, slightly knobbly new potato.

**Jersey Royal (usually grown as 'International Kidney'):** the classic new potato, but it does taste different when grown outside Jersey!

**Red Duke of York:** a good, easy, tasty red-skinned early.

### Second earlies
**Linzer Delikatess:** a fantastic but little-known salad variety bred in Austria.

**Nicola:** well known, and deservedly so; especially good in salads.

### Maincrop
**King Edward:** a famous all-rounder.

**Lady Balfour:** another good all-rounder, easy to grow, stores well.

**La Ratte:** sometimes tricky to grow but a wonderful salad potato.

### Purple, blue and red fleshed potatoes
**Highland Burgundy Red:** deep russet red skin, thin outer layer of white flesh, wonderful burgundy inside.

**Vitelotte, Salad Blue:** dark blue/purple skin, blue flesh that stays bright even when cooked.

## Rhubarb

**Champagne Early:** pretty, and possibly the best-tasting variety.

**Glaskin's Perpetual:** easy and quick to grow from seed.

**Timperley Early:** good for forcing.

**Victoria:** an old reliable variety, late spring cropping.

## Squash

### Summer squash
**Courgettes (see page 392).**

**Sunburst:** pattypan squash with shape like a bright yellow UFO.

**Tiger Cross:** typical marrow, high-yielding.

**Trombolino:** amazing curly trombone shape.

### Winter squash
**Chieftain:** butternut squash, great flavour, high-yielding but compact plants.

**Crown Prince:** one of the best tasting squashes, steel-grey skin, orange flesh.

**Marina di Chioggia:** wonderful flavour, large and knobbly, stores really well.

**Musquée de Provence:** orange flesh, large, ribbed, great flavour.

**Rolet:** gem squash, cricket-ball-sized, perfect for roasting.

**Turk's Turban:** best eaten young, amazing shape.

### Pumpkins
**Atlantic Giant:** grows really big; a fun one for the kids.

**Rouge Vif d'Etamps:** old French variety, lovely ribbed orange fruit, good flavour.

## Summer salad leaves

### Butterhead lettuce
**Avondefiance:** very good resistance to aphids and mildew.

**Marvel of Four Seasons:** stunning, fast-growing red and green heirloom variety.

### Cos lettuce (also known as romaine)
**Bionda:** classic Caesar salad variety.

**Kendo:** crunchy cos-type with distinct and very ornamental red blush to the outer leaves.

### Loose-leaf and oakleaf lettuce
**Bijou:** lovely dark reddish-purple leaves; usually grown as a cut-and-come-again crop.

**Salad Bowl:** frilly red or green leaves.

**Valdai:** a really dark red oak-leaf type; looks good and is resistant to bolting and mildew.

### Radicchio and endive
**Saladini:** a mixture that includes many easy varieties plus a little lettuce.

### Rocket
**Skyrocket:** a great variety.

**Wild Rocket:** slower-growing, with finer-cut leaves and more of a kick.

### Sorrel
**Buckler Leaf:** fast-growing, with a zingy citrus tang.

### Other fun salad ingredients
Look out for amaranth, perilla, nasturtium, beet, chard, orache, fennel, oriental leaves, dandelion, cress, mustards, baby spinach, baby kales and lovely extras like pea-shoots and edible flowers. Some seed suppliers offer amazing mixtures of varieties.

### Swede

**Brora:** good for winter use.

**Marian:** a reliable variety.

### Tomatoes

### Guaranteed favourites
**Gardener's Delight:** small sweet cherry-sized fruits.

**Marmande:** big, beefy, well-flavoured, easy and productive.

**Moneymaker:** popular round medium-sized red tomato.

### A few fun varieties!
**Auriga:** medium orange, tangy flavour.

**Black Krim:** also known as Black Russian, odd colour but still tasty.

**Brandywine:** considered by many to be the best flavoured of all.

**Chocodel:** small dark red, almost brown fruits, fabulous flavour.

**Costoluto Fiorentino:** big, meaty, misshapen red fruits.

**Green Zebra:** yellow-green, darker stripes when ripe; stunning flavour.

**Lemon Boy:** large yellow tomato with a hint of lemon.

**Matt's Wild Cherry:** tiny red fruits, full of flavour.

**Prudens Purple:** large dark pinky-purple fruit.

**San Marzano:** popular plum tomato, good for pasta sauces.

**Yellow Pear:** small pear-shaped yellow fruits, hugely productive.

### Turnips

**Golden Ball:** tender yellow flesh.

**Milan Purple:** white flesh, easy and reliable.

**Oasis:** amazing turnip, can be eaten raw like an apple, crunchy and juicy.

### Turnip tops
**Namenia, Cima di Rapa:** special Italian types grown for their tasty leaves and flowering shoots.

### Winter salad leaves

**Grumolo Verde:** lovely deep green colour, very hardy.

### Corn salad/Lamb's lettuce
**D'Olanda:** winter-hardy green leaves full of vitamins and minerals.

**Verte de Cambrai:** old French variety.

### Kale
**Cavalo Nero, Red Russian:** sown in autumn, will give good crops of baby leaves for cutting all winter.

### Mustard leaves
**Giant Red Mustard:** deep red/purple leaves, quite hot!

**Mustard Green Frills:** green version of Red Frills, below.

**Mustard Red Frills:** amazingly frilly, finely cut red leaves that look delicate but are really hardy.

### Radicchio
**Rossa di Treviso:** pointed leaves, heads in autumn, deep red outside, pink and white inside.

**Rossa di Verona:** rounded tight heads in winter, deep red outside, paler inside.

**Variegata di Chioggia:** lovely speckled red, green and white heads in winter.

### Winter radish
**Mantanghong:** green/white skin hides amazing magenta flesh; lovely raw.

**Mooli:** amazingly long white roots; mild peppery taste, lovely crunchy texture.

### Other leaves
**Chervil:** grows well over winter, even though it looks really delicate; anise-like taste.

**Land cress, American cress:** looks and tastes like watercress, easy to grow; can be cut, carefully, all winter.

**Mizuna:** lovely frilly leaves, crunchy and mild.

**Rocket:** will crop all winter if sown in autumn and given some shelter.

**Spinach:** winter-hardy varieties, small leaves great for winter salad.

**Winter Purslane/Miners' Lettuce:** very easy hardy leaf salad.

**Winter Saladini:** wonderful mix of winter-hardy 'cutting' leaves. Sown in autumn and if given some protection will provide baby salad leaves all winter.

# Fruit

## Apples

**Ashmead's Kernel (dessert):** aromatic russet green with yellow brown flush; stores well.

**Ellison's Orange (dessert):** good flavour with a tinge of aniseed.

**Lord Lambourne (dessert):** greenish yellow with red flushed stripes; crisp and sweet.

**The Queen (cooking):** large pale yellow, crimson flushed; good for baking and much sought after in Essex!

## Pears

**Conference:** long dark green fruit ripening to a yellowish brown russet colour; flesh creamy, often tinged pink.

**Doyenne du Comice:** large golden/pale green fruit with some russeting; superb flavour; likes a sheltered site.

## Plums, gages, damsons

**Cambridge Gage:** green/yellow fruit, sweet and juicy; ideal for eating raw, cooking and making preserves.

**Marjorie's Seedling:** deep purple skin, yellow flesh; good either raw or cooked.

**Victoria:** an old favourite with superb flavour; best eaten raw or cooked when slightly underripe.

**Cherry plums**
**Gipsy Mirabelle:** large red fruit with an amazing flavour.

**Golden Sphere Mirabelle:** large fruit, like apricots; good eaten raw, superb for jam and preserves.

## Strawberries

**Cambridge Favourite (hybrid):** reliable, mid-season strawberry with good flavour.

**Elvira (hybrid):** early fruiting, heavy yield, lovely flavour.

**Fragaria vesca:** the true 'wild strawberry', sensational flavour.

**Mara de Bois (wild/hybrid):** the flavour of wild strawberries but the size of traditional English hybrids; fruits all summer … my favourite!

**Rhapsody (hybrid):** late summer cropping, good flavour.

## Where to buy them

**Association Kokopelli**
Ripple Farm
Crundale
Canterbury
Kent
CT4 7EB
Tel: 01227 731815
**www.kokopelli-seeds.com**
Old variety veg seeds you won't easily find elsewhere.

**Gourmet Woodland Mushrooms**
Beacon Hill
North Lane
Welwick
Hull
HU12 0SL
Tel: 01964 631868
**www.gourmetmushrooms.co.uk**
Great for mushroom growing kits.

**Jekka's Herb Farm**
Rose Cottage
Shellards Lane
Alveston
Bristol
BS35 3SY
Tel: 01454 418878
**www.jekkasherbfarm.com**
Best supplier of organically grown herbs in Britain.

**The Organic Gardening Catalogue**
Riverdene Business Park
Molesey Road
Hersham
Surrey
KT12 4RG
Tel: 0845 130 1304
**www.organiccatalog.com**
Very good range of veg seed and fruit trees. Huge range of useful organic-gardening-based sundries.

**Ragman's Lane Farm**
Lydbrook
Gloucestershire
GL17 9PA
Tel: 01594 860244
**www.ragmans.co.uk**
Everything you need for growing mushrooms at home.

**Seeds of Italy**
C3 Phoenix Industrial Estate
Rosslyn Crescent
Harrow
Middlesex
HA1 2SP
Tel: 020 8427 5020
**www.seedsofitaly.com**
Good range of fruit, veg and herb seeds, specializing in Italian varieties. Also supplies mushrooms and 'truffle trees'.

**Suffolk Herbs**
Monks Farm
Kelvedon
Colchester
Essex
CO5 9PG
Tel: 01376 572456
**www.suffolkherbs.com**
Good range of organic veg and herb seeds plus wildflower seeds.

**Tamar Organics**
Cartha Martha Farm
Rezare
Launceston

Cornwall
PL15 9NX
Tel: 01579 371087
**www.tamarorganics.co.uk**
For all your favourite organic veg seeds, fruit plants and trees.

**Tuckers Seeds**
Edwin Tucker & Sons Ltd
Brewery Meadow
Stonepark
Ashburton
Newton Abbot
Devon
TQ13 7DG
Tel: 01364 652233
**www.tuckers-seeds.co.uk**
Good range of seeds, plants and sundries; particularly organic seed potatoes.

# Other good addresses and websites

**Battery Hen Welfare Trust**
North Parks
Chumleigh
Devon
EX18 7EJ
**www.thehenshouse.co.uk**
This is where I got my rescued battery chickens from. They're fit and healthy and laying like the clappers!

**The Hen House Garden Company**
Oak Cottage
Thwaite Road
Thorndon
Eye
Suffolk
IP23 7JJ
Tel: 01379 678085
**www.hen-house.co.uk**
Makers of fantastic custom-built henhouses.

**Implementations**
PO Box 2568
Nuneaton
Warwickshire
CV10 9YR
Tel: 024 7639 2497
**www.implementations.co.uk**
Amazing Austrian hand-made copper garden tools that also repel slugs and snails.

**Omlet Ltd**
Tufthill Park
Wardington
Oxfordshire
OX17 1SD
Tel: 0845 4502056
**www.omlet.co.uk**
Suppliers of modern 'eglus' for chickens and other small animals (housing/runs).

**Rooster**
Greenvale Farms Limited
Orchard Close
Middleton Tyas
North Yorkshire
DL10 6PE
Tel: 01325 339971
**www.rooster.uk.com**
Really good organically certified fertilizer made from organically reared chicken manure. Available from good garden centres.

**Sylvantutch**
Unit 10
Corris Craft Centre
Corris, Nr. Machynlleth
Mid Wales
SY20 9RF
Tel: 01654 761614
**www.sylvantutch.co.uk**
Amazing hand-built, recycled wooden benches and seats. Perfect for the garden.

**Wolf Tools**
Tel: 0845 241 7413
**www.worldofwolf.co.uk**
Very useful range of garden tools, especially for growing vegetables. (Also available at most good garden centres.)

And check out these great websites too:

**www.agroforestry.co.uk**

**www.allotment.org.uk**

**www.annforfungi.co.uk**

**www.gardenorganic.org.uk**

**www.nvsuk.org.uk**

**www.permaculture.co.uk**

**www.seercentre.org.uk**

**www.soilassociation.org**

**www.wewantrealfood.co.uk**

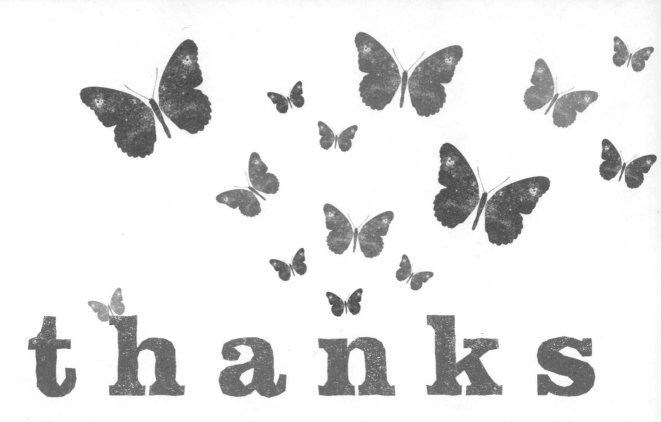

# thanks

To Jools, Poppy and Daisy for making my life so beautiful. And to Mum, Dad and all the family. xxx

To my much-loved food team for all their hard work: my fantastic mentor, Gennaro Contaldo, the inspirational Peter Begg, my amazing style girls Ginny Rolfe and Anna Jones, and the lovely Bobby Sebire. And last but not least, thanks so much to Georgie Socratous and Lizzie Cope for all their brilliant recipe-testing work.

On words, thanks to my editorial team: my editor the lovely Lindsey Evans, and to the superb Suzanna de Jong and Sophia Brown.

And to the rest of the team back at the office – thanks for everything.

A special thanks to the best food photographer in the world – Lord David Loftus (www.davidloftus.com). Well done, mate. And to his assistants Rosie, Abi, Rebecca and Alicia.

To John Hamilton, my Art Director at Penguin – nice one, mate! And to Chris Callard (www.beachstone.co.uk), a freelance text designer and a top boy who's worked on a few of my books now. Let's have more of those *montagés*! Thanks to Matt and Brad at the design company The Plant for all their lovely illustrations in the book (www.theplant.co.uk). Great job, guys!

A massive thank you to my long-term publishers, Penguin. Most especially to Tom Weldon, Keith Taylor, Juliette Butler, Sophie Brewer, Jessica Jefferys, Rob Williams, Tora Orde-Powlett, Naomi Fidler, Clare Pollock and the rest of their teams who work so damn hard! Check out www.penguin.co.uk. And a particularly big thanks to Annie Lee.

I'd like to say thanks to the lovely people at Fresh One Productions (www.freshone.tv): Jo Ralling, Zoe Collins and Andrew Conrad (who left halfway through, you bastard! xxx), and a particular thanks to the director, my darling mate Helen Downing, who totally got it from the very beginning, and big love to the best crew ever. Thanks to the boys: Luke Cardiff, Louis Caulfield, Toby Ralph, Godfrey Kirby, Mike Sarah. Thanks to the girls: Ginny and Anna, Lizzie, Abigail and Harrie. And the rest of the

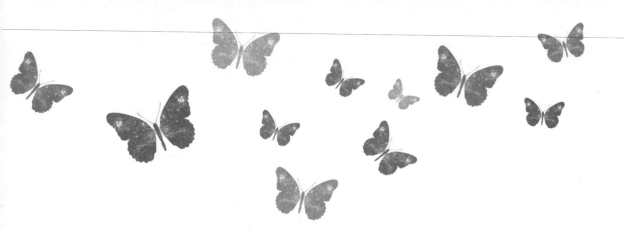

production team: Emily, Hannah, Jemma, Dan, Mo, Leigh, Daniel, Simon, Craig, Guy, Rod and Matt. Thanks also to Rob and Tom from Chalk and Cheese Catering (07931 389038) for feeding us lovely food during shooting – these boys are both ex-students of mine. And thanks to the guys at Hello Charlie who did all the graphics for the programme.

Back at home I grow quite a lot of stuff for Fifteen restaurant in London, as well as having my own veg garden, and I'm lucky enough to work with some beautiful people – Brian Skilton, who appears in the TV series, and an amazing talent, Pete Wrapson. These boys also helped me with the gardening pages in this book. Also, big thanks to Beth, Zoot and Bill, who help to make everything happen.

Thanks to Geoff Garrod, the gamekeeper at Audley End House in Essex, for his knowledge and inspiration.

Thanks to my great suppliers: Tony at Booths at Borough Market, Gary and all the guys at Moen's butchers and Daphne Tilly at Elwy Valley Lamb. To the Lacquer Chest gang – Gretchen, Viv, Ewan, Agnes, Merly – for all their patience and kindness. Please make sure we get all the good stuff first!

So much testing goes into putting a good cookbook together, and there are a few companies that always provide us with kit to do this. Many thanks to: Luc, Florence and the Tefal team, David, Helen and the Royal Worcester team, Michael and Oscar at Merison, Nick and everybody at William Levene, Simon Kinder from Magimix and Simon Boniface from Kenwood. Also to the lovely people at the St Lucia Coalpot Company.

Last but not least, there are a couple of people who directly or indirectly helped me get a derelict old garden that hadn't been loved for thirty years sorted out. One is my good mate Jekka McVicar, who helped me with the herb garden and various other areas of the garden (www.jekkasherbfarm. com). Look out for the brand new reissue of her classic book *Jekka's Complete Herb Book*. And Roger Platts – a fantastic garden designer who runs a nursery in Kent (www.rogerplatts.com).

# index

Page references in **bold** indicate an illustration
v indicates a vegetarian recipe

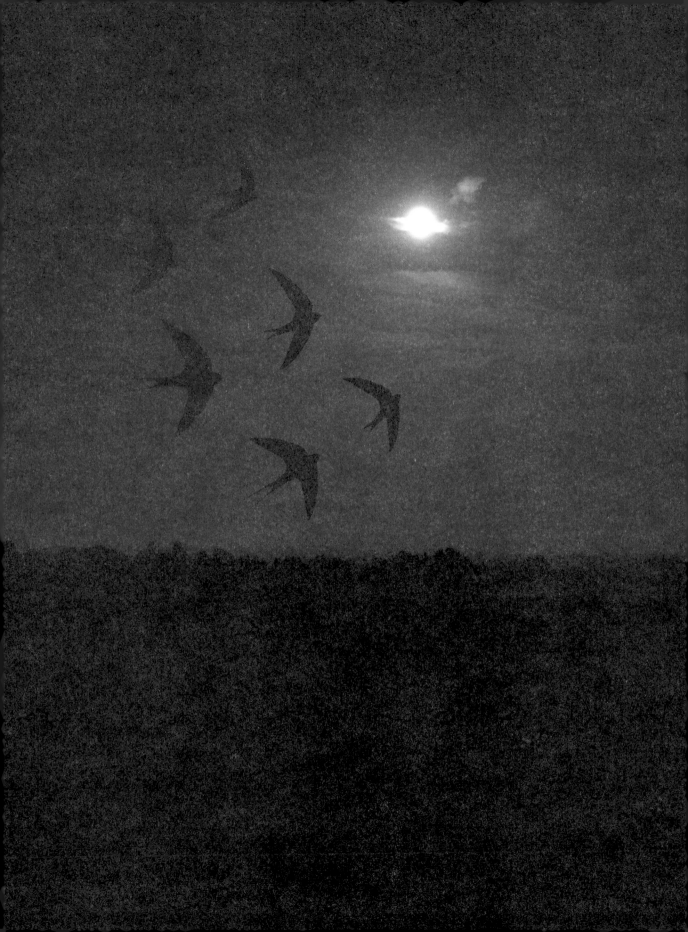